Transplantation
NURSING
Acute and Long-Term Management

Transplantation NURSING
Acute and Long-Term Management

Marie T. Nolan, RN, DNSc
Nurse Researcher
The Johns Hopkins Hospital
Assistant Professor of Nursing
Johns Hopkins University
Baltimore, Maryland

Sharon M. Augustine, RN, MS, CANP, CCTC
Coordinator
Heart and Lung Transplant Programs
The Johns Hopkins Hospital
Baltimore, Maryland

APPLETON & LANGE
Norwalk, Connecticut

Copyright © 1995 by Appleton & Lange
A Simon & Schuster Company

95 96 97 98 / 10 9 8 7 6 5 4 3 2 1

Prentice Hall International (UK) Limited, *London*
Prentice Hall of Australia Pty. Limited, *Sydney*
Prentice Hall Canada, Inc., *Toronto*
Prentice Hall Hispanoamericana, S. A., *Mexico*
Prentice Hall of India Private Limited, *New Delhi*
Prentice Hall of Japan, Inc., *Tokyo*
Simon & Schuster Asia Pte. Ltd., *Singapore*
Editora Prentice Hall do Brasil Ltda., *Rio de Janeiro*
Prentice Hall, *Englewood Cliffs, New Jersey*

Library of Congress Cataloging-in-Publication-Data
Transplantation nursing / [edited by] Marie T. Nolan, Sharon M.
  Augustine.
      p. cm.
    Includes index.
    ISBN 0-8385-8989-8
    1. Transplantation of organs, tissues, etc.—Nursing.   I. Nolan,
  Marie T.   II. Augustine, Sharon M.
    [DNLM: 1. Organ Transplantation—nursing.   WY 161 T772 1995]
  RD129.8.T73   1995
  617.9′5—dc20
  DNLM/DLC
  for Library of Congress   94-31323
                                                           CIP

Editor-in-Chief: Sally J. Barhydt
Production Editor: Jennifer Sinsavich
Designer: Michael J. Kelly

PRINTED IN THE UNITED STATES OF AMERICA

ISBN 0-8385-8989-8

90000

Contents

Preface

The age of transplantation has placed nurses at the cutting edge of the technological revolution in health care. Although the complexity of the care required by these patients can be daunting, nurse clinicians of the past have faced equally daunting challenges and have risen to the occasion. At the turn of the century, the scourge of tuberculosis fell on both urban and rural America. While surgical removal of the lung was of benefit, the "cure" became professional nursing care. Working together, nurses in the hospital, sanatorium, and home eradicated the tubercle bacilli through innovations in infection control. These innovations, coupled with nursing's holistic consideration for the impact of the illness on the patient and family, brought a nation back to life.

Professional nursing care is again part of the cure for patients undergoing transplantation. While incorporating innovations in immunology, pharmacology, and technology into their care, transplant nurses have retained their predecessors' holistic view of the patient and family. *Transplantation Nursing* is offered in the same spirit of our early nurse leaders. Readers will find the latest innovations in the nursing care of patients undergoing heart, lung, liver, small bowel, renal, bone marrow, and corneal transplantation. Each organ-related chapter contains a discussion of the evaluation process, a brief description of the surgical techniques used during transplantation, and a review of nursing management in the immediate and later postoperative periods.

Nurses involved in either the critical care or general care of transplant patients will find the nursing care plans offered at the end of each chapter to be useful guidelines for the complex care these patients require. The pattern of health and illness experienced by many patients in long-term followup is also addressed. This information can be shared with patients who are deciding whether to undergo transplantation, ensuring truly informed consent. Further, nurses who care for patients in the pretransplantation phase may find this information useful as a source for preoperative teaching.

Chapters 1 and 2, devoted to transplantation immunology and infectious disease, undergird nursing assessment and interventions for the complications of rejection and infection. These chapters will be valuable to the student nurse, staff nurse, clinical nurse specialist, and transplant coordinator seeking to master the complex physiology of transplantation care. Chapter 3 covers the stressors and coping methods of patients and their families. This chapter gives insight into the experience of waiting for a donor organ and hoping for a second chance at life. Chapters on legislative issues, organ donation, and ethical implications of transplantation provide the larger framework under which transplantation nursing is practiced. Finally, Chapter 14, Nursing Research in Transplantation, provides a look at the future of the science of transplantation nursing. It is our belief that scientific inquiry will define the advanced practice of nursing in the future of transplantation. With continued innovations and a holistic approach to patient care, transplantation nursing will claim a place in health care history and continue the extraordinary advances of this century.

The editors would like to thank the contributing authors for their expertise and the commitment they brought to this project. We also thank Nancy Polvinale for her secretarial support in the preparation of this manuscript.

Marie T. Nolan
Sharon M. Augustine

Contributors

Myrlin O. Agunod, RN, MAS
Liver, Kidney and Pancreas Transplant
  Patient Care Specialist
Department of Surgery
The Johns Hopkins Hospital
Baltimore, Maryland

Kathy A. Altieri, RN, BSN, CCTC
Pediatric Transplant Coordinator
Pittsburgh Transplantation Institute
University of Pittsburgh Medical Center
Pittsburgh, Pennsylvania

Sharon M. Augustine, RN, MS,
  CANP, CCTC
Coordinator
Heart and Lung Transplant Programs
The Johns Hopkins Hospital
Baltimore, Maryland

Denise Burrell-Diggs, RN, BSN
Liver, Kidney and Pancreas Transplant
  Patient Care Coordinator
Department of Surgery
The Johns Hopkins Hospital
Baltimore, Maryland

Fred H. Cate, J. D.
Associate Professor of Law
Annenberg Senior Fellow
Indiana University School of Law
Bloomington, Indiana

JoAnn Coleman, RN, MS, CS, OCN
Clinical Nurse Specialist
Gastrointestinal Surgery
The Johns Hopkins Hospital
Baltimore, Maryland

Sandra A. Cupples, RN, DNSc, CCRN
Cardiovascular Clinical Specialist
Director, Cardiac
  Rehabilitation Program
National Naval Medical Center
Bethesda, Maryland

Jacqueline K. Darmody, RN, BSN
Liver, Kidney and Pancreas Transplant
  Patient Care Coordinator
Department of Surgery
The Johns Hopkins Hospital
Baltimore, Maryland

Mimi Funovitz, RN, BS, CCTC
Small Intestine Transplant
    Clinical Coordinator
Pittsburgh Transplantation Institute
University of Pittsburgh Medical Center
Pittsburgh, Pennsylvania

Janet L. Hanson, RN, MS
Bone Marrow Transplant Clinical
    Nurse Specialist
The Johns Hopkins Oncology Center
Baltimore, Maryland

Mary Jo Holechek, RN, MS, CNN
Liver, Kidney and Pancreas Lead
    Transplant Coordinator
The Johns Hopkins Hospital
Baltimore, Maryland

Cynthia A. Kaczmarek, RN, MS
Liver, Kidney and Pancreas Transplant
    Patient Care Coordinator
The Johns Hopkins Hospital
Baltimore, Maryland

Judith A. Kovalak, RN, MSN
Clinical Transplant Coordinator
Pittsburgh Transplantation Institute
University of Pittsburgh Medical Center
Pittsburgh, Pennsylvania

Anne Nicholson Macdonald, RN,
    MS, CCTC
Cardiothoracic Transplant Coordinator
Department of Surgery
University of Arizona
Tucson, Arizona

Maryhelen Masiello Miller, RN,
    MSN, CS
Clinical Case Manager
Department of Cardiac Surgery
The Johns Hopkins Hospital
Baltimore, Maryland

Melinda Mendoza, RN, MS
Liver, Kidney and Pancreas Transplant
    Clinical Nurse Specialist
The Johns Hopkins Hospital
Baltimore, Maryland

Victoria B. Navarro, RN, MAS
Director
Clinical Services
The Wilmer Ophthalmological Institute
The Johns Hopkins Hospital
Baltimore, Maryland

Marie T. Nolan, RN, DNSc
Nurse Researcher
The Johns Hopkins Hospital
Assistant Professor of Nursing
Johns Hopkins University
Baltimore, Maryland

Karen V. Ohly, RN, MSN
Autologous Bone Marrow Transplant
    Clinical Nurse Specialist
The Johns Hopkins Oncology Center
Baltimore, Maryland

Sharon G. Owens, RN, MSN, MPH
Nurse Manager
Cardiac Surgical Intensive Care Unit
Department of Surgical Nursing
The Johns Hopkins Hospital
Baltimore, Maryland

Kathleen S. Rohrer, RN, MS
Nurse Educator
Department of Surgical Nursing
The Johns Hopkins Hospital
Baltimore, Maryland

Jane C. Shivnan, RN, MScN
Nurse Manager
Bone Marrow Transplant
The Johns Hopkins Oncology Center
Baltimore, Maryland

**Sandra M. Staschak-Chicko,
  RN, CCTC**
Clinical Administrator
Pittsburgh Transplantation Institute
University of Pittsburgh
  Medical Center
Pittsburgh, Pennsylvania

Julie Mull Strange, RN, CCRN, CPTC
Executive Director
Transplant Resource Center of
  Maryland, Inc.
Baltimore, Maryland

David C. Taylor, RN
Clinical Coordinator
Organ Recovery Coordinator
Transplant Resource Center of
  Maryland, Inc.
Baltimore, Maryland

Frances M. Tolley, RN, BSN
Nurse Manager, The Wilmer Nursing
  and Trauma Center
The Wilmer Ophthalmological Institute
The Johns Hopkins Hospital
Baltimore, Maryland

Janice M. Wallop, RN, MSN
Clinical Case Manager
Cardiac Surgery
Department of Surgical Nursing
The Johns Hopkins Hospital
Baltimore, Maryland

Barbara V. Wise, RNC, MS
Clinical Nurse Specialist
Pediatric Surgery
The Johns Hopkins Hospital
Baltimore, Maryland

Foreword

Organ transplantation remains one of the more exciting and scientifically interesting success stories in medicine that has evolved during the 20th century. Transplantation has a short history dating to 1954 when the first kidney transplant between identical twins was performed successfully at the Peter Bent Brigham Hospital in Boston. The introduction of the immunosuppressive drug, 6-mercaptopurine, in 1960 and the subsequent development of azathioprine led to the initial success of cadaver kidney transplantation beginning in the early 1960s. Remarkable progress in understanding the immunology of transplantation, organ preservation, and the development and use of increasingly more specific immunosuppressive drugs has resulted in the emergence of heart, liver and lung transplantation as a realistic and viable approach to patients with end-organ disease refractory to other medical or surgical management.

The clinical availability of cyclosporine in 1983 resulted in an exponential rise in the number of organ transplants throughout the world. Within one year of its introduction, the survival rate of patients undergoing heart transplantation was 80 percent compared with 60 percent previously obtained using steroids, azathioprine, and antithymocyte globulin. Increased survival and less morbidity is now observed in transplant recipients of all organs. Application of the various procedures has been extended to neonates, children, and increasingly older adults.

Although there is much justified optimism, considerable problems exist for many of our transplant patients. The donor shortage remains a significant issue. Approximately 30,000 recipients are listed on transplant waiting lists throughout the United States. Infections, drug toxicities and the need for retransplantation remain significant problems for our transplant patients.

Although newer immunosuppressive medications and better methods for the diagnosis of rejection have contributed to increased patient survival and reduced morbidity, significant credit should go to the coordinated team approach in the care of the transplant recipient. These patients require intensive support and care in the early postoperative period as well as continued surveillance and followup for the rest of their lives. The transplant nurse, whether in the intensive care unit, the recovery floor, or involved in the long-term postoperative care, has played a critical role in the trans-

plantation success story. The care of these patients has become increasingly complicated and requires the detailed approach provided by nurses, physicians, and other
important health care providers involved in transplantation.

In this book, Marie Nolan and Sharon Augustine provide state of the art information and practical management issues for all nurses, students, and transplant coordinators involved in the early and/or long-term care of transplant patients. The editors
are to be congratulated on providing a book which is both detailed and easily read-
able. Their dedication to both nursing and transplantation is evident in the breadth of
knowledge and conduct of care seen in each chapter.

The future of transplantation remains bright. Evolving techniques of molecular
biology will undoubtedly lead to the eventual ability to transplant across species barriers. Newer immunosuppressive drugs will provide the recipient with increasing
longevity and a reduction in significant side-effects. This transplantation nursing book
will be the benchmark for further books dealing with nursing management issues involved in the care of transplant patients.

William A. Baumgartner, MD
Professor of Surgery
Cardiac Surgeon-in-Charge
The Johns Hopkins University School of Medicine
Baltimore, Maryland

Transplantation
NURSING
Acute and Long-Term Management

Transplantation Immunology

Kathleen S. Rohrer

THE NORMAL IMMUNE SYSTEM

The immune system protects the body against invasion by foreign substances. Transplanted organs are seen as foreign by the body, and the immune system is activated to destroy, or reject, this invader. The more similar the transplanted organ is to the recipient's tissue, the less the immune system will respond. The goal of transplantation is to minimize the immune response by implanting a donor organ that is as similar to the recipient's tissue as possible and then suppressing the immune response through immunosuppressive therapy.

Familiarity with the normal functions of the immune system is essential to understand how the body reacts to an implanted donor organ. The major components of the immune system are the physiologic defenses of protective body structures and the cellular defenses of the white blood cell (WBC) system.

Physiologic Defense

Body structures and secretions compose the first line of defense of the immune system, a barrier defense. The skin and mucous membranes protect the internal environment of the body from entrance of foreign organisms and substances. Bacterial colonization of the skin is checked by the low pH of the surface and the process of normal skin cell turnover. Nasal hairs and secretions, cilia, and the cough reflex trap and remove organisms from the respiratory system. Organisms can be eliminated from the body through the gastrointestinal tract or destroyed in the low pH of the stomach and urinary system. Sphincters also prevent entrance of organisms from the external environment into the gastrointestinal and urinary tracts (Drutz & Mills, 1987; Male & Roitt, 1989; Morton, 1989).

Other protective immune structures include the lymph nodes and tissues, the tonsils, the appendix, and the spleen (Griffin, 1986; Morton, 1989; Smith, 1990). The lymph system acts as a filter and removal system for foreign particles and dead or damaged cells. The strategic locations of these tissues impedes the movement of substances into the central core of the body. Axillary and femoral lymph nodes drain the extremities, and the tonsils offer protection from organisms that enter through the oropharynx. Collections of lymph tissue around the intestines, called Peyer patches, and the appendix remove organisms and cell debris from food passages. The spleen is essential in the development of the cellular components of the immune system, and it also functions as a lymph organ by collecting organisms and cell debris as blood passes through its circulation (Gurka, 1989).

Cellular Defense

The WBCs (leukocytes) provide the immune system with both nonspecific and specific responses to substances recognized as foreign by the body (Table 1–1). The nonspecific defense provides natural or nonspecific immunity by responding to any invader that enters the body. This defense mechanism is also known as the inflammatory response (Gurevich, 1989; Male & Roitt, 1989; Morton, 1989). The response is the same regardless of the organism or stressor that has entered or injured the body. Cellular components of natural immunity are granulocytes and monocytes, two of the three major groups of WBCs. Complement proteins and mediator substances such as bradykinin and histamine enhance this inflammatory response (Smith, 1990).

Lymphocytes, the third category of WBCs, provide the specific immune responses known as acquired immunity. Lymphocytes are programmed during formation to respond to only specific invaders, such as bacteria, virus, or foreign tissue.

Natural Immunity

All three groups of leukocytes are derived from stem cells that mature and differentiate in the bone marrow and lymph system (Figure 1–1). The cells are classified by their appearance under a microscope. The granulocytes are named for the granules that are seen in the cells (Allen, 1993; Guyton, 1991). They also have a multilobed nucleus. Granulocytes also may be called polymorphonuclear leukocytes (PMNs), polys, or

TABLE 1–1. CELLULAR DEFENSES

	Response	
	Nonspecific (Inflammatory)	*Specific (Immune)*
Action	Responds to any foreign substance	Responds only to targeted substances
Cells involved	Granulocytes	B lymphocytes
	Monocytes	T lymphocytes

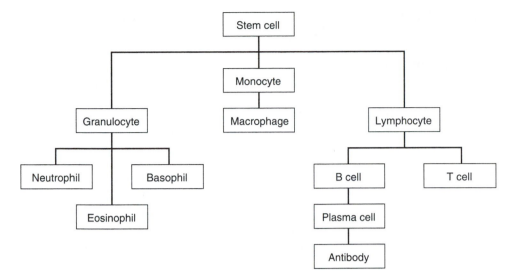

Figure 1–1. Cellular defenses.

segs. Even though they are similar in appearance, the three groups of granulocytes have different functions.

Neutrophils account for 50 to 70% of the total leukocyte count (Dressler, 1993; Griffin, 1986; Gurevich, 1989). They are the primary phagocytic component of the nonspecific inflammatory response, and they are the first cells to encounter an invading organism. Phagocytosis is the ability of a cell to surround and destroy an organism. Immature neutrophils known as bands are produced and released from the bone marrow in response to a foreign substance. Historically, the more immature forms of a cell are printed from the left side of a WBC differential report (Allen, 1993; Gurevich, 1989). The increase in bands in response to an infection is seen on the left side of the report and has become known as a shift to the left. Only the mature neutrophils are phagocytic, and administration of steroids decreases the number and effectiveness of neutrophils, impairing the inflammatory response (Allen, 1993; Seller & Owen, 1993).

Eosinophils and basophils are the remaining groups of granulocytes (Dressler, 1993; Griffin, 1986; Smith, 1990). Eosinophils constitute 2 to 4% of the total leukocyte count. They are slightly phagocytic and are most responsive in allergic reactions and in the presence of parasitic infections. Basophils compose less than 1% of the total leukocyte count and have little phagocytic activity. Basophils participate in allergic reactions and release heparin and histamine to increase vascular permeability.

Monocytes provide nonspecific protection. These cells compose 4 to 7% of the leukocyte count (Auger & Ross, 1992; Dressler, 1993; Werb, 1987). The monocytes are also phagocytic and are found in large numbers in the lymph system and most body compartments. When the monocytes move out of the vascular space into the tissues, they are called macrophages. Monocytes are effective against bacteria and efficient in cleaning up cellular debris at the site of infection.

Acquired Immunity

Acquired immunity is provided by the lymphocytes, which make up 20 to 30% of the total WBC count (Gurka, 1989; Seller & Owen, 1993). The lymphocytes are divided into two groups, known as B lymphocytes and T lymphocytes. Both groups of lymphocytes contribute to the specific, or immune, response when they are stimulated by an antigen.

Immunoglobulins. The B-lymphocyte system is also known as humoral immunity, and the cells produce antibodies when they are stimulated (Flye, 1989; Huffer et al, 1986). B lymphocytes arise from the stem cell differentiation that produces all of the leukocyte types. The cells were designated as B lymphocytes because their development was first discovered in the bursa of Fabricius in birds (Flye, 1989; Griffin, 1986). In humans, the B lymphocytes develop initially in the fetal liver; after birth they develop in the bone marrow (Levitt & Cooper, 1987; Lydyard & Grossi, 1989). The B cells then migrate primarily to the tissues of the lymph system, where further differentiation takes place.

B lymphocytes mediate the immune response by the production of immunoglobulin or antibody. The primary response occurs the first time an antigen is introduced to a B lymphocyte. The lymphocytes are activated to produce plasma cells, which in turn produce a specific antibody (Figure 1–2). Other leukocytes are also essential for antibody production: Macrophages present an antigen to B lymphocytes, which causes a plasma cell response, and helper T lymphocytes stimulate antibody production (Griffin, 1986; Seller & Owen, 1993; Smith, 1990). Plasma cells release antibody until the antigen is destroyed. After this primary antigen–antibody response, B memory cells remain a part of the immune system and provide a faster secondary response if the antigen is encountered again. An advantage of humoral immunity is

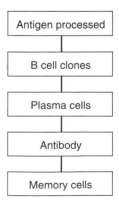

Figure 1–2. Antibody development.

that it can be transferred by serum between people by immunization or maternal–fetal transfer (Seller & Owen, 1993; Shumway, 1990).

Antibodies are divided into five different categories (Table 1–2). Immunoglobulin M (IgM) is the first antibody formed in response to an antigen. It provides a great deal of protection during a primary encounter. Immunoglobulin G (IgG) is the largest immunoglobulin pool. It is the predominant antibody produced during a secondary response to an antigen. IgG is capable of crossing the placental barrier, and it helps provide immune system protection for a fetus until production of IgM begins. Antibodies other than IgM are present during fetal life, but IgM provides the major response (Goodman, 1987; Stobo, 1987). Immunoglobulin A (IgA) is found predominantly in body secretions, where it complements the physiologic defenses at body entry portals. Immunoglobulin E (IgE) is less than 1% of the serum immunoglobulin pool, but it is found on basophils and mast cells, where it is associated with allergic reactions (Dawson, 1991; Turner, 1989). The function of immunoglobulin D (IgD) is unknown. It is found on the surface of many B lymphocytes, which suggests that it may facilitate the differentiation of the types of cells (Goodman, 1987; Turner, 1989). All of the antibody types are present before birth, but the full adult immune response does not develop for several years (Stobo, 1987).

T lymphocytes. T lymphocytes are important to transplant immunology because they are primarily responsible for acute rejection of solid organ grafts (Allen, 1993; Flye, 1989). The T-lymphocyte system is also known as cellular immunity. In contrast to humoral immunity, cellular immunity cannot be transferred in the serum between people. The lymphocytes originate in the bone marrow from stem cells and become functionally mature in the thymus gland (Guyton, 1991; Seller & Owen, 1993). During thymic development, the T cells develop the ability to differentiate self from non-self through the expression of antigen receptors. They leave the thymus and move into the lymphoid tissues and bloodstream as immunocompetent cells (Stobo, 1987). T lymphocytes provide immunity against most viruses and fungi, slow-developing bacteria such as those that cause tuberculosis, cancer cells, and transplanted organs (Allen, 1993; Flye, 1989; Griffin, 1986).

TABLE 1–2. ANTIBODY CATEGORIES

Category	Percent of Total	Function
IgM	10	Initial immune response to most antigens
IgG	75	Responsible for secondary response Only immunoglobulin that crosses placenta; provides protection during first few months of life
IgA	15	Found in body secretions; believed to protect at mucous sites
IgD	<1	Not yet determined
IgE	<1	Part of allergic response

Four subgroups of T lymphocytes provide cellular immunity: killer (cytotoxic), memory, helper, and suppressor cells. The subgroups are identified by molecules expressed on the cells and designated CD (Male, 1991; Shumway, 1990). Cytotoxic T cells are designated as CD8. They destroy invading cells directly or through the production of lymphokines. Interleukins and interferon are two of the many lymphokines that mediate the immune response. The major functions of lymphokines are the recruitment and activation of macrophages, production of antiviral proteins within the cell, and stimulation of T-cell proliferation (Dawson, 1991; Drutz & Mills, 1987; Rook, 1989; Smith, 1990; Stobo, 1987). Memory cells are also produced when the lymphocytes are stimulated by an antigen. The presence of the memory cells provides for an accelerated secondary response when the lymphocyte system encounters the antigen again.

In addition to the effector functions, the T lymphocytes contribute two regulatory functions, helper and suppressor. Helper T cells assist B cells in producing antibody; they also produce lymphokines. T helper cells are designated CD4. Suppressor T cells act to balance both the B- and T-cell responses by inhibiting B-cell antibody production and cytotoxic T-cell effects (Smith, 1990; Stobo, 1987).

HISTOCOMPATIBILITY

Transplantation requires suppression of the normal immune functions to prevent rejection of the graft. The more alike the donor and recipient tissues are, the less rejection is likely to occur. Histocompatibility testing is the evaluation of donor antigens with recipient antibodies.

Two antigen systems that have a considerable impact on transplantation have been identified on red blood cells and tissue cells. These are the ABO and human leukocyte antigen (HLA) systems. The rhesus (Rh) factor, a concern in blood transfusions, does not impact organ transplantation because the Rh antigens are not found on endothelial tissues (Smith, 1990).

ABO

The A and B antigens are located on red blood cells and vascular endothelium; they determine blood type. Type A blood has the A antigen and type B, the B antigen. Type AB has both the A and B antigens, and type O has neither antigen. Naturally occurring antibodies are present in the sera when a particular antigen is lacking on the cells. Anti-A antibodies are found in people who do not have the A antigen (blood types B and O), and anti-B antibodies are found in those without the B antigen (A and O types). People with type AB blood have both antigens, so they have neither antibody (Table 1–3). Type A has been divided into A_1 and A_2 on the basis of different responses to some antibodies (Marcus, 1989).

ABO grouping is the primary determinant for solid organ transplantation. The same compatibility rules that apply to blood transfusion apply to transplantation. Table 1–3 identifies proportions of the caucasian population by blood type and potential organ donors according to ABO type (Garovoy et al, 1987; Arcus, 1989). The

TABLE 1–3. ABO SYSTEM

Type	Antigen	Antibody	Percent of Population	Potential Donor
A	A	Anti-B	41	A or O
B	B	Anti-A	9	B or O
AB	A & B	None	3	Any
O	None	Anti-A and B	47	O only

frequency of blood types and other antigens differs among world populations depending on region (ethnicity) and race (Bollinger & Sanfilippo, 1989).

Human Leukocyte Antigen

The major histocompatibility complex (MHC) is a group of genes located on one chromosome that is involved in the immune response, particularly graft rejection. In humans, this group is located on chromosome 6 and is called human leukocyte antigen. The name recognizes that the antigens were first discovered on WBCs (Bartucci & Seller, 1990; Bollinger & Sanfilippo, 1989; Dawson, 1991; Male, 1991; Marboe et al, 1990). The HLA system differentiates self from non-self and recognizes the introduction of foreign tissue into the body. If the antigens on the donor graft are not present in the recipient, rejection occurs (Flye, 1989).

There are four gene sites, or loci, on chromosome 6 that are important in transplantation: A, B, C, and DR (Table 1–4). These sites express different antigens, and each site may consist of one of many different gene forms, or alleles (Bartucci & Seller, 1990; Schwartz, 1987). A worldwide consensus group has identified more than 100 antigens on these four sites, as shown in Table 1–5: 23 on the A site, 50 on B, 11 on C, and 18 on the DR site (Bartucci & Seller, 1990; Hart, unpublished, 1991; Schwartz, 1987).

The four gene sites are divided into class I antigens, consisting of A, B, and C, and class II antigens, the DR category. Class I antigens are expressed on all body cells with a nucleus and are recognized by CD8 lymphocytes, which are the cytotoxic T cells (Marboe et al, 1990). The class I antigens present the major target for antibody and T-cell reactions to transplanted grafts (Bartucci & Seller, 1990; Bollinger & Sanfilippo, 1989; Dawson, 1991). Class II antigens (DR) have limited distribution in the tissues. They are expressed on macrophages, B lymphocytes, and activated T lymphocytes.

TABLE 1–4. GENE SITES (LOCI)

Chromosome Number 6

Gene site A	Gene site B	Gene site C	— —	Gene site DR

Class I antigens are on sites A, B, and C. Class II antigens are on site DR.

TABLE 1–5. POTENTIAL ANTIGENS BY SITE

Class I Antigens							Class II Antigens	
A		B				C	DR	
A2	A29	B5	B35	B50	BW63	CW1	DR1	DRW10
A3	A30	B7	B37	BW51	BW64	CW2	DR2	DRW11
A9	A31	B8	B38	BW52	BW65	CW3	DR3	DRW12
A10	A32	B12	B39	BW53	BW67	CW4	DR4	DRW13
A11	AW33	B13	B40	BW54	BW70	CW5	DR5	DRW14
A19	AW36	B14	BW41	BW55	BW71	CW6	DR6	DRW15
A23	AW43	B15	BW42	BW56	BW72	CW7	DR7	DRW16
A24	AW66	B16	B44	BW57	BW73	CW8	DR8	DRW17
A25	AW68	B17	B45	BW58	BW75	CW9	DR9	DRW18
A26	AW69	B18	BW46	BW59	BW76	CW10		
A28	AW74	B21	BW47	BW60	BW77	CW11		
A29		B22	BW48	BW61				
		B27	B49	BW62				

The rejection response is determined in part by the lack of match between class I or class II antigens in the donor and recipient tissues (Bollinger & Sanfilippo, 1989; Garovoy et al, 1987; Marboe, et al, 1990).

The complex of the four histocompatibility genes is known as haplotype and is usually inherited as a unit (Bollinger & Sanfilippo, 1989; Schwartz, 1987). Offspring inherit one of each parent's haplotypes to produce their own set of haplotypes. The genes at these sites are codominant, so both sets of inherited antigens are present on the cells of the offspring. Each child has a 50% chance of sharing one haplotype with a sibling and a 25% chance of sharing either both or neither haplotype (Figure 1–3).

HLA typing is used primarily in living-related kidney transplantation. Bollinger and Sanfilippo (1989) reported that the antigens at sites A, B, and DR have been demonstrated to be the most important in predicting successful kidney transplantation. A perfect donor–recipient relationship would produce a six-antigen match based on these three sites. In a parent–child pair there is always a three-antigen match from the inherited haplotype. Siblings have a 50% chance of having a three-antigen match and a 25% chance of having either no antigens match or a perfect six-antigen match. The more antigens that match, the less severe is the problem of rejection. The potential for a six-antigen match with an unrelated donor is very rare. It is also important to remember that ABO blood type must be compatible for solid-organ transplantation.

Not all graft tissues or substances induce the same allogenic reaction, that is, rejection (Goodman, 1987; Welsh & Male, 1989). The antigens expressed by the cells

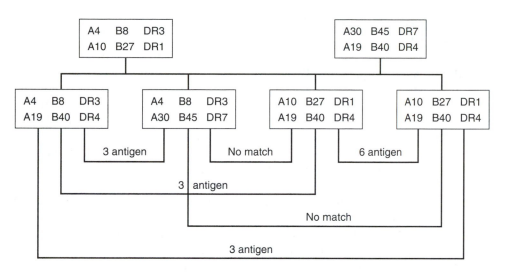

Figure 1–3. Haplotypes shared among siblings.

vary with different tissues, and some tissues may not have cells that present the antigens for processing. Bone marrow has the greatest capability of inducing a reaction, followed by the skin, heart, kidney, and the liver, which has the least allogenic potential (Welsh & Male, 1989).

HLA typing is performed using a technique called microlymphocytoxicity testing. Typing reagents to the four antigen types (A, B, C, and DR) are human sera obtained primarily from multiparous women who have produced antibodies during pregnancy to the antibodies of the fetus that originated from the father (Bollinger & Sanfilippo, 1989; Hart, unpublished, 1991). The specific antibody reagents are combined with lymphocytes, and a dye is added. If the lymphocyte expresses the antigen for the antibody, the cell is lysed and the dye enters the cell. The number of lysed cells are counted using a microscope, and a determination is made of the HLA type (Schwartz, 1987; Smith, 1990).

Histocompatibility Testing

To produce optimum results, particularly with kidney transplants, histocompatibility testing is done to observe for interaction of donor and recipient cells. Histocompatibility testing is most helpful with a living donor to predict compatibility, but it also may be used with a cadaveric donor to predict rejection potential and to assist with immunosuppressive therapy (Bollinger & Sanfilippo, 1989; Smith, 1990).

Three separate matching procedures can be performed. A WBC cross-match reveals if there are preformed antibodies to the lymphocytes of a potential donor (Bartucci & Seller, 1990; Garovoy et al, 1987; Smith, 1990). The presence of preformed antibodies provides a warning of hyperacute rejection and is a contraindication to transplantation from that donor. The sera of the donor and recipient are incubated, and a marker for cell death is added. Death of more than 10% of the cells is considered a positive cross-match, and the transplant is not done (Garovoy et al, 1987). The test requires about 6 hours.

A mixed leukocyte reaction detects class II antigens and can predict compatibility at the DR site (Smith, 1990). This test requires several days, so it is useful only for living-related donors as a pretransplant tool.

Repetitive antibody testing is beneficial for ongoing screening, particularly for patients waiting for a kidney transplant. Approximately once a month the sera of the potential recipient is cross-matched against a pool of lymphocyte samples from random donors. The percentage of samples to which the recipient reacts is known as the panel reactive antibody or PRA (Bollinger & Sanfilippo, 1989; Garovoy et al, 1987; Smith, 1990). The percentage is viewed as the risk of reaction with a random donor. A PRA of 90% indicates that the recipient reacted with 90% of the sample pool and would therefore be expected to react with most random donors. These results, in combination with ABO type, can help predict how long a patient may have to wait for a suitable donor. For example, a potential kidney recipient with a 95% PRA and blood type O might have to wait years for a good match from an unrelated donor. Another potential recipient with a PRA of 10% and blood type A may have a very short wait. The antibody screening is repeated monthly because antibody titers change over time.

HLA matching is most important in kidney and bone marrow transplantation and has shown some importance in pancreatic grafts (Bollinger & Sanfilippo, 1989; Garovoy et al, 1987). Histocompatibility testing is performed on potential heart recipients, but the information is used retrospectively because of the limitation of available grafts and the successful use of immunosuppressive drugs to limit rejection (Bollinger & Sanfilippo, 1989; Garovoy et al, 1987; Marboe et al, 1990). HLA matching is not used for the liver, which seems able to tolerate antigen products (Garovoy et al, 1987; Smith, 1990).

REJECTION

Rejection is the recognition and response to foreign donor antigens by the recipient's immune system. The antigens can be part of the ABO system, HLA antigens, or antigens that to which humans are exposed in daily life. The three classifications of rejection are hyperacute, acute, and chronic.

Hyperacute Rejection

Hyperacute rejection occurs within minutes to hours after graft transplantation. Preformed antibodies in the recipient react quickly to ABO or class I HLA (A, B, or C) antigens from the donor tissue (Ascher et al, 1989; Flye, 1989; Garovoy et al, 1987). Antibodies are more prevalent in recipients who have had multiple transfusions, multiple pregnancies, or a prior transplant.

The kidney is at greatest risk because the antibodies attach to vascular endothelium, initiating a cascade of events that results in activation of the clotting mechanism and massive intravascular coagulation in the glomerular vessels, causing tissue necrosis. The process can occur fast enough to be seen while the patient is still on the operating table.

There is no treatment of hyperacute rejection, but improved cross-matching techniques and careful screening have essentially eliminated the complication. This type of rejection is not seen in the liver. It is believed that the liver is used to the circulation of waste products and absorbs the antibodies (Smith, 1990). Hyperacute rejection in cardiac transplantation is rare (Welsh & Male, 1989).

Acute Rejection

In the first few days after transplantation a normal immune response is initiated. Acute rejection is usually seen from a week to a year after transplantation, but infrequently it may occur after a year (Shumway, 1990; Smith, 1990). Cellular immunity, the T-cell response, is thought to be primarily responsible for acute rejection, although the antibody system also participates (Welsh & Male, 1989). Antigens from the graft tissue are processed by the recipient's antigen processing cells (APCs) and presented to helper T cells, which stimulate interleukin production and T-cell proliferation (Ascher et al, 1989; Flye, 1989; Garovoy et al, 1987). Interleukins recruit other inflammatory cells, such as macrophages, and activate cytotoxic cells, which invade and destroy the graft if not checked. Memory T cells are also produced, which would lead to an accelerated rejection if the recipient ever required another transplant and the same antigen were present in the graft (Flye, 1989). Both interleukin and helper T cells stimulate antibody production, increasing the overall immune response against the graft (Ascher et al, 1989; Garovoy et al, 1987). Immunosuppressive therapy depresses the inflammatory and immune responses, preventing or minimizing rejection.

Rejection of most grafts is identified by laboratory studies that indicate deterioration in function, such as increased blood urea nitrogen (BUN), creatinine, or liver enzyme levels. Cardiac transplantation depends on regular biopsies to determine rejection; symptoms of decreased function do not appear until the process is too advanced to treat effectively. The extent of rejection is determined by the recipient's response to immunosuppressive therapy (Garovoy et al, 1987).

Chronic Rejection

Chronic rejection occurs over months to years after transplantation. There is gradual decrease in organ function caused by progressive fibrotic changes in the vascular supply of the graft (Flye, 1989; Garovoy et al, 1987). The actual cause is unknown, but it may be T-cell action and the multitude of mediators such as interleukins and other lymphokines that are part of the immune response. The only treatment of chronic rejection is retransplantation, with the exception of renal transplants, for which dialysis can be resumed.

The rejection process results in the presence of infiltrates of inflammatory cells and vascular and tissue damage that lead to organ failure (Ascher et al, 1989; Bartucci & Seller, 1990; Garovoy et al, 1987). The nonspecific changes of inflammation, such as fever, malaise, and tenderness or swelling around the graft site, may be present. Recognition of rejection is specific to the graft type. A decrease in function accompanied by altered laboratory studies can be seen in the kidney and liver. A biopsy can confirm the diagnosis. Chronic rejection of a cardiac graft is recognized by the development of atherosclerotic changes in the coronary arteries observed at cardiac catheterization (Garovoy et al, 1987).

Graft-versus-host disease (GVHD) is a rejection complication of bone marrow transplantation (Shelton, 1993). GVHD occurs when immunocompetent donor T cells respond to the recipient's tissues as foreign (Clark & Webster, 1990; Hawthorne, 1993). Acute and chronic forms of GVHD exist and are recognized by dysfunction of organ systems populated by immune system cells. Clinical findings may include skin rashes, blisters, loss of skin layers, elevated liver enzyme levels, gastrointestinal malabsorption, gastrointestinal bleeding, and fluid and electrolyte imbalance (Clark & Webster, 1990; Hawthorne, 1993).

INFECTION

The use of immunosuppressants to prevent graft rejection leads to a delicate balancing act with the prevention of infection. Drugs used to depress the immune response to the foreign tissue also depress the ability to fight other invading and infective organisms. All of the cellular responses are affected by corticosteroid therapy. Basophils, monocytes, and lymphocytes decrease in number. The number of neutrophils increases in response to corticosteroids, but the ability to participate in the inflammatory response decreases (American Hospital Formulary Service [AHFS], 1993; Hooks, 1990). Azathioprine decreases the activity of all types of immune system cells and suppresses the total WBC count. Other drugs, including the most commonly used, cyclosporine, target the lymphocytes, especially the T cells (AHFS, 1993; Bartucci, 1993; Hooks, 1990).

With a decrease in the number or effectiveness of the immune system cells, the body is vulnerable to attack by infecting organisms. Opportunistic infections are the most important cause of death among immunocompromised patients (Smith, 1990). Opportunistic organisms are typically present in the environment or have already colonized the graft recipient. Suppression of the immune system prevents the normal defenses from eliminating or controlling the organisms. Recipients can be infected by bacteria, viruses, or fungi that they encounter, normal resident flora, or reactivation of latent organisms. Herpes simplex virus (HSV) and cytomegalovirus (CMV) are common infecting viruses.

Infections are related to the type and extent of immunosuppression and the presence of environmental organisms. It is important to remember that recipients may be predisposed to infection by their preoperative condition, nosocomial factors, the presence of hospital organisms resistant to multiple drugs, invasive procedures, antibiotic use, and immunosuppression. The risk of infection is always present in immunosuppressed patients, and nursing must provide adequate protection and surveillance.

Prevention of infection should be a nursing priority. Hand-washing remains the best prevention technique. Maintenance of a clean environment is essential. Skin and mucous membranes should be protected. Mouth care should be provided frequently to prevent drying and cracking. Invasive devices should be limited as much as possible to preserve skin integrity. Surveillance for signs of infection must be an ongoing process.

Recipient and graft survival depends on the balance of immunosuppression to prevent rejection and the presence of an immune system capable of preventing infection. Knowledge of how the immune system works and of the actions of the immunosuppressant drugs helps the nurse recognize the development of rejection or infection in transplant recipients.

THE FUTURE

The ability to further understand and manipulate the immune system will determine the future of transplantation. Specific monoclonal antibodies that target the lymphocyte groups responsible for the rejection response are under development and in clinical trials (Crandall, 1990; Hourmant et al, 1994; Morris, 1991). Other immunosuppressive drugs such as FK506 and rapamycin are also being investigated for the prevention and treatment of rejection. Some organs, especially the liver, are more tolerant of transplantation than others. Studies are underway to induce tolerance to grafts by pretreating the recipient with donor antigens (Morris, 1991; Starzl, 1993). The antigens are administered as cells or a blood transfusion and lessen the likelihood or severity of rejection.

Xenografts, or the transplantation of organs or tissues from other species, are being studied as both permanent grafts or bridges until an appropriate human organ can be obtained (Cooper, 1992; Hammer et al, 1992; White & Wallwork, 1993). The major immunologic obstacle is the presence of natural human cytotoxic antibodies against other species. Bioartificial organs attempt to avoid problems with the immune system by enclosing cells or organs in a selectively permeable membrane or capsule (Galletti, 1992). The membrane allows the use of both allograft and xenograft tissues. This technology is the farthest in the future, but it is fascinating to consider this and other transplantation breakthroughs that may be seen in the 21st century.

REFERENCES

Allen MA (1993). The immune system. In: Wright JE, Shelton BK, eds. *Desk Reference for Critical Care Nursing.* Boston: Jones and Bartlett, 1091–1116.

American Hospital Formulary Service (AHFS) (1993). Bethesda: American Society of Hospital Pharmacists.

Ascher NL, Hanto DW, Simmons RL (1989). Immunobiology of allograft rejection. In: Flye MW, ed. *Principles of Organ Transplantation.* Philadelphia: Saunders, 91–104.

Auger MJ, Ross JA (1992). The biology of the macrophage. In: Lewis CE, McGee JO, eds. *The Macrophage.* New York: Oxford University Press, 3–12.

Bartucci MR (1993). Organ donation In: Clochesy JM, et al, eds. *Critical Care Nursing*. Philadelphia: Saunders, 1102-1115.

Bartucci MR, Seller MC (1990). The immunology of transplant rejection. In: Sigardson-Poor KM, Haggerty LM, eds. *Nursing Care of the Transplant Recipient*. Philadelphia: Saunders, 35-52.

Bollinger RR, Sanfilippo F (1989). Immunogenetics of transplantation. In: Flye MW, ed. *Principles of Organ Transplantation*. Philadelphia: Saunders, 47-71.

Clark JC, Webster JS (1990). Bone marrow transplantation. In: Smith SL, ed. *Tissue and Organ Transplantation: Implications for Professional Nursing Practice*. St. Louis: Mosby, 312-337.

Cooper DKC (1992). Is xenotransplantation a realistic clinical option? *Transplant Proc.* 24:2393-2396.

Crandall B (1990). Immunosuppression. In: Sigardson-Poor KM, Haggerty LM, eds. *Nursing Care of the Transplant Recipient*. Philadelphia: Saunders, 53-85.

Dawson MM (1991). *Lymphokines and Interleukins*. Boca Raton: CRC Press, 1-32.

Dressler DK (1993). Hematologic physiology. In Clochesy JM, et al eds. *Critical Care Nursing*. Philadelphia: Saunders, 1047-1054.

Drutz DJ, Mills J (1987). Immunity and infection. In: Stites DP, Stobo JD, Wells JV, eds. *Basic & Clinical Immunology,* 6th ed. Norwalk: Appleton & Lange, 167-185.

Flye MW (1989). Transplantation immunobiology. In: Flye MW, ed. *Principles of Organ Transplantation*. Philadelphia: Saunders, 18-45.

Galletti PM (1992). Bioartificial organs. *Artif Organs.* 16:55-60.

Garovoy MR, Melzer JS, Gibbs VC, Bozdech M (1987). Clinical transplantation. In: Stites DP, Stobo JD, Wells JV, eds. *Basic & Clinical Immunology,* 6th ed. Norwalk: Appleton & Lange, 420-434.

Goodman JW (1987). Immunoglobulins. I. Structure and function. In Stites DP, Stobo JD, Wells JV, eds. *Basic & Clinical Immunology,* 6th ed. Norwalk: Appleton & Lange, 27-36.

Griffin JP (1986). *Hematology and Immunology: Concepts for Nursing*. Norwalk: Appleton-Century-Crofts, 28-53.

Gurevich I (1989). *Infectious Diseases in Critical Care Nursing: Prevention and Precautions.* Rockville, Md: Aspen, 15-34.

Gurka AM (1989). The immune system: Implications for critical care nursing. *Crit Care Nurs.* 9:24-35.

Guyton AC (1991). *Human Physiology and Mechanisms of Disease,* 8th ed. Philadelphia: Saunders, 356-389.

Hammer C, Suckfüll M, Saumweber D (1992). Evolutionary and immunological aspects of xenotransplantation. *Transplant Proc.* 24:2397-2400.

Hawthorne JL (1993). Immunocompromised patients. In: Clochesy JM, et al, eds. *Critical Care Nursing*. Philadelphia: Saunders, 1116-1134.

Hooks MA (1990). Immunosuppressive agents used in transplantation. In: Smith SL, ed. *Tissue and Organ Transplantation: Implications for Professional Nursing Practice*. St. Louis: Mosby, 48-80.

Hourmant M, Le Mauff B, Cantarovich D et al (1994). Prevention of acute rejection episodes with an anti-interleukin 2 receptro monoclonal antibody. *Transplantation.* 57:204-207.

Huffer TL, Kanapa DJ, Stevenson GW (1986). *Introduction to Human Immunology*. Boston: Jones and Bartlett, 75-80.

Levitt D, Cooper MD (1987). Lymphocytes. II. B cells. In: Stites DP, Stobo JD, Wells JV, eds. *Basic & Clinical Immunology,* 6th ed. Norwalk: Appleton & Lange, 72-81.

Lydyard P, Grossi C (1989). Development of the immune system. In: Roitt IM, Brostoff J, Male DK, eds. *Immunology,* 2nd ed. Philadelphia: Lippincott, 14.2-14.9.

Male D (1991). *Immunology An Illustrated Outline,* 2nd edition. New York: Gower Medical.

Male D, Roitt I (1989). Adaptive and innate immunity. In: Roitt IM, Brostoff J, Male DK, eds. *Immunology,* 2nd ed. Philadelphia: Lippincott, 1.1–1.9.

Marboe CC, Buffaloe A, Fenoglio JJ Jr (1990). Immunologic aspects of rejection. *Prog Cardiovasc Dis.* 32:419–431.

Marcus DM (1989). The ABO, Hh, secretor, and Lewis systems. In Litwin SD, ed. *Human Immunogenetics: Basic Principles and Clinical Relevance.* New York: Marcel Dekker, 685–695.

Morris PJ (1991). Prospects in transplantation. *Transplant Proc.* 23:2133–2137.

Morton PG (1989). *Health Assessment in Nursing.* Springhouse, Pa: Springhouse, 553–581.

Rook G (1989). Cell-mediated immune responses. In: Roitt IM, Brostoff J, Male DK, eds. *Immunology,* 2nd ed. Philadelphia: Lippincott, 9.2–9.12.

Schwartz BD (1987). The human major histocompatibility HLA complex. In: Stites DP, Stobo JD, Wells JV, eds. *Basic & Clinical Immunology,* 6th ed. Norwalk: Appleton & Lange, 50–62.

Seller MC, Owen DC (1993). Physiologic response to infection. In: Clochesy JM et al, eds. *Critical Care Nursing.* Philadelphia: Saunders, 1075–1101.

Shelton BK (1993). Bone marrow transplantation. In: Wright JE, Shelton BK, eds. *Desk Reference for Critical Care Nursing.* Boston: Jones and Bartlett, 1212–1243.

Shumway S (1990). Basic immunologic concepts involved in organ transplantation. In: Baumgartner WA, Reitz BA, Achuff SC, eds. *Heart and Heart-Lung Transplantation.* Philadelphia: Saunders, 15–24.

Smith SL (1990). Immunologic aspects of transplantation. In: Smith SL, ed. *Tissue and Organ Transplantation: Implications for Professional Nursing Practice.* St. Louis: Mosby, 15–47.

Starzl TE (1993). Cell migration and chimerism: A unifying concept in transplantation; with particular reference to HLA matching and tolerance induction. *Transplant Proc.* 25:8–12.

Stobo JD (1987). Lymphocytes. In: Stites DP, Stobo JD, Wells JV, eds. *Basic & Clinical Immunology,* 6th ed. Norwalk: Appleton & Lange, 65–81.

Turner M (1989). Molecules which recognize antigen. In: Roitt IM, Brostoff J, Male DK, eds. *Immunology,* 2nd ed. Philadelphia: Lippincott, 5.1–5.11.

Welsh K, Male D (1989). Transplantation and rejection. In: Roitt IM, Brostoff J, Male DK, eds. *Immunology,* 2nd ed. Philadelphia: Lippincott, 24.1–24.10

Werb Z (1987). Phagocytic cells: Chemotaxis & effector functions of macrophages & granulocytes. In: Stites DP, Stobo JD, Wells JV, eds. *Basic & Clinical Immunology,* 6th ed. Norwalk: Appleton & Lange, 96–113.

White D, Wallwork D (1993). Xenografting: Probability, possibility, or pipe dream? *Lancet.* 342:879–880.

2

Infectious Disease in the Organ Transplant Patient

Sharon M. Augustine
Anne Nicholson Macdonald

As the field of solid organ transplantation expands each year because of improvements in procurement and preservation of donor organs as well as in surgical technique, infection remains an important cause of morbidity and mortality (Anderson et al, 1973; Baumgartner et al, 1979; Hofflin et al, 1987; Martin et al, 1991a; Corti et al, 1991; Keating et al, 1992). Fortunately, there has been a reduction in the incidence and severity of infections for the following reasons: the introduction of cyclosporine (Kahan, 1985; Gentry & Zeluff, 1986; Mora et al, 1991); experience with clinical patterns (Horn & Bartlett, 1990; Ho et al, 1990; Rubin & Tolkoff-Rubin, 1991; Keating et al, 1992); a decrease in the empiric use of steroids; improved diagnostic aids; and new antimicrobial agents (Horn & Bartlett, 1990). Nursing staff and clinical coordinators play an important role in the prevention, recognition, and treatment of infectious diseases in transplant patients.

FACTORS PREDISPOSING TO INFECTION: IMMUNOSUPPRESSIVE AGENTS AND SECONDARY RISK FACTORS

The factor most responsible for the development of infection in a transplant recipient is the use of pharmacologic immunosuppression. Additional predisposing factors include disruption of the skin or mucous membranes, chronic illness, poor nutritional status, and extremes in age. The manipulation of immunosuppressive agents to find a balance between the prevention of rejection and the development of infection, remains a challenge. The net state of immunosuppression and the subsequent incidence and severity of infection is related to the level, type, and duration of immunosuppressive agents used (Linder, 1988; Rubin & Tolkoff-Rubin, 1991). In general, immunosuppressive medications suppress cellular and humoral immunity, resulting in an increased risk of opportunistic infections. Overall, however, infections associated with cyclosporine-based immunosuppression occur less frequently than and are less severe than infections associated with conventional immunosuppression with azathioprine and prednisone alone (Copeland, 1988; Horn & Bartlett, 1990; Linder, 1988). Although immunosuppressive regimens vary among institutions, triple therapy with cyclosporine, prednisone, and azathioprine is commonly used. Quadruple therapy adds anti-thymocyte (ATG) or anti-lymphocyte (ALG) globulins (ATG, ALG) for the prophylaxis or management of acute rejection (Rubin & Tolkoff-Rubin, 1991).

Cyclosporine, a potent immunosuppressive agent, is a cyclic polypeptide produced from the fungus Tolypocladium inflatum (Hooks, 1990). Released for general use by the United States Food and Drug Administration (FDA) in 1983, cyclosporine dramatically improved immunosuppressive regimens through its selective action on lymphocytes. Cyclosporine specificity is primarily on the T helper–inducer lymphocyte subpopulation; the minimal effect is on B lymphocytes. The drug inhibits T-lymphocyte responsiveness to and production of interleukin-2 (IL-2) and interleukin-1 (IL-1) (Hooks, 1990; Van Der Meer, 1988).

Corticosteroids have broad immunosuppressive and anti-inflammatory effects. Cell-mediated immunity is depressed, and antibody production suppressed when the drugs are used in high doses (Whitman & Hicks, 1988). The anti-inflammatory response is suppressed by stabilization of the lysosomal membrane. The anti-inflammatory effect of corticosteroids inhibits fibrin deposition, phagocytic activity, capillary dilatation, and edema (Bass, 1986). Corticosteroids also inhibit the leukocyte mobilization that affects peripheral blood leukocytes; neutrophil counts increase and lymphocyte, monocyte, and basophil counts decrease (Hooks, 1990).

Azathioprine, an antimetabolite, inhibits purine synthesis. The antipyrine effects interfere with synthesis of RNA and DNA, resulting in decreased stimulation and proliferation of T cells (Crandall, 1990). ALG polyclonal preparations suppress cell-mediated immunity by causing pan-T-lymphocyte depletion (Crandall, 1990). Monoclonal antibodies, such as muromonab-CD3, block the function of T lymphocytes by specifically reacting with the T3 antigen complex (Hooks, 1990). The use of monoclonal antibodies eliminates the lot variability of immunosuppressive effects that can be found in polyclonal preparations.

In addition to immunosuppressive agents, multiple secondary risk factors predispose transplant recipients to infection. The skin and mucous membranes provide excellent first-line barriers to infection. Skin integrity, however, is disrupted by surgical incisions and invasive lines and tubes, providing a pathway for infection. Normal body flora and secretory IgA in the respiratory, gastrointestinal (GI), and genitourinary tracts provide protection against infection under normal circumstances. In addition, blood and body fluid pH levels inhibit the growth of organisms (Whitman & Hicks, 1988). Respiratory barriers to infection, such as the cough reflex, mucous production, and ciliary action can be impaired by intubation, anesthesia, smoking, and chronic lung disease. The normal intestinal flora, GI motility, and gastric acids can be altered by surgical intervention and medications (Smith, 1990). Urinary tract infections, the most common nosocomial infection, are commonly caused by the use of indwelling Foley catheters.

Chronic illnesses that predispose transplant recipients to infection include diabetes mellitus, hepatic dysfunction (eg, hepatitis, cirrhosis), renal disease with uremia, and disruption of splenic function (splenectomy) (Brayman et al, 1992; Dunn & Najarian, 1990; Smith, 1990). Nutritional deficiencies, often complicated by steroid use, can further predispose transplant recipients to infection (Weil & Rovelli, 1990). Extremes in age also increase susceptibility to infection. Neonates are compromised because their host defense mechanisms are immature. Elderly patients have atrophy and drying of the skin and mucous membranes and increased risk for trauma and degeneration of repair mechanisms. Humoral and cellular immunity are reduced in the elderly (Van Der Meer, 1988).

PREVENTION AND SURVEILLANCE

Pretransplant Assessment

Assessment for the likelihood of posttransplant infection is essential at the time of evaluation for the transplant. A detailed history of past infections, especially recurrent infections such as pneumonia, sinusitis, or urinary tract infections, should be obtained. Environmental, occupational, and travel-related exposures should be documented, as should immunization history and drug allergies (Keating et al, 1992). Serologic testing is done to establish a baseline regarding the patient's status of latent infection and to ensure the absence of a life-threatening latent virus such as the human immunodeficiency virus (HIV), which should exclude the patient from transplantation. The enzyme-linked immunosorbant assay (ELISA) is used to screen for HIV. Although this test is sensitive, it is not specific, that is, there is an attendant high percentage of false-positive results. The western blot, is a standard rapid test required to confirm any positive ELISA (Horn & Bartlett, 1990). Serologic tests are also performed to detect agents of latent infection that might be reactivated during immunosuppression. Routine serologic tests include those for cytomegalovirus (CMV), herpes simplex virus (HSV), varicella-zoster virus (VZV), Epstein–Barr virus (EBV), *Toxoplasma gondii*, hepatitis B virus (HBV), and hepatitis C virus (HCV). Some centers also test for tuberculosis and pathogenic fungi (histoplasmosis and coccidioidomycosis in endemic areas (Horn & Bartlett, 1990; Keating et al, 1992). Viral blood cultures for CMV and HSV are done at some centers, as are urine, stool, and sputum cultures to detect colonizing or infecting bacteria or fungi. Table 2–1 summarizes these tests.

Serologic tests are performed on donor serum to document agents that may be transmitted by the donor organ (Horn & Bartlett, 1990; Gottesdiener, 1989). The usual tests include CMV, *T gondii*, HBV, HCV, and HIV. Donors who have serologic evidence of HBV or HIV, or donors with a history of high-risk behaviors for HIV are excluded (Horn & Bartlett, 1990; Keating et al, 1992). Currently, there is not total agreement on the acceptability of donors who are seropositive for HCV (Mizrahi et al,

TABLE 2–1. PRETRANSPLANT ASSESSMENT FOR INFECTIOUS DISEASES

Thorough history and physical examination

Serologic tests
  Cytomegalovirus
  Herpes simplex virus
  Varicella-zoster virus
  Epstein-Barr virus
  Hepatitis B
  Hepatitis C
  Human immunodeficiency virus
  Toxoplasma gondii IgG

Pathogenic fungi

Tuberculin test

Viral or bacterial cultures

1991). Some centers have accepted carefully selected organs of donors with bacterial infections (Lammermeier et al, 1990).

Prophylaxis

Perioperative prophylactic antibiotic regimens vary according to the organ transplanted and center preference. These agents are used to combat postoperative nosocomial infections, such as pneumonia, line sepsis, and drain-related infections. Antibiotics are also used for infections specific to the site of the operation, such as mediastinitis, peritonitis, or urinary tract infections. Postoperatively, many centers use nystatin to prevent oral thrush in the immediately postoperative period. Long-term prophylaxis with trimethoprim–sulfamethoxazole (TMP–SMX) is advocated by many authorities to prevent common opportunistic infections, including those caused by *Pneumocystis carinii, Legionella, Listeria, Nocardia* and *Streptococcus pneumoniae,* and *T gondii* (Bartlett JG, personal communication, November 1992; Maki et al, 1992).

Prevention of Viral Infections. Viral infections, especially due to the herpesvirus group—CMV, EBV, HSV and varicella-zoster virus (VZV)—may be primary or reactivated. Reactivation occurs when a virus exists in a patient and becomes reactivated after transplantation. Primary infections occur as new infections after transplantation from an exogenous source such as a donated organ or transfused blood. Although it is not feasible to match CMV status between donors and recipients because of the paucity of donor organs, serologic testing of the donor and of the recipient preoperatively is important to establish a baseline.

Dental Prophylaxis. Before transplantation, any question concerning the oral cavity as a potential site of infection requires dental consultation. After transplantation, dental problems should be kept in mind as a potential source of fever. All dental work on a transplant recipient should be preceded by antibiotic therapy (Wade & Schimpff,

1988). Most centers use the standards set by the American Heart Association (Dajani et al, 1990) as follows:

Standard Dental Prophylaxis Regimen for Patients at Risk

Amoxicilin 3.0 g orally 1 hour before dental procedure, then 1.5 g 6 hours after initial dose

For patients allergic to amoxicillin and penicillin:

Erythromycin ethylsuccinate 800 mg or erythromycin stearate 1.0 g orally 2 hours before procedure, then one-half dose 6 hours after the initial administration

or

Clindamycin 300 mg orally 1 hour before procedure and 150 mg 6 hours after initial dose

Alternative Prophylactic Regimens for Dental or Oral Respiratory Tract Procedures on Patients at Risk

For patients unable to take oral medications:

Ampicillin 2.0 g IV or IM 30 minutes before procedure then 1.0 g IV or IM

or

Amoxicillin 1.5 g orally 6 hours after initial dose

For patients allergic to ampicillin, amoxicillin, and penicillin unable to take oral medications:

Clindamycin 300 mg IV 30 minutes before procedure and 150 mg IV or orally 6 hours after initial dose

For patients considered to be at high risk who are not candidates for the standard regimen:

Ampicillin 2.0 g IV or IM plus gentamicin 1.5 mg/kg IV or IM (not to exceed 80 mg) 30 minutes before procedure followed by amoxicillin 1.5 g orally 6 hours after the initial dose. Alternatively, the parenteral regimen may be repeated 8 hours after the initial dose.

For patients allergic to amoxicillin, ampicillin, and penicillin considered to be at high risk:

Vancomycin 1.0 g IV administered over 1 hour, starting 1 hour before the procedure. No repeat dose is necessary.

Vaccination

Transplant recipients as immunocompromised hosts are considered to be at high risk for influenza; therefore, transplant patients and their care providers, should receive influenza vaccine annually (Centers for Disease Control [CDC], 1984). The efficacy of most influenza vaccines varies with the season; it is estimated at 50 to 70% for prevention. Patients who acquire influenza despite the vaccine usually have a mild course. Immunocompromised patients who have been exposed to influenza and who have not been vaccinated may be given the vaccine along with amantadine 100 mg orally prophylactically for 2 weeks during the time required for the serologic response. Amantadine (200 mg/day) is recommended for treatment; patients with renal failure may require reduced dosages. Pneumococcal vaccine with the 23 valent preparation is advocated. This vaccine is given once, preferably before the transplant (Horn & Bartlett, 1990; Health and Public Policy Committee, American College of Physicians, 1986). Revaccination should be strongly considered after 6 years (CDC, 1993). Neither the influenza vaccine nor the pneumococcal vaccine contains live viruses; therefore, they may be given at any time either before or after transplantation.

Vaccines containing live attenuated viruses should not be given to an immunosuppressed patient because viral replication may be facilitated. Live vaccines to be avoided are measles–mumps–rubella (MMR); bacille Calmette-Guérin (BCG); smallpox vaccine, and the oral polio vaccine (OPV) (Horn & Bartlett, 1990; Soave, 1986; Redfield et al, 1987). OPV should not be used to immunize immunocompromised patients or close contacts (household contacts or nursing personnel in close contact with patients); enhanced inactivated polio vaccine (IPV) is recommended for such people. "If OPV is inadvertently administered to a household or intimate contact (regardless of prior immunization status) of an immunocompromised patient, close contact between the patient and the recipient of OPV should be avoided for approximately one month after vaccination, the period of maximum excretion of vaccine virus" (CDC, 1993, p 5). Transplant recipients should avoid all contact with the stool of a child who has received OPV for 1 month after the vaccination, or the child should receive IPV (Horn & Bartlett, 1990).

Isolation

Experience has suggested that there is no benefit to strict isolation procedures over various simplified procedures, including hand-washing only (Gamberg et al, 1987; Miller & Lough, 1987; Hess et al, 1985; Clark & Joy, 1985; Crow, 1983; CDC Guidelines, 1983). Differences among centers vary according to philosophies and experiences of the transplant team within the guidelines of infection control departments. Regardless of particular policies, good hand-washing should be emphasized.

POTENTIAL FOR RISKS TO NURSES AND OTHER HEALTH CARE PROVIDERS

Nurses and other health care providers are often concerned about the risk of contracting infections from their patients. With good hand-washing and attention to routine barriers regarding skin and mucous membrane exposure, however, nurses need not fear personal susceptibility (CDC Guidelines, 1983). The infections to which health care providers are susceptible are tuberculosis, salmonellosis, cryptosporidiosis, HSV infection, and VZV infection (Bartlett J, MD, personal communication, June 1993). Many of the late infections for which patients are readmitted are due to opportunistic organisms that invade immunocompromised hosts but not people with intact immune systems.

A common fear for pregnant women is exposure to patients with CMV disease. A study comparing health care workers caring for newborns and infants with groups of young women in the community concluded that no precautionary measures other than good personal hygiene and routine precautionary procedures for handling potentially contaminated material are required (Dworsky et al, 1983). Lipscomb and associates (1984) reported "no association between seropositivity and either current or past exposure to 'high risk' patients, such as infants and immunosuppressed individuals" after evaluating the prevalence of serum antibodies to CMV among nursing personnel working in various areas of a hospital. The study suggested that hospital nursing is not a major risk factor for acquiring CMV infection.

TIMING OF INFECTIONS

The most common infections observed during the first month after transplantation are similar to those acquired by any postoperative patient (Tolkoff-Rubin & Rubin, 1992; Bia & Flye, 1989). Examples are wound infections, line and drain infections, and urinary tract infections.

One to six months after transplantation is the time of greatest risk for life-threatening infection. The duration rather than the actual quantity of immunosuppressant medications contributes to the net state of immunosuppression (Rubin & Tolkoff-Rubin, 1989). One month after transplantation, the patient's host defenses are considerably compromised. Serious viral infections, especially by the herpesviruses and hepatitis viruses, tend to present during this period. Viral infections produce an immunosuppressed state that further compromises patients and leaves them at increased risk for superinfection by opportunistic organisms (Tolkoff-Rubin & Rubin, 1988; Bia & Flye, 1989; Rubin & Tolkoff-Rubin, 1991). After the first 6 months, the patient remains susceptible to opportunistic organisms in addition to community-acquired pathogens (Tolkoff-Rubin & Rubin, 1988, 1992; Bia & Flye, 1989).

Although it is helpful to use the timing of various syndromes as a diagnostic aid, infections do not always fall in line with this timetable. For example, it is important to remember that patients who have been treated with immunosuppressive agents before transplantation may experience an earlier onset of opportunistic infections than patients who have not received pretransplant therapy (Horn & Bartlett, 1990).

SITES AND TYPES OF INFECTIONS

Central Nervous System Infections

Infections of the central nervous system (CNS) are a serious cause of morbidity and mortality in transplant recipients. Infections can result in meningitis, meningoencephalitis, and brain abscesses (Miksits et al, 1991). The clinical presentation can be subtle even though serious. Symptoms may include headache, fever, malaise, nausea and vomiting, seizures, nuchal rigidity, and altered levels of consciousness or changes in mental status. The most common presentation is headache with or without fever (Horn & Bartlett, 1990). Neurologic findings may be focal or diffuse.

Even nonspecific clinical findings deserve prompt attention in the compromised host. The diagnosis is made with a careful physical examination followed by several diagnostic tools. Lumbar puncture is performed to examine the cerebrospinal fluid (CSF). Computed tomography (CT) with contrast enhancement and magnetic resonance imaging (MRI) are also important methods of diagnosis. A biopsy of the brain, if necessary, may be performed on focal lesions.

The most common CNS pathogens found in transplant recipients are *Listeria monocytogenes, Aspergillus fumigatus, Cryptococcus neoformans, Nocardia asteroides, T gondii*, and HSV (Ho et al, 1990; Horn & Bartlett, 1990; Ristuccia, 1985).

Bacterial Infections. *L monocytogenes*, a gram-positive rod, is the most common bacterial cause of CNS infections. *L monocytogenes* causes meningitis or cerebritis. The infection may present with minimal symptoms, such as a headache, or with a fever or a change in mental status. Patients with *L monocytogenes* bacteremia, even in the absence of CNS symptoms, should be evaluated with lumbar puncture because of the morbidity of the disease. The diagnosis is generally made with positive cultures from the CSF or blood and pleocytosis in the CSF (Ho et al, 1990). The treatment of choice is ampicillin, with or without an aminoglycoside (Armstrong & Polsky, 1988; Dunn & Najarian, 1990). TMP–SMX is an alternative treatment for patients who have penicillin allergies.

N. asteroides is a gram-positive rod that characteristically causes single or multiple brain abscesses. Thus, patients with pulmonary *Nocardia* infections should undergo CT of the head. The lungs are the primary site of infection. The definitive diagnosis is usually made by CT-guided needle aspiration. In general, long-term sulfonamide therapy (sulfisoxazole or sulfadiazine) is the treatment of choice (Armstrong & Polsky, 1988). Alternative agents include TMP–SMX, minocycline, amikacin, and cephalosporins (Ho et al, 1990). Other bacterial organisms that cause CNS infection in immunocompromised hosts include *Mycobacterium tuberculosis, S pneumoniae, Haemophilus influenzae, Neisseria meningitis, Staphylococcus aureus, Staphylococcus epidermidis*, and *Pseudomonas aeruginosa* (Ristuccia, 1985).

Fungal Infections. Fungi are a common cause of CNS infections in transplant recipients. For many types of fungal infections (eg, those due to *Cryptococcus, Aspergillus*, and *Coccidioides*), the lung is the primary site of infection, and the infection disseminates to the CNS. The drug of choice of most fungal infections is amphotericin B. New triazole antifungal agents have become available as therapeutic alternatives. Fluconazole has been used effectively for cryptococcal and candidal infections. In preliminary use, itraconazole has been used for *Aspergillus* infections (Rubin & Tolkoff-Rubin, 1991). These new treatment regimens are promising; however, for the purpose of this discussion standard treatment regimens are reviewed.

C neoformans is the second most common agent of CNS infection, after *L monocytogenes* (Armstrong & Polsky, 1988; Ristuccia, 1985). As seen with *L monocytogenes* meningitis, the clinical presentation may initially be subacute with a headache, fever, and malaise. Focal deficits are unusual. Lumbar puncture should be performed even with subtle clinical findings. *C neoformans* can be visualized by antigen assay in blood with 95% sensitivity and in CSF with 100% sensitivity. India ink preparations or Gram stains demonstrate the organism in the CSF (Armstrong & Polsky, 1988; Dunn & Najarian, 1990). The usual initial treatment is with amphotericin B and 5-fluorocytosine (Horn & Bartlett, 1990). Fluconazale may be used for oral maintenance therapy.

Aspergillus species (*flavus*, *fumigatus*, and *niger*) infections of the CNS are serious and often fatal. *Aspergillus*, like *N asteroides*, can cause single or multiple brain abscesses. The patient may exhibit focal neurologic findings, seizures, and disorientation (Ho et al, 1990). The diagnosis is generally confirmed by CT and biopsy aspiration. Treatment may include drainage or resection if feasible and long-term amphotericin B (Dunn & Najarian, 1990).

Less common etiologic agents of fungal infections in the CNS include *Candida* species, *Coccidioides immitis*, *Mucoraceae*, and *Histoplasma capsulatum* (rare) (Armstrong & Polsky, 1988; Ho et al, 1990; Ristuccia, 1985).

Protozoan Infections. *T gondii* is a protozoan parasite that can cause encystment in organs or tissues. Transmission can occur through the transplanted organ or blood products, or it can be a reactivation of a latent infection in the recipient. In the CNS, *T gondii* can cause focal abscesses and diffuse encephalitis (Rubin & Tolkoff-Rubin, 1991). The clinical presentation may include a headache, visual disturbances, photophobia, seizures, and focal neurologic findings (Ho et al, 1990). The diagnosis is generally made by serologic titers from the donor and recipient. Disseminated disease is common; therefore, a lung biopsy or needle aspiration or heart biopsy may provide a tissue diagnosis. Treatment of choice is with a sulfonamide (eg, sulfisoxazole) and pyrimethamine. For patients who are allergic to sulfonamides, the combination of clindamycin and pyrimethamine can be used. Another parasitic organism that may cause CNS infection in transplant recipients is *Strongyloides stercoralis*.

Viral Infections. Viral infections involving the CNS are commonly caused by members of the herpesvirus family. HSV types 1 and 2 (HSV-1, HSV-2) can cause encephalitis, but rarely. VZV infections result from dermatomal dissemination. The definitive diagnosis of HSV and VZV infections is rarely made from the CSF and usually requires a brain biopsy. VZV infection, however, can usually be recognized by CSF involvement with pleocytosis. The drug of choice is acyclovir. Less common causes of CNS infection include CMV and papovaviruses (Ristuccia, 1985).

Pulmonary Infections

The lungs are a frequent site of infection for all transplant recipients. Heart and lung transplant recipients, however, have a higher rate of pulmonary infections than recipients of other solid organs. Heart recipients may be increasingly susceptible to pulmonary infections secondary to pulmonary edema from congestive heart failure or prolonged intubation (Miller, 1991). The incidence of infection, however, is highest in heart-lung and lung recipients because of decreased mucociliary clearance, lack of a cough reflex, intubation, and an increased frequency of rejection resulting in increased immunosuppression (Maurer et al, 1992; Stewart & Cary, 1991).

TABLE 2–2. DIFFERENTIAL DIAGNOSIS OF FEVER AND PULMONARY INFILTRATES IN THE PATIENT WITH MALIGNANT DISEASE[a]

Chest x-ray abnormality	Etiology	
	Acute	*Subacute-chronic*
Consolidation	Bacterial	Fungal
	Thromboembolic	Nocardial
	Hemorrhage	Tuberculous
	(Pulmonary edema)	Tumor
		(Viral, pneumocystis, radiation, drug-induced)
Interstitial infiltrate	Leukoagglutinin reaction	Viral
	Pulmonary edema	*Pneumocystis*
	(Bacterial)	Radiation
		Drug-induced
		(Fungal, nocardial, tuberculous, tumor)
Nodular infiltrate[b]	(Bacterial, pulmonary edema)	Tumor
		Fungal
		Nocardial
		Tuberculous

[a]According to radiographic abnormality and the rate of progression of symptoms. An acute illness is defined as one developing and requiring medical attention in a matter of a relatively few hours (<24). A subacute-chronic process is one which develops over several days to weeks. Note that unusual causes of a process are placed in parentheses.

[b]A nodular infiltrate is defined as one or more large (>1 cm² on chest x-ray) focal defects with well-defined, rounded edges, surrounded by ae rated lung. Multiple tiny nodules of smaller size, as are sometime caused by an agent such as VZV or CMV, are not included here.

(Reprinted with permission from Rubin RH et al (1982). Current Clinical Topics in Infectious Diseases.

The clinical manifestations of pulmonary infections include pulmonary infiltrates or nodules (diffuse or focal), fever, cough (productive or nonproductive), dyspnea, fatigue, and malaise. It is often difficult to distinguish between symptoms of infection and those of rejection in heart-lung and lung recipients. The presentation and duration of an infection, in addition to the chest radiographic pattern can provide characteristic markers for identification of infection (Table 2–2 Ho et al, 1990; Horn & Bartlett, 1990). A short onset of illness with severe symptoms and a brief duration suggest a bacterial cause of the infection. A subacute onset may suggest a viral or opportunistic pathogen. Localized or focal infiltrates on a chest radiograph may be characteristic of bacterial or opportunistic pathogens such as *Nocardia* or *Aspergillus*. Diffuse infiltrates suggest a viral infection, as by CMV or HSV, or *Pneumocystis* infection.

Diagnostic procedures include a complete physical examination and history followed by baseline and serial chest radiographs. Diagnostic procedures should be instituted aggressively, beginning with less invasive procedures if the patient's condition is stable, such as obtaining sputum cultures or a transtracheal aspirate. Bronchoscopy with bronchoalveolar lavage (BAL) or brushings, however, is commonly used because of its high diagnostic yield and low associated morbidity (Linder, 1988). CT and MRI are helpful in detecting and delineating the anatomic features of pulmonary lesions. CT or fluoroscopy-guided needle biopsy is useful in the detection and diagnosis of nodular or localized peripheral lesions (Gentry & Zeluff, 1988a). Transbronchial lung biopsy is helpful in distinguishing between pulmonary rejection and infection; however, it is associated with risk of hemorrhage. Open lung biopsy is generally reserved for seriously ill patients with rapidly progressing symptoms when a definitive diagnosis is needed immediately. This invasive procedure requires thoracotomy and postoperative chest tube placement. Open lung biopsy, however, is particularly useful in the diagnosis of diffuse or multifocal infiltrates (Rubin & Greene, 1988).

Bacteria are the most common cause of pulmonary infections but are associated with the lowest mortality (Ettinger & Trulock, 1991; Maurer et al, 1992). The early postoperative period (1 month or less after transplantation) is dominated by bacterial nosocomial infections, whereas in the late postoperative period, the incidence of opportunistic infections, such as CMV, *Pneumocystis*, and fungal infections, increases (Miller, 1991). CMV is the most frequent pulmonary infection seen in transplant recipients. Additional common pathogens include nosocomial bacteria, including, *Legionella* and *Nocardia*; *Aspergillus*; *Cryptococcus*; *Candida*; *C immitis*; *H capsulatum*; and *Pneumocystis*.

Bacterial Infections. The predominant bacterial pathogens causing pneumonia in the early postoperative period are gram-negative bacilli, such as *P aeruginosa*, *Klebsiella pneumoniae*, and *Enterobacter* species. Gram-positive organisms, such as *S aureus* also may be seen (Gentry & Zeluff, 1988b; George et al, 1992; Maurer et al, 1992; Saint-Vil et al, 1991). Nosocomial bacterial pneumonias are related to intubation, atelectasis, and aspiration (Ettinger & Trulock, 1991).

Legionella, a gram-negative bacillus, may occur epidemically from nosocomial environmental sources, such as aerosolized contaminated water supplies in hospitals. The clinical manifestations of legionellosis vary, but they may include a characteristic presentation of high fever, dry cough, dyspnea, and pleuritic chest pain. Headache, diarrhea and changes in mental status may be present. Chest radiographs usually reveal patchy alveolar infiltrates, more commonly unilateral than bilateral, that increase and consolidate over time. Nodular infiltrates and cavitation can occur (Ampel & Wing, 1988).

The diagnosis, although not extremely sensitive, can be made from respiratory secretions by culture and direct fluorescent antibody staining and urinary antigen assay. Empiric antibiotic therapy with erythromycin is instituted as soon as legionellosis is suspected, because a definitive diagnosis is often difficult or delayed and the mortality, even with treatment, among this patient population is high (Dummer et al, 1988; Gentry & Zeluff, 1988a).

Nocardia species (primarily *N asteroides*) is a gram-positive rod, found in soil. *Nocardia* has been associated with environmental infections, presumably from contaminated air, water, or dust (Sahathevar et al, 1991). *N asteroides* is a serious opportunistic pathogen that infects the lungs primarily. The signs and symptoms of the illness can be nonspecific or absent (Simon, 1988). *Nocardia* infection characteristically produces focal or nodular infiltrates on chest radiographs (Miller, 1991).

Nocardia infection has been associated with infections by numerous other organisms, such as mycobacterial infections (Dunn & Najarian, 1990). The diagnosis is generally made by Gram and acid-fast stains and cultures of sputum and other respiratory studies, such as transtracheal aspiration, BAL, and percutaneous needle biopsy. The treatment of choice is with sulfonamides (eg, sulfisoxazole) or TMP–SMX. Additional agents include minocycline and amikacin (Horn & Bartlett, 1990; Simon, 1988).

Fungal Infections. Fungi that cause pulmonary infections include invasive opportunistic fungi, such as *Aspergillus* species (*niger*, *fumigatus*, and *flavus*), and *C neoformans*, and endemically restricted fungi, such as *C immitis* (southwest and western United States) and *H capsulatum* (midwestern US), (Dunn & Najarian, 1990; Rubin & Tolkoff-Rubin, 1991). The lung is the primary site of infection for most of these organisms, and dissemination (eg, to the CNS, joints, sinuses, and skin) may occur. These infections are also commonly associated with or superimposed on other viral or bacterial infections.

Aspergillus species, a deadly opportunistic pathogen, often is found in environmental sources, such as hospital construction (Gentry & Zeluff, 1988b; Weil & Rovelli, 1990). Pulmonary aspergillosis usually affects the lung parenchyma, but it also has been reported to cause ulcerative tracheobronchitis in heart-lung and lung transplant patients (Kramer et al, 1991). The presentation of aspergillosis can be subacute and characterized by fever, malaise, a nonproductive cough, pleuritic pain, and dyspnea (Dunn & Najarian, 1990). Pulmonary involvement may produce focal or diffuse infiltrates on a chest radiograph. The most characteristic lesion is a pleural cavitary lesion.

The early diagnosis of fungal infections is often difficult because of minimal symptoms, difficulty in obtaining a specimen, and slow culture growth. Diagnostic techniques include BAL and, if necessary, an open lung biopsy for histologic examination and culture. Rapid diagnosis has been demonstrated with the use of antigen assays for *Cryptococcus* and *Histoplasma* and Giemsa stain of respiratory secretions. Some patients may require percutaneous transthoracic fine-needle aspiration cytologic testing for localized lesions (McCalmont et al, 1991).

The treatment of choice of most pulmonary fungal infections is with amphotericin B, with or without 5-fluorocytosine. As in CNS infections, triazole antifungal agents, such as ketoconazole, fluconazole, and itraconazole, are also being used in the treatment of some cases of aspergillosis, cryptococcosis, histoplasmosis, and coccidiomycosis.

Protozoan Infections. The predominant protozoan infection causing pneumonia in the transplant population is *P carinii*. *T gondii* also can cause pneumonitis; however, it is relatively uncommon (Dunn & Najarian, 1990; Horn & Bartlett, 1990).

The clinical presentation of *P carinii* pneumonia (PCP) typically includes fever, a dry cough, and progressive dyspnea, which can lead to severe hypoxia (Gentry & Zeluff, 1988a; Rubin & Tolkoff-Rubin, 1991). A chest radiograph reveals diffuse bilateral interstitial infiltrates, which are often difficult to distinguish from CMV pneumonia (Bia & Flye, 1989; Horn & Bartlett, 1990). In addition, PCP commonly coexists with CMV pneumonia (Ettinger & Trulock, 1991).

Diagnostic procedures include bronchoscopy with BAL and transbronchial biopsy. Rapid diagnosis can be made with methenamine silver stain or direct fluorescent antibody staining of cytospun smears of BAL fluid (Dummer et al, 1988). Open lung biopsy is warranted if the patient's condition is critical and a diagnosis is needed immediately.

Because of the progressive and serious nature of PCP, empiric parenteral (TMP–SMX) therapy should be instituted while awaiting the diagnosis (Dunn & Najarian, 1990). Parenterally administered TMP–SMX is the treatment of choice for PCP; intravenous pentamidine can be used, but it has more adverse side effects than TMP–SMX (Horn & Bartlett, 1990). Prophylaxis with TMP–SMX, aerosolized pentamidine, or dapsone is used routinely to prevent PCP (Maurer et al, 1992; Rubin & Tolkoff-Rubin, 1991).

Viral Infections. CMV infection is an important cause of morbidity and mortality in all types of organ transplantation (Alessiani et al, 1991; Smyth et al, 1991). Pulmonary involvement resulting in CMV pneumonitis is the most common serious presentation of CMV disease (Calhoon et al, 1992).

The clinical presentation of CMV pneumonitis with cough and dyspnea also can be associated with the generalized mononucleosis-like symptoms of CMV, such as fever, malaise, hepatitis, and leukopenia. A chest radiograph typically reveals diffuse bilateral, primarily lower lobe infiltrates (Gentry & Zeluff, 1988a). CMV also may be associated with pulmonary superinfection caused by opportunistic organisms, such as *P carinii*, bacterial infections (such as those due to *P aeruginosa*), and fungal infections (Grattan et al, 1989; Rand et al, 1978; Smyth et al, 1991).

The diagnosis of CMV infection is usually made by bronchoscopy with BAL and transbronchial biopsy. Lung tissue can demonstrate characteristic CMV inclusion bodies or a positive culture. CMV antibody serologic titers may support a diagnosis of CMV infection, but they usually are not considered helpful (Dunn & Najarian, 1991). Treatment of CMV infections is controversial. Many authors believe the immunologic response is the most important problem, and that it accounts for the relatively poor response to standard antiviral agents such as ganciclovir or foscarnet. Some studies suggest ganciclovir plus CMV immune globulin is a superior form of treatment (Frank & Friedman, 1988; Icenogle et al, 1987; Keay et al, 1988; Ross et al, 1991; Smyth et al, 1991).

HSV, although rarely, can cause pneumonia (Ho et al, 1990; Maurer et al, 1992). HSV pneumonia, like CMV pneumonia, usually presents a diffuse interstitial pattern on a chest radiograph. Treatment is with intravenous acyclovir.

Cardiovascular Infections

Infectious complications of the heart, though not common, do occur. Bacteria are the most likely cause of cardiac infections, but they do not differ greatly from the bacteria in people who have not had transplants. *T gondii* and CMV can cause cardiac infections that result in myocarditis. These organisms are most often transmitted by donor-infected organs or in blood from seropositive donors to seronegative recipients. Reactivation of a latent infection in the recipient can occur. The diagnosis can be made with examination of endomyocardial tissue, but infection may be confused with rejection or may coexist with rejection (Stewart & Cary, 1991). Toxoplasmosis is more common in heart transplant recipients than in recipients of other organs because of predilection of the parasite for muscle (Dunn & Najarian, 1990; Gottesdiener, 1989). Therapy for toxoplasmosis consists of pyrimethamine and sulfadiazine. Seronegative recipients of hearts from seropositive donors should receive prophylactic pyrimethamine (Gentry & Zeluff, 1988a).

Gastrointestinal Infections

There are several difficulties in the diagnosis and management of GI complications in patients receiving organ transplants. These include the masking effect of immunosuppression, the preoperative metabolic state, the associated toxicity of immunosuppressive drugs, and the graft itself in recipients of renal, hepatic, and pancreatic allografts (Augustine et al, 1991; Dunn & Najarian, 1990).

Careful preoperative evaluation of patients with a history of ulcer disease is important. However, not all patients who have GI ulceration after transplantation have a history of GI problems. Corticosteroids have been implicated in duodenal ulceration and bleeding by disrupting the cytoprotective gastric mucosal barrier (Dayton et al, 1987; Hadjiyannakis et al, 1971; Messer et al, 1983). In addition, there may be an immunosuppression-associated reduction in gastric-associated lymphoid tissue, which would predispose the GI system to bacterial invasion, subsequent local infection, ischemia, and necrosis. Perforation may be the result of necrotizing enterocolitis (Dunn & Najarian, 1990).

Hypercalcemia due to tertiary hyperparathyroidism has been reported to induce upper GI bleeding after renal transplantation in patients with normal renal function (Saylor et al, 1984). Once ulceration or perforation occurs, superinfection with opportunistic organisms may follow.

Liver transplantation leaves a patient particularly susceptible to abdominal infections, because of the length and technical difficulties of the operation, the anastomosis to nonsterile sites, and the frequency of heavy bleeding. Patients with liver disease often suffer particularly from poor nutrition and metabolic deficiencies. Technical aspects of the operation itself may pose specific risks. For example, a choledochojejunostomy with anastomosis of the biliary duct to a Roux-en-Y jejunal loop is associated with a higher incidence of fungal infection than is a choledochocholedochostomy with anastomosis to the common bile duct (Ho et al, 1990).

Abdominal infection in pancreatic transplantation, varies depending on the method of pancreatic exocrine secretion. Anastomosis of the ampulla of Vater to the urinary bladder has a low incidence of deep wound infection because of the reduced intraoperative enteric contamination (Ho et al, 1990).

Diagnosis may be difficult, especially for patients who have not had recent abdominal operations, after which infection may be anticipated. Aggressive evaluation of even mild or vague symptoms, such as a low-grade fever and abdominal tenderness without leukocytosis, guarding, or rebound tenderness, is imperative (Augustine et al, 1991; Hubbard et al, 1980; Sterioff et al, 1974). These may be the only clues to intra-abdominal catastrophe in patients receiving steroids. Abdominal radiographs to look for air-fluid levels, endoscopy, upper and lower GI radiographic series, or colonoscopy should be initiated without delay. Stool cultures for routine pathogens should be performed early in persistent diarrhea, as should endoscopic or colonoscopic biopsies to look for CMV. Ultrasonography, CT, or MRI may demonstrate intra-abdominal abscesses.

Bacterial Infections

Bacterial infections are predominantly due to enterococci, gram-negative intestinal organisms, and anaerobes. In addition, staphylococci are often associated with peritonitis and abscesses. Radiographic studies of the biliary tract, such as T-tube cholangiography or endoscopic retrograde cholangiopancreatography (ERCP) may predispose the patient to cholangitis, abscess formation, and bacteremia. Therefore, prophylactic antibiotics are recommended (Rubin, 1988). *Clostridium* is the most common cause of diarrhea, but other causes include *Salmonella, Giardia,* and rotaviruses (Augustine et al, 1991).

Fungal Infections. *Candida albicans,* which causes thrush of the oral cavity, is commonly seen in immunosuppressed patients. Prophylactic or immediate treatment with oral nystatin is usually successful (Horn & Bartlett, 1990). Endoscopy or colonoscopy with biopsy may be required for diagnosis. Localized *Candida* infections may be treated with ketoconozole (Horn & Bartlett, 1990).

Viral Infections. HSV is seen frequently in the oral cavity, especially in the early post-transplant period but may be encountered at any time. It is the main cause of ulcers and vesicles, which may be painful. Treatment or prevention may be accomplished with acyclovir or ganciclovir, but foscarnet may be required for resistant cases. Acyclovir is usually sufficient, but prompt or frequent recurrences may require treatment followed by suppressive doses. The diagnosis is often delayed if there is no evidence of herpes stomatitis. Small ulcers on the oral mucosa can be difficult to see, even on thorough examination with appropriate lighting. The observation of concomitant thrush, which is relatively easy to see, often terminates the examination prematurely. To avoid extending the time patients may have to endure painful lesions, viral cultures or Tzanck tests should be obtained whenever possible if a patient complains of a sore or painful area in the mouth, even in the presence of obvious thrush. Herpetic esophagitis may occur and may require intravenous acyclovir therapy.

Although uncommon, HSV-1 hepatitis has been reported, as has hepatitis due to herpesvirus hominis and VZV (Elliott et al, 1980; Anuras & Summers, 1976; Holdsworth et al, 1976; Mozes et al, 1978). Hepatitis also may be caused by hepatitis A virus (HAV), HBV, HCV, or CMV. In liver transplant recipients, the diagnosis is particularly difficult because of the similar symptoms of rejection. Patients who receive liver or kidney transplants are more likely to develop hepatitis, reflecting the large number of blood transfusions required by recipients of livers and the long-term hemodialysis needed by kidney recipients. Recurrence of hepatitis B is manifested by elevated liver enzyme levels accompanied by malaise, nausea, and jaundice. It typically occurs 2 months after transplantation (Smith & Ceferni, 1990; Demitris et al, 1986). Serologic testing should be done for hepatitis B surface (HBsAg) and hepatitis core (HB c AG) antigens. The presence of hepatitis delta virus (HDV) before a transplant may signal increased risk for recurrence of hepatitis B (Smith & Ceferni, 1990; Colledan et al, 1987; Mason & Taylor, 1991; Rizzetto et al, 1991). Initially, there are only minimal changes in liver function. In the long-term, however, these patients may present with signs and symptoms of far-advanced cirrhosis and hepatocellular carcinoma (Rizzetto et al, 1991; Demetris et al, 1986).

The recent identification of HCV (Choo et al, 1989) has established HCV as the most important cause of posttransfusion and nonendemic non A, non B hepatitis (Martin et al, 1991b). Liver and kidney recipients are again at greater risk for this infection because of the frequency of blood transfusions and hemodialysis. The clinical course is variable, and patients with anti-HCV seropositivity before a transplant occasionally have recurrences, but de novo seroconversion appears to be uncommon (Martin et al, 1991b).

CMV tissue invasion can be identified by CMV inclusion bodies on tissue samples obtained by upper GI endoscopy, colonoscopy, or liver biopsy. CMV infection of the upper GI tract (esophagitis, gastritis, duodenitis, ileitis) has been reported to be associated with nausea, a sense of abdominal fullness, emesis, and dysphagia. Van Thiel and co-authors (1992) demonstrated enhanced gastric retention in these patients. Lower GI involvement (colitis) usually causes diarrhea, fever, and cramps. GI bleeding or even massive GI hemorrhage, perforation, multiple system failure, and death can occur (Sutherland et al, 1979; Dunn & Najarian, 1990, 1991). Furthermore, as Dunn and associates (1984) noted, in renal transplant recipients, concurrent HSV and CMV infections are associated with a higher allograft loss rate and patient mortality than CMV infection alone. Prophylaxis or early treatment with ganciclovir is therefore essential for patient survival and, in the case of liver transplantation, for graft survival.

It should be emphasized that a high degree of awareness and an aggressive evaluation may be required. The role of ganciclovir in treating CMV colitis is unclear. Severe GI infection may be seen in transplant recipients, for whom the masking effects of immunosuppression tend to lead to presentation with vague or deceptively mild symptoms.

Genitourinary Infections

Although they occur in all immunocompromised patients, urinary tract infections are seen most often and are more clinically significant in renal transplant patients than in others (Dunn & Najarian, 1990; Ho & Dummer, 1990).

Bacterial Infections. The predominant organisms that cause genitourinary infections in transplant recipients are those seen in the general population, including *Escherichia coli, Klebsiella,* Enterobacteriaceae, *P aeruginosa,* and enterococci. Early treatment with appropriate antibiotics is important. Any patient with dysuria should have a urine culture before treatment is started. Patients who have a fever without obvious cause but no other symptoms or patients who are diabetic with an unexplained rise in blood sugar levels should have urine cultures. Broad-spectrum antibiotics may be started after the culture specimen is obtained provided results are checked carefully so that switching to the organism-sensitive antibiotic can be accomplished promptly. Correction of stricture or other anatomic problems is also important. Infections of the urinary tract were once a major source of fatal bacteremia (Myerowitz et al, 1972; Anderson et al, 1973), but with more effective antibiotics and more awareness of the need to carefully monitor aminoglycosides (Tofte et al, 1982), mortality and morbidity have decreased.

Viral Infections. Papovaviruses are the usual source of viral infection after renal transplantation. The infections may be primary or reactivated. Although viral infections are not uncommon, they are frequently symptomatic and may be detected by viral culture, cytologic examination, or rises in antibody titers (Ho et al, 1990; Hogan et al, 1980; Gardner et al, 1984).

Fungal Infections. *Candida* is the predominant fungus seen in urinary tract infections, but other unusual pathogens have been reported, including *Mycoplasma hominis* and *Mycobacterium tuberculosis* (Ho et al, 1990). Treatment is controversial; it consists of local amphotericin B or fluconazole.

Infections of the Skin

The incidence of wound infections varies widely. It is reported to be highest among liver recipients, lower in heart and lung recipients, and lowest in kidney and bone marrow recipients. The most common pathogen is *S aureus.* Sternal wound infections in heart and heart-lung recipients may be most life-threatening if they result in mediastinitis (Ho et al, 1990; Steffenson et al, 1987).

An important skill in the prompt diagnosis of skin and soft-tissue infections is recognition of a characteristic localization and morphologic appearance. Therefore, early consultation with a dermatologist or infectious disease specialist or both is important. The definitive diagnosis often depends on culture results. Cultures of open or purulent lesions are usually productive, but contamination is a problem. Unfortunately, aspiration of inflammatory lesions such as cellulitis has a low yield. Because of an increasing problem with methicillin-resistant *S aureus,* identification is even more important, especially in immunocompromised patients (Feingold & Hirschman, 1992). Occasionally, surgical biopsy of involved tissue may be required.

The most common viral pathogens are VZV, HSV-1 and HSV-2, which may cause mucocutaneous lesions in the oral and perineal area, and VZV. Mild cases in which the patient shows no symptoms of systemic disease are usually successfully treated with acyclovir in oral doses. Severe and disseminated disease requires hospitalization for high-dose intravenous therapy. Herpetic iritis may cause partial or total blindness and severe pain; prompt referral to an ophthalmologist is important.

TABLE 2–3. COMMON SKIN PATHOGENS IN TRANSPLANT RECIPIENTS

Staphylococcus aureus
Herpes simplex virus
Varicella-zoster virus
Papilloma virus
Dermatophytes
Candida species

(From Ho M, et al (1990). Infections in solid organ transplant recipients. In: Mandell GL, et al, eds. Principles and Practice of Infectious Diseases, 3rd edition. New York: Churchill Livingstone, 2294–2303.)

Ho and co-authors (1990) point out that "the skin is often a target organ for many systemic infections. Systemic bacterial, candidal, cryptococcal, aspergillus, nocardial, atypical mycobacteria, and CMV infections may present with skin manifestations. As a rule, one should be aggressive about investigating any new or unusual skin lesion by biopsies in transplant recipients."

Infections of the Bloodstream

Sources of septicemia, like other infections, often reflect the type of transplantation. Catheter-associated sepsis is also a common source in the early postoperative period or whenever readmission includes insertion of an intravenous line. Depending on the organism, catheters placed by tunneling procedures often may be left in place and treated with antibiotics for most pathogens other than *P aeruginosa* and *C albicans* (Horn & Bartlett, 1990).

Other common sites of bacteremia include the lung, urinary tract, abdomen, biliary tract, skin, and soft tissues. Uncommon sources include upper airway structures, the sinuses, bone, and the CNS (Ho et al, 1990). In states of severe leukopenia, translocation of bacteria across the intestine may occur (Dunn & Najarian, 1990).

Detection of CMV in the blood does not have a high positive predictive value for disease; many patients are found to have positive CMV blood cultures. However, clinically significant CMV disease seldom occurs in the absence of CMV viremia (Ho et al, 1990).

DIFFICULTIES IN DIAGNOSIS AND TREATMENT

A thorough history, physical examination, and comprehensive laboratory testing are crucial to the diagnosis of infection in all patients. In spite of a prompt and aggressive diagnostic evaluation, transplant recipients present several unique circumstances that further challenge the transplant team.

The anti-inflammatory effects of steroids restrict the ability to produce pyrogens, therefore they often mask a fever. Medications that contain antipyretics should be ad-

TABLE 2–4. COMMON DIAGNOSTIC PROBLEMS IN SOLID ORGAN TRANSPLANTATION

Masking effects of steroids
Coexistent rejection
Multiple coexistent infections
Confusing or misleading laboratory results
Opportunistic infections
Subtle clinical presentation

ministered with caution, and patients should be clear about the nature of the drugs before discharge. An aggressive fever evaluation should be performed for temperatures greater than 38.5 °C. Nursing responsibilities often include obtaining proper specimens without contamination, collecting them in the proper container and medium, and ensuring delivery to the appropriate laboratory within a specified time (Gurevich, 1987). Initially, patients may not feel ill, because of steroid-induced euphoria, the blunting of symptoms, or both.

Rejection of some organs may cause confusing symptoms. Unless care providers have a high degree of awareness, early signs and symptoms of infection may be attributed to rejection. Furthermore, multiple infections may coexist.

Laboratory test results may be confusing or misleading. Elevated white blood cell (WBC) counts may be partially attributable to steroids, whereas low WBC counts could be a side effect of azathioprine or the result of a viral infection. Other medications, such as allopurinol or TMP–SMX, may suppress WBCs, making management of concomitant problems difficult. Treatment of rejection in the presence of infection can be problematic, increasing the patient's susceptibility to infection. Common diagnostic problems unique to transplantation are listed in Table 2–4.

Cyclosporine may cause nephrotoxicity and many antimicrobial agents synergistically exacerbate this problem. Moreover, because cyclosporine is metabolized almost completely by the cytochrome P-450 enzyme system in the liver (Van Buren, 1986), other medications using this system interfere with cyclosporine metabolism, leading to an increase or decrease in serum levels. Table 2–5 summarizes the common antimicrobial drugs that may affect cyclosporine levels.

SPECIAL INFECTIOUS COMPLICATIONS

Cytomegalovirus Infections

CMV infection is considered the most common serious infection impacting solid organ transplantation (Dunn & Najarian, 1991; Rubin, 1988). CMV infection is common in people with normal immunity and is usually subclinical; however, in immunosuppressed transplant recipients, CMV can cause serious disease. The primary risk factors for development of a CMV infection include: receiving an organ or blood products from a CMV seropositive donor and augmented immunosuppression (Pillay et al, 1992). There are three types of CMV infections: primary, reactivation, and super-infection (reinfection) (Lauzurica et al, 1992; Migliori & Simmons, 1988; Pollard, 1988; Pillay et al, 1992; Tolkoff-Rubin & Rubin, 1988).

Primary infections are infections of a seronegative recipient by a seropositive donor organ or blood products. Reactivation infections are caused by a latent virus in a seropositive recipient. Reactivation infections are commonly associated with aug-mented immunosuppression (Calhoon et al, 1992; Pollard, 1988; Smyth et al, 1991). Superinfection or reinfection occurs with infection transmitted from a seropositive donor organ or blood product to a seropositive recipient. Reactivation can involve transmission of different viral strains (Rocha et al, 1991). Approximately 66% of transplant patients at risk for primary infection, 20% at risk for reactivation infection, and 20 to 40% at risk for CMV superinfection become clinically ill. More than 90% of these illnesses occur 3 weeks to 4 months after transplantation (Rubin & Tolkoff-Rubin, 1993).

Primary infections in seronegative recipients are generally more severe than re-activation infections (Pollard, 1988; Weimar et al, 1991), but the incidence may be similar (Rocha et al, 1991). Seronegative recipients with seropositive donors are at highest risk for the development of CMV disease (Dunn & Najarian, 1991). The group at least risk for infection is seronegative recipients of organs from seronegative donors (Rocha et al, 1991; Smyth et al, 1991).

CMV can cause a generalized syndrome of fever, malaise, myalgia or leukopenia in addition to the following organ-specific syndromes: retinitis, pneumonitis, esophagitis, gastritis, colitis, glomerulitis, hepatitis, and pancreatitis (Calhoon et al, 1992; Keay et al, 1988; Rubin & Tolkoff-Rubin, 1991; Van Thiel et al, 1992).

The relation between CMV and rejection has severe consequences in transplant recipients. CMV is believed to modulate the immune system and is associated with acute and chronic rejection (Grattan et al, 1989; Weimar et al, 1991). CMV infection and disease have been associated with acute rejection and graft atherosclerosis in heart transplant recipients, obliterative bronchiolitis in heart-lung and lung transplant recipients, glomerulopathy in renal transplant recipients, and chronic rejection (van-ishing bile duct syndrome) in liver transplant patients (Grattan et al, 1989; Keenan et al, 1991; McDonald et al, 1989; O'Grady et al, 1988; Richardson et al, 1981; Weimar et al, 1991).

Clinical signs and symptoms can guide the diagnosis of CMV, but the definitive diagnosis is made with histopathologic examination or culture. CMV culture speci-mens include tissue, blood, urine, or nasopharyngeal throat swabbings. The use of the shell vial culture technique allows rapid identification of the virus (Dunn & Najarian, 1991). Tissue examination also can reveal the presence of CMV inclusion bodies.

The use of seronegative blood products and, when feasible, seronegative donor-recipient organ matching, prevents primary CMV infections. Numerous agents have been studied for prophylactic use. These include ganciclovir, acyclovir, foscarnet, im-munoglobulin, live attenuated CMV vaccine, and human leukocyte interferon. The ef-ficacy of these agents is not conclusive; however, the combined use of ganciclovir and immunoglobulins is most promising (Calhoon et al, 1992; Lauzurica et al, 1992). Treat-ment of CMV is with intravenous ganciclovir, foscarnet, or ganciclovir plus CMV hy-

TABLE 2–5. COMMON ANTIMICROBIAL AGENTS THAT MAY AFFECT CYCLOSPORINE LEVELS

Agent	Action	Affect
Aminoglycosides	Nephrotoxic agent	Increased nephrotoxicity
Amphotericin B	Nephrotoxic agent	Increased nephrotoxicity
Acyclovir	Nephrotoxic agent	Increased nephrotoxicity
Cephalosporins	—	No effect (animal studies)
Erythromycin	Impaired CyA metabolism	Elevated CyA blood concentration with and without nephrotoxicity
	Impaired biliary excretion	Elevated CyA blood concentrations with and without nephrotoxicity
	Increased absorption	Elevated CyA blood concentrations with and without nephrotoxicity
Imipenem	Increased CyA metabolism	Decreased CyA blood concentrations (animal studies)
	Unknown	Enhanced neurotoxicity (animal studies)
Itraconazole	Impaired CyA metabolism	Elevated CyA blood concentrations (conflicting data)
Josamycin	Impaired CyA metabolism	Elevated CyA blood concentrations
Ketoconazole	Impaired CyA metabolism	Elevated CyA blood concentrations with and without nephrotoxicity
Nafcillin	Increased CyA metabolism	Decreased CyA blood
Sulfamethoxazole and/ or Trimethoprim		Decreased CyA blood concentrations with
IV	Unknown	associated rejection episodes
PO	Tubular effect on creatinine	Increased serum creatinine
Isoniazid	Increased CyA metabolism	Decreased CyA blood concentrations with associated rejection of transplanted organs
Rifampin	Increased CyA metabolism	Decreased CyA blood concentrations with associated rejection of transplanted organs

(Adapted with permission from, Lake KD (1988). Cyclosporine drug interactions: A review. Cardiac Surgery: State of the Art Reviews. Philadelphia: Hanley & Belfus, p 618.)

perimmune globin (Icenogle et al, 1987; Keay et al, 1988; Ross et al, 1991; Smyth et al, 1991).

Epstein-Barr Virus Infection

EBV infections are associated with a mononucleosis-like syndrome and often fatal B-cell lymphoproliferative disease (Bia & Flye, 1989). Primary and reactivation infections occur, as in CMV infections. The overall rate of EBV infections, including primary infections and reactivation, is 41%, however, most infections are clinically silent (Ho et al, 1988).

The patients at highest risk for posttransplant lymphoproliferative disease (PTLD) are patients who have primary EBV infections after transplantation (Armitage et al, 1991). The frequency of EBV-associated PTLD is highest in the pediatric population since they are more likely to be seronegative at transplant and develop a primary infection after transplantation. The incidence of PTLD in pediatric transplant recipients is 4% compared with 0.8% in adults (Ho et al, 1988). The incidence of PTLD appears to be higher in heart and lung transplant recipients than other solid organ transplant groups. Armitage and associates (1991) found the incidence of PTLD in heart transplantation to be 3.4% and 7.9% after lung transplantation.

The diagnosis of EBV-associated PTLD is based on histologic tissue evaluation and EBV serologic titers performed before the transplant and compared with titers at the time of the diagnosis of PTLD. The occurrence of PTLD appears to be related to high levels of immunosuppression (Bia & Flye, 1989). Therapy for PTLD includes a reduction in immunosuppressive therapy and, in some cases, the use of acyclovir (Ho et al, 1988; Tolkoff-Rubin & Rubin, 1988). In some cases, surgical excision, chemotherapy, and radiation therapy are also used (Armitage et al, 1991).

CONCLUSION

Infection is a serious problem for immunosuppressed transplant patients. Infectious organisms are separated into four categories: bacteria, fungi, protozoa, and viruses. The sites of infections include the CNS, lung, heart, GI tract, genitourinary tract, skin, and bloodstream. The site of infection often corresponds to the transplanted organ.

Aggressive diagnosis and treatment are critical. The unique nature of the transplant recipients, because of susceptibility to or the coexistence of rejection, multiple infections, the subtle clinical presentation of infections, and the masking effects of steroids, makes diagnosis and treatment challenging. The incidence of infectious complications will be reduced by improved immunosuppressive agents and their combinations, improved antimicrobial regimens, and advances in diagnostic procedures. Clinical research and practice will focus on problematic areas such as CMV infection and its association with rejection and EBV-related lymphoproliferative disease.

REFERENCES

Alessiani M, Kusne S, Fung J, et al (1991). CMV infection in liver transplantation under cyclosporine or FK 506 immunosuppression. *Transplant Proc.* 23:3035-3037.

Ampel N, Wing F (1988). In: Rubin R, Young L, eds. *Clinical Approach to Infection in the Compromised Host*, 2nd ed. New York: Plenum, 305-324.

Anderson RJ, Schafer LA, Olin DB, Eickhoff TC (1973). Septicemia in renal transplant recipients. *Arch Surg.* 106:692-694.

Anuras S, Summers R (1976). Fulminant herpes simplex hepatitis in an adult: Report of a case in renal transplant recipient. *Gastroenterology.* 70:425–428.

Armitage J, Kormos R, Stuart R, et al (1991). Posttransplant lymphoproliferative disease in thoracic organ transplant patients. *J Heart Lung Transplant.* 10:877–887.

Armstrong D, Polsky B (1988). Central nervous system infections in the compromised host. In: Rubin R, Young L, eds. *A Clinical Approach to Infection in the Compromised Host,* 2nd ed. New York: Plenum, 165–191.

Augustine SM, Yeo CJ, Buchman TG, et al (1991). Gastrointestinal complications in heart and in heart-lung transplant patients. *Journal Heart Lung Transplant.* 10:547–556.

Bass M (1986). Common complications of immunosuppression in the renal transplant patient. *ANNA J.* 13:196–199.

Baumgartner WA, Reitz BA, Oyer PE, et al (1979). Cardiac homotransplantation. *Curr Probl Surg.* 16:1–61.

Bia MJ, Flye MW (1989). Infectious complications in renal transplant patients. In: Flye MW, ed. *Principles of Organ Transplantation.* Philadelphia: Saunders, 294–306.

Brayman K, Stephanian E, Matas A, et al (1992). Analysis of infectious complications occurring after solid-organ transplantation. *Arch Surg.* 127:38–48.

Calhoon J, Nichols L, Davis R, et al (1992). Single lung transplantation: Factors in postoperative cytomegalovirus infection. *J Thorac Cardiovasc Surg.* 103:21–26.

CDC (1984). Prevention and control of influenza: Recommendation of the immunization practices committee. *Ann Intern Med.* 101:218–222.

CDC (1993). Recommendations of the Advisory Committee on Immunization Practices (ACIP): Use of vaccines and immune globuline in persons with altered immunocompetence. *MMWR.* 42(RR–4):1–18.

CDC Guidelines (1983). Section 4: Modification of isolation precautions. *Infect Control.* 4:324–325.

Choo QL, Kuo G, Weiner AJ, et al (1989). Isolation of a cDNA clone derived for a blood-borne non-A, non-B viral hepatitis genome. *Science.* 244:359–362.

Colledan M, Gislon M, Doglia M, et al (1987). Liver transplantation in patients with B viral hepatitis and delta infection. *Transplant Proc.* 14:4037–4076.

Copeland J (1988). Cardiac transplantation. *Curr Probl Cardiol.* 13:163–224.

Corti A, Sabbadini D, Pannacciulli E, et al (1991). Early severe infections after orthotopic liver transplantation. *Transplant Proc.* 23:1964.

Crandall B (1990). Immunosuppression. In: Sigardson K, Haggerty L, eds. *Nursing Care of the Transplant Recipient.* Philadelphia: Saunders, 53–85.

Crow S (1983). Nursing care of the immunosuppressed patient. *Infect Control.* 4:465–467.

Dajani AS, Bisno AL, Chung JK, et al (1990). Prevention of bacterial endocarditis: Recommendations by the American Heart Association. *JAMA.* 264:2919–2922.

Dayton MT, Kleckner SC, Brown DK (1987). Peptic ulcer perforation associated with steroid use. *Arch Surg.* 122:376–380.

Demitris AJ, Sheahan DG, Burnham J, et al (1986). Recurrent hepatitis B in liver allograft recipients: Differentiation between viral hepatitis B and rejection. *Am J Pathol.* 125:161–172.

Dummer J, Ho M, McMahon D, et al (1988). Infectious complications in heart and heart-lung transplant recipients: Incidence and management. In: Gallucci V, et al, eds. *Heart and Heart-Lung Transplantation Update.* Venice, Italy: Uses Edizioni Scientifiche Firenze, 159–173.

Dunn DL, Matas AJ, Fryd DS, et al (1984). Association of concurrent herpes simplex virus and cytomegalovirus with detrimental effects after renal transplantation. *Arch Surg.* 119:812–817.

Dunn DL, Najarian JS (1990). Infectious complications in transplant surgery. In: Shires GT, Davis J, eds. *Principles and Management of Surgical Infections.* Philadelphia: Lippincott, 426–464.

Dunn DL, Najarian JS (1991). New approaches to the diagnosis, prevention, and treatment of cytomegalovirus infection after transplantation. *Am J Surg.* 161:250–255.

Dworsky ME, Welch K, Cassady G, Stagno S (1983). Occupational risk for primary cytomegalovirus infection among pediatric health-care workers. *N Engl J Med.* 309:950–953.

Elliott WC, Houghton DC, Bryant RE, et al (1980). Herpes simplex type 1 hepatitis in renal transplantation. *Arch Intern Med.* 140:1656–1660.

Ettinger N, Trulock E (1991). Pulmonary considerations of organ transplantation. *Am Rev Respir Dis.* 146:1386–1405.

Feingold DS, Hirschmann JV (1992). Approach to the patient with skin or soft tissue infection. In: Gorbach SL, et al, eds. *Infectious Diseases.* Philadelphia: Saunders, 1064–1066.

Frank I, Friedmann HM (1988). Progress in the treatment of cytomegalovirus pneumonia. *Ann Intern Med.* 109:769–771.

Gamberg P, Miller JL, Lough ME (1987). Impact of protective isolation on the incidence of infection after heart transplantation. *J Heart Transplant.* 6:147–149.

Gardner SD, MacKenzie EF, Smith C, Porter AA (1984). Prospective study of the human polyomaviruses BK and JC and cytomegalovirus in renal transplant recipients. *J Clin Pathol.* 37:578–586.

Gentry LO, Zeluff BJ (1988a). Infection in the cardiac transplant patient. In: Rubin R, Young L, eds. *Clinical Approach to Infection in the Compromised Host.* New York: Plenum, Medical Book Company, 623–648.

Gentry LO, Zeluff BJ (1988b). Nosocomial and other difficult infections in the immunocompromised cardiac transplant patient. *J Hosp Infect.* 11(Suppl A):21–28.

Gentry LO, Zeluff BJ (1986). Diagnosis and treatment of infection in cardiac transplant patients. *Surg Clin North Am.* 66:459–465.

George D, Arnow P, Fox A et al (1992). Patterns of infection after pediatric liver transplantation. *Am J Dis Child.* 146:924–929.

Gottesdiener KM (1989). Transplanted infections: Donor-to-host transmission with the allograft. *Ann Intern Med.* 110:1001–1016.

Grattan M, Moreno-Cabral C, Starnes V, et al (1989). Cytomegalovirus infection is associated with cardiac allograft rejection and atherosclerosis. *JAMA.* 261:3561–3566.

Gurevich I (1987). The cardiothoracic patient with infection: Effective collection of specimens. *Cardiothorac Nurse.* 5:5–8.

Hadjiyannakis EJ, Evans DB, Smellie WA, Calne RY (1971). Gastrointestinal complications after renal transplantation. *Lancet.* 2:781–785.

Health and Public Policy Committee, American College of Physicians (1986). Pneumococcal vaccine. *Ann Intern Med.* 104:118–120.

Hess N, Brooks-Brunn J, Clark D, Joy K (1985). Complete isolation: Is it necessary? *Heart Transplant.* 4:458–459.

Ho M, Dummer JS (1990). Risk factors and approaches to infections in transplant recipients. In: Mandel GL, et al, eds. *Principles and Practice of Infectious Disease,* 3rd ed. New York: Churchill Livingstone, 2284–2291.

Ho M, Dummer JS, Peterson PK, Simmons RL (1990). Infections in solid organ transplant recipients. In: Mandell GL, et al, eds. *Principles and Practice of Infectious Diseases,* 3rd ed. New York: Churchill Livingstone, 2294–2303.

Ho M, Jaffe R, Miller G, et al (1988). The frequency of Epstein-Barr virus infection and associated lymphoproliferative syndrome after transplantation and its manifestations in children. *Transplantation.* 45:719–727.

Hofflin JM, Potasman, I, Baldwin JC, et al (1987). Infectious complications in heart transplant recipients receiving cyclosporine and corticosteroids. *Ann Intern Med.* 106:209–216.

Hogan TF, Borden EC, McBain JA, et al (1980). Human polyomavirus infections with JC virus and BK virus in renal transplant patients. *Ann Intern Med.* 92:373–378.

Holdsworth SR, Atkins RC, Scott DF, Hayes K (1976). Systemic herpes simplex infection with fulminant hepatitis post-transplantation. *Aust NZ J Med.* 6:588–590.

Hooks MA (1990). Immunosuppressive agents used in transplantation In: Smith SL, ed. *Tissue and Organ Transplantation: Implications for Professional Nursing Practice.* St. Louis: Mosby Year Book, 48–80.

Horn JE, Bartlett JG (1990). Infectious complications following heart transplantation. In: Baumgartner WA, et al, eds. *Heart and Heart and Lung Transplantation.* Philadelphia: Saunders, 220–236.

Hubbard SG, Bivins BA, Lucas BA, Litvak AS (1980). Acute abdomen in the transplant patient. *Am Surg.* 46:116–120.

Icenogle T, Peterson E, Ray G, et al (1987). DHPG effectively treats CMV infection in heart and heart-lung transplant patients: A preliminary report. *J Heart Transplant.* 6:199–203.

Kahan BD (1985). Cyclosporine: The agent and its actions. *Transplant Proc.* 17 (Suppl 1):5–18.

Keating MR, Wilhelm MP, Walker RC (1992). Strategies for prevention of infection after cardiac transplantation. *Mayo Clin Proc.* 67:676–684.

Keay S, Petersen E, Icenogle T, et al (1988). Ganciclovir treatment of serious cytomegalovirus infection in heart and heart-lung transplant recipients. *Rev Infect Dis.* 10:S563–S572.

Keenan R, Lega M, Dummer S, et al (1991). Cytomegalovirus serologic status and postoperative infection correlated with risk of developing chronic rejection after pulmonary transplantation. *Transplantation.* 51:433–438.

Kramer M, Denning D, Marshall S, et al (1991). Ulcerative tracheobronchitis after lung transplantation. *Am Rev Respir Dis.* 144:552–556.

Lake KD (1988). Cyclosporine drug interactions: A review. *Cardiac Surgery: State of the Art Review.* 4:617–630 (monograph).

Lammermeier DE, Sweeney MS, Haupt HE, et al (1990). Use of potentially infected donor hearts for cardiac transplantation. *Ann Thorac Surg.* 50:222–225.

Lauzurica R, Borras M, Serra A, et al (1992). Reinfection or reactivation of cytomegalovirus infection in renal transplantation. *Transplant Proc.* 24:85–86.

Linder J (1988). Infection as a complication of heart transplantation. *J Heart Transplant.* 7:390–394.

Lipscomb JA, Linnemann CC Jr, Hurst PF, et al (1984). Prevalence of cytomegalovirus antibody in nursing personnel. *Infect Control.* 5:513–518.

Maki DG, Fox BC, Kuntz J, et al (1992). A prospective, randomized, double-blind study of trimethoprim–sulfamethoxazole for prophylaxis of infection in renal transplantation: Side effects of trimethoprim–sulfamethoxazole. *J Lab Clin Med.* 119:11–24.

Martin M, Kusne S, Alessiani M, et al (1991a). Infections after liver transplantation: Risk factors and prevention. *Transplant Proc.* 23:1929–1930.

Martin P, Munoz SJ, DeBisceglie AM, et al (1991b). Recurrence of hepatitis C virus infection after orthotopic liver transplantation. *Hepatology.* 13:719–721.

Mason WS, Taylor JM (1991). Liver transplantation: A model for the transmission of hepatitis delta virus. *Gastroenterology.* 101:1741–1743.

Maurer J, Tulles E, Grossman R, et al (1992). Infectious complications following isolated lung transplantation. *Chest.* 101:1056–1059.

McCalmont T, Silverman J, Geisinger K (1991). Cytologic diagnosis of aspergillosis in cardiac transplantation. *Arch Surg.* 126:304–306.

McDonald K, Rector T, Braunlin E, Olivari M (1989). Cytomegalovirus infection in cardiac transplant recipients predicts the incidence of allograft atherosclerosis. *J Am Coll Cardiol.* 13:213A.

Messer J, Reitman D, Sacks HS, et al (1983). Association of adrenocorticosteroid therapy and peptic-ulcer disease. *N Engl J Med.* 309:21–24.

Myerowitz RL, Medeiros AA, O'Brien TF (1972). Bacterial infection in renal homotransplant recipients: A study of fifty-three bacteremic episodes. *Am J Med.* 53:308–314.

Migliori R, Simmons R (1988). Infection prophylaxis after organ transplantation. *Transplant Proc.* 20:395–399.

Miksits K, Stoltenburg G, Neumayer H, et al (1991). Disseminated infection of the central nervous system caused by nocardia farcinica. *Nephrol Dial Transplant.* 6:209–214.

Miller L (1991). Long-term complications of cardiac transplantation. *Prog Cardiovasc Dis.* 33:229–282.

Mizrahi S, Hussey JL, Hayes DH, Boudreaux JP (1991). Organ transplantation and heptitis C virus infection. *Lancet.* 337:1100.

Mora NP, Cofer JB, Solomon H, et al (1991). Analysis of severe infections (INF) after 180 consecutive liver transplants: The impact of amphotericin B prophylaxis for reducing the incidence and severity of fungal infections. *Transplant Proc.* 23:1528–1530.

Mozes MF, Ascher NL, Balfour HH Jr, et al (1978). Jaundice after renal allotransplantation. *Ann Surg.* 188:783–790.

O'Grady J, Alexander G, Sutherland S, et al (1988). Cytomeglovirus infection and donor/recipient HLA antigens: Interdependent co-factors in pathogenesis of vanishing bile duct syndrome after liver transplantation. *Lancet.* 2:302–305.

Pillay D, Charman H, Burroughs A, et al (1992). Surveillance for CMV infection in orthotopic liver transplant recipients. *Transplantation.* 53:1261–1265.

Pollard R (1988). Cytomegalovirus infections in renal, heart, heart-lung and liver transplantation. *Pediat Infect Dis J.* 7(Suppl 5):97–102.

Rand K, Pollard R, Merigan T (1978). Increased pulmonary superinfections in cardiac transplant recipients undergoing primary CMV infection. *N Engl J Med.* 298:951–953.

Redfield RR, Wright DC, James WD, et al (1987). Disseminated vaccinia in a military recruit with human immunodeficiency virus (HIV) disease. *New Engl J Med.* 316:673–676.

Richardson W, Colvin R, Cheeseman S, et al (1981). Glomerulopathy associated with cytomegalovirus viremia in renal allographs. *N Engl J Med.* 305:57–63.

Ristuccia P (1985). Microbiologic aspects of infection in the compromised host. *Nurs Clin North Am.* 20:171–179.

Rizzetto M, Recchia S, Salizzoni M (1991). Liver transplantation in carriers of the HBsAg. *J Hepatol.* 13:5–7.

Rocha E, Campos H, Rouzioux C, et al (1991). Cytomegalovirus infections after kidney transplantation: identical risk whether donor or recipient is the virus carrier. *Transplant. Proc.* 23:2638–2640.

Ross C, Beynon H, Savill J, et al (1991). Ganciclovir treatment for cytomegalovirus infection in immunocompromised patients with renal disease. *Q J Med.* 81:929–936.

Rubin RH (1982). The cancer patient with fever and pulmonary infiltrates. In: Remington J, Swartz M, eds. *Current Clinical Topics in Infectious Disease.* New York: Mcgraw-Hill, 298.

Rubin R (1988). Infection in the renal and liver transplant patient. In: Rubin R, Young L, eds. *Clinical Approach to Infection in the Compromised Host,* 2nd ed. New York: Plenum, 557–621.

Rubin R, Greene R (1988). Etiology and management of the compromised patient with fever and pulmonary infiltrates. In: Rubin R, Young L, eds. *Clinical Approach to Infection in the Compromised Host,* 2nd ed. New York: Plenum, 131–163.

Rubin RH, Tolkoff-Rubin N (1989). Infection: The new problems. *Transplant Proc.* 21:1440–1445.

Rubin RH, Tolkoff-Rubin N (1991). The impact of infection on the outcome of transplantation. *Transplant Proc.* 23:2068–2074.

Rubin RH, Tolkoff-Rubin N (1993). Antimicrobial strategies in the care of organ transplant recipients. *Antimicrob Agents Chemother.* 37:619–624.

Sahathevan M, Harvey F, Forbes G, et al (1991). Epidemiology, bacteriology and control of an outbreak of *Nocardia asteroides* infection on a liver unit. *J Hosp Infect.* 18 (Suppl A):473–480.

Saint-Vil D, Luks F, Lebel P, et al (1991). Infectious complications of pediatric liver transplantation. *J Pediatr Surg.* 26:908–913.

Saylor RP, Sarosdy MF, Wright LF, Banowsky LH (1984). Hypercalcemia-induced upper gastrointestinal bleeding after renal transplantation. *Urology.* 24:337–339.

Simon H (1988). Mycobacterial and nocardial infections in the compromised host. In: Rubin R, Young L, eds. *Clinical Approach to Infection in the Compromised Host,* 2nd ed. New York: Plenum, 221–251.

Smith S (1990). Immunologic aspects of transplantation. In: Smith, SL, ed. *Tissue and Organ Transplantation: Implications for Professional Nursing Practice.* St. Louis: Mosby Year Book, 15–47.

Smith SL, Ciferni M (1990). Liver transplantation. In: Smith SL, ed. *Tissue and Organ Transplantation: Implications for Professional Nursing Practice.* St. Louis: Mosby Year Book, 273–300.

Smyth R, Scott J, Borysiewicz L, et al (1991). Cytomegalovirus infection in heart-lung transplant recipients: Risk factors, clinical associations, and response to treatment. *J Infect Dis.* 164:1045–50.

Soave R (1986). The immunocompromised host. In: Reese RE, Douglas RG Jr, eds. *A Practical Approach to Infectious Disease,* 2nd ed. Boston: Little, Brown, 514–544.

Steffenson DO, Dummer JS, Granick MS, et al (1987). Sternotomy infections with *Mycoplasma hominis. Ann Intern Med.* 106:204–208.

Sterioff S, Orringer MB, Cameron JL (1974). Colon perforations associated with steroid therapy. *Surgery.* 75:56–58.

Stewart S, Cary N (1991). The pathology of heart and heart and lung transplantation: An update. *J Clin Pathol.* 44:803–811.

Sutherland DE, Chan FY, Foucar E, et al (1979). The bleeding cecal ulcer in transplant patients. *Surgery.* 86:386–398.

Tofte RW, Canafax DM, Simmons RL, Peterson PK (1982). Aminoglycoside dosing in renal transplant patients. *Ann Surg.* 195:287–293.

Tolkoff-Rubin NE, Rubin RH (1988). Infection in the organ transplant recipient. In: Cerilli GJ, ed. *Organ Transplantation and Replacement*, Philadelphia: Lippincott, 445–461.

Tolkoff-Rubin NE, Rubin RH (1992). Infection in organ transplant recipients. In: Gorbach SL, Bartlett JG, Blacklow NR, eds. *Infectious Diseases.* Philadelphia: Saunders, 1040–1047.

Van Buren CT (1986). Cyclosporine: Progress, problems, and perspectives. *Surg Clin North Am.* 66:435–449.

Van Der Meer J (1988). Defects in host-defense mechanisms. In: Rubin R, Young L, eds. *Clinical Approach to Infection in the Compromised Host,* 2nd ed. New York: Plenum, 41–73.

Van Thiel DH, Gavaler JS, Schade RR, et al (1992). Cytomegalovirus infection and gastric emptying. *Transplantation.* 54:70–73.

Wade JC, Schimpff SC (1988). Epidemiology and prevention of infection in the compromised host. In: Rubin R, Young L, eds. *Clinical Approach to Infection in the Compromised Host,* 2nd ed. New York: Plenum. 5–40.

Weil M, Rovelli M (1990). Infectious disease and transplantation. In: Sigardson K, Haggerty L, eds. *Nursing Care of the Transplant Recipient* Philadelphia: Saunders, 88-113.

Weimar W, Balk A, Metselaar H, et al (1991). On the relation between cytomegalovirus infection and rejection after heart transplantation. *Transplantation,* 52:162-164.

Whitman G, Hicks L (1988). Major nursing diagnoses following cardiac transplantation. *J Cardiovasc Nurs.* 2:1-10.

3

Stress and Coping Among Transplant Patients and Their Families

Sandra A. Cupples

The purpose of this chapter is to discuss stressors commonly encountered by transplant patients and their families and the strategies employed by these people in coping with their stressors. The discussion begins with a consideration of stress and coping in general and of family stress and coping theory. Two models of family coping are presented. The section following the general discussion consists of a review of the literature pertaining to particular stressors and coping strategies associated with various types of transplants: bone marrow, liver, lung, kidney, and heart.

THEORETIC ISSUES

Stress and Coping Theory

Definition of Stress. Lazarus and Folkman (1984) define psychological stress as a transaction between an individual and the environment that is appraised by that individual as taxing or exceeding his or her resources and endangering his or her well-being. "Cognitive appraisal is an evaluative process that determines why and to what extent a particular transaction or series of transactions between the person and the environment is stressful" (Lazarus & Folkman, 1984, p 19). Through this process, all the facets of a given transaction are evaluated with respect to their significance for well-being. There are two types of appraisals—primary and secondary.

Primary Appraisal. A primary appraisal asks, "Does this transaction or encounter affect me, and if so, in what way and what is at stake?" Lazarus and Folkman (1984) distinguish three types of primary appraisal. An irrelevant appraisal occurs when a transaction has no implication for one's well-being. A benign-positive appraisal occurs when the outcome of the transaction is interpreted as positive in that it maintains or enhances one's well-being. A stress appraisal occurs when a transaction involves danger to one's well-being.

Secondary Appraisal. Secondary appraisal is a process of evaluating one's coping resources and options. One asks, "What can be done in this particular situation?" "[Secondary appraisal] is a complex evaluative process that takes into account which coping options are available, the likelihood that a given coping option will accomplish what it is supposed to, and the likelihood that one can apply a particular strategy or set of strategies effectively" (Lazarus & Folkman, 1984, p 35).

Reappraisal. A reappraisal is a change in one's original appraisal as a result of new information or feedback from the environment. It is a subsequent appraisal that follows and modifies an initial appraisal of the same episode or encounter.

Definition of Coping. Coping is defined as " . . . constantly changing cognitive and behavioral efforts to manage specific external and/or internal demands that are appraised as taxing or exceeding the resources of the person" (Lazarus & Folkman, 1984, p 141). The manner in which one appraises a given encounter affects both the coping process itself and one's emotional reactions to the encounter. The role of emotions is central to Lazarus' theory. Emotions are, in part, the products of cognitive appraisal. Once generated, however, emotions can in turn affect the appraisal process. Furthermore, both cognition and emotions have an interdependent relationship with behavior. Thus, coping involves managing not only the demands of the stressful person–environment transaction, but also the emotions generated by that transaction (Lazarus & Folkman, 1984).

Types of Coping. Lazarus (1966) and others (George, 1974; Mechanic, 1962, 1974; Murphy, 1974; Pearlin & Schooler, 1978) have identified two major types of coping efforts. Problem-focused coping is directed at managing or changing the problem that is causing the distress. Emotion-focused coping is aimed at controlling the emotional response to the problem (Lazarus & Folkman, 1984).

Problem-focused Coping. Problem-solving coping strategies are typically used when a stressful event is appraised as amenable to change. These strategies can be directed at the environment (ie, the stressor) or they can be directed inward toward the self. Strategies directed at the environment are similar to problem-solving strategies. They include defining the problem, thinking of possible solutions, weighing alternatives, and selecting an alternative and acting on it. Problem-focused coping directed toward the self helps the person manage the problem and employs such motivational or cognitive strategies as finding alternative sources of gratification or learning new skills and behaviors. Most inward-directed strategies involve cognitive reappraisals that are problem-focused (Lazarus & Folkman, 1984; Kahn et al, 1964).

Emotion-focused Coping. As its name implies, emotion-focused coping is directed at managing the emotional response to the stressor. This type of coping behavior is more likely to be used when a person has concluded that nothing can be done to change the stressful situation.

Emotion-focused strategies can be directed at decreasing or increasing emotional distress. Strategies directed at decreasing emotional distress include such defensive cognitive processes as avoidance, distancing, selective attention, denial, and minimization. Emotion-focused coping strategies directed at increasing emotional distress attempt to mobilize the individual for action. Athletes who "psych themselves up" before a competitive event use such a strategy.

Emotion-focused coping strategies can also be used to minimize a stressful event by changing its meaning. Statements such as "I realized that there are more important things to worry about" or "I decided that things could be much worse" are examples of emotion-focused coping strategies designed to reappraise the manner in which the event is conceptualized. The degree of threat is lessened by changing the meaning of the situation without changing the situation itself.

It is important to note that emotion-focused and problem-focused coping strategies can be used simultaneously. Moreover, emotion-focused and problem-focused coping can either facilitate or impede each other when used simultaneously. In the following example, these two coping strategies are mutually facilitative:

> A student beginning a major exam experiences great anxiety. The anxiety abates when attention is turned to taking the exam. In this instance, turning to the task (problem-focused coping) results in a reduction of emotional distress (Lazarus & Folkman, 1984, p 153).

The following is an example of how emotion-focused and problem-focused coping strategies can impede each other:

> A person with a recently diagnosed illness perseveres in gathering and evaluating information, the acquisition of which contributes to uncertainty and increased anxiety. He gets trapped in a cycle of problem-focused coping (information-gathering and -evaluating) which exacerbates his emotional distress and interferes with mechanisms such as avoidance that might otherwise be used to reduce stress (Lazarus & Folkman, 1984, p 154).

Family Stress and Coping Theory

Rodgers (1964, p 264) defines a family as a "semiclosed system . . . which is composed of interrelated positions and roles defined by the society of which it is a part as unique to that system." Family crisis has been defined as a disruption in the routine operation of the family system (McCubbin et al, 1982). Numerous family stress and coping studies were initiated in the 1930s to determine the impact of the Great Depression on the family unit. Since that time, the effects of other stressors, such as war separation, bereavement, and alcoholism, have been investigated.

The ABCX Model. In 1958, Hill articulated the ABCX model of family stress and coping (Hill, 1958). This model posits that X (the amount of crisis experienced by a family) is determined by the following factors:

A. The stressful event that causes a change in the family social system
B. The family's resources to deal with the stressful event
C. The family's perception of the stressful event; that is, the family's subjective appraisal of the severity of change caused by the stressful event.

The Double ABCX Model. Later social scientists theorized that family stress and coping are more complicated than Hill's original ABCX model. Using Lazarus' (1966, p 27) concept of stress as " . . . a generic term for the whole area of [physiologic, sociologic, and psychological] problems that includes stimuli producing stress reactions, the reactions themselves and the various intervening processes," these later family theorists identified normative and non-normative family stressors.

Normative Stressors. Normative stressors are predictable developmental changes that occur over the lifespan of individual family members and in the family unit as a whole. The first type of normative stressors are the human developmental changes postulated by Erikson (1950) and other developmental psychologists. These major stages of human development are prenatal to infancy; infancy to childhood; childhood to puberty and adolescence; adolescence to adulthood; adulthood to middle age; middle age to old age; old age to death.

The second type of normative changes are the stages of family development: establishment of the marriage; birth of the first child; entrance of the first child into school; families with adolescents; families in the launching stage; families without the children (the empty nest); retirement.

Thus, "the family unit is called upon to adapt to individual changes (human development) and family system changes (roles, relationships, organization, etc.) as a natural consequence of performing its function of evolving [as] a family unit *over time*" (McCubbin et al, 1982, p xii).

Non-normative Stressors. Non-normative stressors are unanticipated events that the family experiences. These events usually thrust the family into a state of relative instability and require a degree of creative coping efforts. Examples of non-normative stressors are illness of or injury to a family member, loss of employment, or hospitalization of a family member (McCubbin et al, 1982).

The double ABCX Model (McCubbin & Patterson, 1982) extends Hill's original model by taking into consideration both the normative and non-normative stressors that confront families over a life time. The double A represents not only the initial stressor event, but also the simultaneous family life changes and the stressors that result from the family's efforts to cope with the initial stressor event. For example, a family coping with the father's prolonged illness (initial stressor) might also have to deal with simultaneous normative changes associated with adolescent children and the consequences of the mother's return to full-time employment.

The double B factor is expanded to include not only the resources already available to the family (ie, resources developed in coping with prior stressors) but also additional personal, family, or social coping resources developed or strengthened in the current crisis. Examples of these additional resources include self-reliance, family integration, and social support (McCubbin & Patterson, 1982).

The double C factor consists of two perceptions. The first is the family's appraisal of the stressor event. The second factor is the family's perception of the crisis. This second factor takes into consideration the pile-up of other concurrent normative stressors as well as the meaning the family attaches to the total family situation.

In McCubbin and Patterson's (1982) model, the X factor is doubled to include not only the amount of crisis experienced by the family but also the family's adaptation to stress over time. This concept of family adaptation over time takes into consideration both normative and non-normative stressors. It represents the extent to which the family is able to preserve family unity and enhance the growth and development of its members. The double X (family crisis and adaptation) is determined by the previous three factors: double A, double B, and double C.

Family Coping. McCubbin et al (1982, p xv) noted that family coping is an active process which " . . . not only deals with the stressor event by eliminating it or reducing its impact, but also with the simultaneous management of other equally critical aspects of family life." "[It] refers to the cognitive and behavioral efforts to master conditions of harm, threat, or challenge when a routine or automatic response is neither readily available nor a natural part of the individual's or family's basic repertoire" (McCubbin et al, 1982, p xiv). Moreover, family coping strategies change over time as the family unit evolves and as the circumstances surrounding the stressor change. Family coping studies have indicated that there is no single coping mechanism that is effective in dealing with every conceivable stressor. Rather, the research seems to indicate that having a variety of coping responses and resources enhances coping effectiveness (Pearlin & Schooler, 1982).

It is salient to consider why it is important to know how families cope with various stressors. Family coping studies suggest that families are more amenable to influence by professionals during times of stress than during stable periods. Therefore, even minor interventions by health care professionals can significantly influence the outcome of a stressful event. Such positive outcomes not only are rewarding for health care professionals, but also, as McCubbin et al (1982, p xvi) noted, "the successful mastery of family life events can constitute an important growth experience" for the family as well.

SPECIFIC TRANSPLANT POPULATIONS

Bone Marrow Transplantation

General Considerations. Bone marrow transplantation is used to treat leukemia and associated bone marrow disorders. There are two types of bone marrow transplants: allogenic and autologous. With an allogenic transplant, bone marrow from a related or non-related donor is infused into a patient with a life-threatening disease. With an autologous bone marrow transplant, the patient's own bone marrow is removed while the disease is in remission and later reinfused. Autologous bone marrow transplantation is also used to treat patients with other types of cancer. Preparation for either type of bone marrow transplantation includes high-dose conditioning chemotherapy, total body irradiation, or both. The actual transplant procedure is followed by a period of isolation in a germ-free environment. Major complications include pneumonitis, cytomegalovirus infection, delayed immunologic reconstruction, and graft-versus-host disease (GVHD) (Wikle et al, 1990). The average hospital stay for a bone marrow recipient is 6 weeks (Futterman et al, 1991). The average length of time between the initial diagnosis and a successful bone marrow transplant is 2 years. Most major bone marrow transplantation centers report a projected 5-year survival rate of 50 to 60% for either type of transplant (Jenkins et al, 1991).

Stressors and Coping Strategies in the Adult Population. In their landmark article, Brown and Kelly (1976) identified several discrete stages of the bone marrow transplantation process. These stages provide a convenient framework for categorizing the stressors associated with the procedure.

Stage 1. The Decision to Undergo Bone Marrow Transplantation: Anticipation. The decision to proceed with a bone marrow transplant constitutes the initial stressor. Popkin and Moldow (1977) noted that both the patient and the family are immediately confronted with the critical nature of the illness. The search for a donor begins. If a related donor is found, family rivalries may develop if some family members feel unimportant because they were not selected. Conversely, the chosen donor may wish that he or she had not been selected. If no related donor is found, the 2-to-3-month donor bank search begins. If this search is futile, the family may feel that they have not searched long enough (Patenaude, 1990).

   Although the number of bone marrow transplantation centers is increasing, the decision to undergo bone marrow transplantation is usually made some distance away from the transplant center. As a result, patients and families often experience a fear of the unknown, because they are unaware of the specific procedures associated with bone marrow transplantation (Brown & Kelly, 1976). Haberman (1988) noted that it is common for referring physicians to cite survival rates that are more optimistic than the accurate survival statistics (national or institutional) provided by the transplant team. On arrival at the transplantation center, patients and families may experience anger and shock on learning these more realistic rates and may question the validity of the decision to undergo the transplant.

   Despite having to read and sign detailed informed consent statements, bone marrow transplant patients often use defense mechanisms such as denial or displacement to decrease their sense of vulnerability. After signing the consent form, such patients typically avoid thinking or talking about serious risks such as death or sterility and may focus instead on relatively unimportant issues such as hair loss (Brown & Kelly, 1976).

Stage 2. Initial Admission Evaluation: Preparation. This outpatient stage is characterized by extensive medical preparation and psychosocial evaluations. Patients may be concerned that a newly diagnosed medical problem will preclude or postpone the transplant. This period is characterized by protracted waiting, first for test results and then for a hospital bed. Patients report feeling "stuck in limbo" (Haberman, 1988).

Patients who have to relocate nearer to the transplant center are confronted with saying good-byes to families and friends, taking at least a temporary leave of absence from work or school, and finding temporary housing. For most patients, details regarding a will, power of attorney, health insurance, finances, and child care must be finalized during this stage (Haberman, 1988).

Coping strategies used by patients and families during this stage include obtaining information from the transplant team, talking to previous bone marrow recipients, maintaining a positive attitude, and reasserting the will to live (Haberman, 1988).

Stage 3. Immunosuppression and Isolation: The Point of No Return. As Buchsel and Kelleher (1989) noted, bone marrow transplantation is the only transplant procedure in which the recipient undergoes high-dose chemotherapy or total body irradiation to eradicate both the immune response and the disease. Patients begin to think of themselves as physically and psychologically exposed and defenseless during or soon after this preparatory immunosuppression phase. This is the point of no return—the patient must proceed with the transplant. As a result, patients may become more concerned about death and dying at this stage (Brown & Kelly, 1976). Physical stressors include nausea and vomiting. Patients with aplastic anemia who had no symptoms up to this point may now question their decision to undergo transplantation. It is also during this stage that patients may begin to doubt how they will handle the rest of the bone marrow transplant experience (Haberman, 1988). Jenkins and colleagues (1991) in a retrospective study of psychosocial morbidity found that 58% of patients who underwent total body irradiation reported temporary but appreciable cognitive impairment during this stage.

It is at this point that patients require protective isolation. Patients are confined to their rooms and often are further restricted by intravenous tubing. Regardless of the type of isolation (life island, laminar air flow room, or reverse isolation room), feelings of loneliness and barriers to touching and closeness are major stressors for both patients and families (Brown & Kelly, 1976; Haberman, 1988; Holland et al, 1977). The restrictions imposed during this stage are usually more stressful for active than for inactive people (Brown & Kelly, 1984).

Patients often attempt to cope with the stressors of isolation and not being able to "turn back" by demanding more attention or more detailed explanations about and increased control over their care. Both patient and family coping can be facilitated by allowing patients to make as many choices as practical, by suggesting that patients use binoculars or telescopes to expand their boundaries (Patenaude, 1990), and by allowing family members to participate in the patient's care as much as possible (Brown & Kelly, 1976).

In their study of bone marrow recipients in reverse isolation, Collins and associates (1989) found that patients' coping mechanisms were highly individualistic. Coping strategies included dividing the day into blocks of activities; keeping a positive attitude; sleeping; and using televisions, video cassette recorders, and radios. Because patients use sleep as a coping mechanism, nurses were encouraged to consolidate nursing tasks so as not to wake patients unnecessarily.

Stage 4. The Transplant Itself. This central event of the entire bone marrow transplantation process consists of a relatively simple intravenous infusion. Because this stage is brief, there are few stressors other than the recipient's concern for the well-being of the donor (Brown & Kelly, 1976; Haberman, 1988).

Stage 5. Graft Rejection or Take: Waiting. This stage constitutes an extended waiting period (6 to 35 days), during which patients wait for engraftment. Stressors related to changes in body image and isolation may continue. The most important psychosocial stressors for both patients and family members during this stage are uncertainty and the proximity of death (Haberman, 1988; Popkin & Moldow, 1977). Coping mechanisms include taking one day at a time and monitoring laboratory values for evidence of successful engraftment (Brown & Kelly, 1976; Haberman, 1988).

Stage 6. Graft-Versus-Host Disease. Solid organ transplant recipients fear organ rejection. Bone marrow recipients fear graft-versus-host disease, a condition in which the transplanted bone marrow attacks the patient's skin, liver, and gastrointestinal tract (Wikle et al, 1990). Episodes of GVHD are stressful for both patients and family members. Patients often become angry and depressed. Their depression may be worsened by the need for continued isolation and immunosuppression. Family members may be overwhelmed by the ongoing crises. It is not uncommon for related donors to mistakenly believe that some deficiency in their bone marrow precipitated the GVHD (Brown & Kelly, 1976).

Stage 7. Preparation for Discharge. During this stage, patients are taught how to care for themselves after discharge. At this point, they also may be concerned about the social stigma of wearing a protective face mask (Haberman, 1988). As Brown and Kelly (1976) noted, patients gradually begin to pick up the pieces of their former lives. As they do, they may have doubts about their ability to resume their roles as wage earner, spouse, or parent. Some may be concerned that their families will be overprotective (Haberman, 1988).

Typically, patients manifest ambivalent feelings during this stage (Hengeveld et al, 1988; Wikle et al, 1990). While they look forward to going home, patients also fear leaving the security of the hospital setting. For example, patients and family members may doubt their ability to detect a serious medical complication. In addition, patients may become depressed as they terminate their relationships with hospital staff. During this stage, it is important to provide specific follow-up instructions and offer continued support (Brown & Kelly, 1976; Haberman, 1988).

Stage 8. Adaptation Outside the Hospital. Stressors associated with this stage include social isolation (up to 1 year) and rehospitalization for problems due to relapse, infection, chronic GVHD, and renal and hepatic dysfunction (Patenaude, 1990). In their study of 17 adult bone marrow recipients, Wolcott and associates (1986) found that 60% of patients reported "feeling like a leper" due to unpleasant social experiences. Other psychosocial stressors involve gonadal dysfunction such as sterility or premature menopause (Buchsel & Kelleher, 1989), sexual adjustment, reentry into the school or work environment, marital and family reintegration, and reestablishment of an identity other than that of transplant recipient (Freund & Siegel, 1986; Patenaude, 1990). Hengeveld et al (1988) noted that bone marrow recipients are often torn between resuming a normal lifestyle and having to obey the rules while looking for signs and symptoms of possible complications.

Both patients and family members may be concerned about whether the bone marrow transplantation process has permanently changed the recipient. It is essential that health care providers reiterate that the patient is the same person he or she was before the transplant and that the special precautions associated with this phase are only temporary.

Death of the Recipient. In addition to the stressors associated with the death of a family member, the person who suggested or encouraged the recipient to undergo bone marrow transplantation may feel or may be held responsible for the patient's death (Brown & Kelly, 1976).

Stressors and Coping Mechanisms in the Pediatric Population. Although stressors and coping strategies in the pediatric population are similar to those in the adult population, there are some notable differences (Pfefferbaum et al, 1978).

Before the Transplant. With respect to informed consent, parental stress may be compounded by the risks to the healthy sibling donor. In rare cases, parental coercion is a potential stressor for the child donor or recipient. Before the transplant, children often fear being a burden to the family (McConville et al, 1990). Preparatory chemotherapy and total body irradiation are extremely stressful for parents as they helplessly watch the child endure the side effects of these procedures. Hanigan (1990) noted that high-dose chemoradiotherapy can be physiologically more stressful for children than adults because of concurrent organ development and the higher metabolic rate of children.

Day of the Transplant. The actual transplant day may be particularly stressful for parents, who must divide their attention between the recipient and the donor sibling.

After the Transplant. During the posttransplant waiting period, parents often are preoccupied with laboratory values. Participating in the care of the child is often a helpful coping mechanism for parents during this stage. Some children may develop stoical attitudes and deny symptoms in an attempt to ward off painful tests and procedures (Gardner et al, 1977).

Children may believe that they are responsible not only for the illness but also for its course. They may assume responsibility for side effects (such as nausea or diarrhea), undesirable laboratory values, or infiltrated intravenous lines. One 12-year-old commented "I know if I let myself get too depressed, the marrow won't take" (Pfefferbaum et al, 1978, p 627).

Children may attempt to cope with the stress of bone marrow transplantation by acting out, passive aggression, and other forms of negative behavior toward staff and family members. Although this type of behavior represents a coping mechanism for the child, it constitutes a stressor for parents who may feel embarrassed and rejected (Gardner et al, 1977; Pfefferbaum et al, 1978).

After Discharge. On discharge, children may have difficulty in relinquishing the special status associated with being a transplant patient (Brown & Kelly, 1976; Pfefferbaum et al, 1978). Confronted with possible social rejection due body image changes (alopecia, cushingoid appearance, wearing a mask), one adolescent remarked "I used to feel special; now I just feel strange" (Pfefferbaum et al, 1978, p 627). Adolescents may also express concerns about their sexual attractiveness and future reproductive capability (McConville et al, 1990). After discharge, siblings may resent the recipient's continued need for attention (McConville et al, 1990).

Sibling Donors. Bone marrow transplantation is especially stressful for sibling donors. They may assume inordinate responsibility for the outcome and experience tremendous guilt should GVHD develop. At the same time, sibling donors may feel jealous and neglected by parents who are preoccupied with the recipient (Gardner et al, 1977).

Death of Recipient. Stressors encountered by families whose children have died include guilt, continued grieving, blaming behavior, and marital and family dissension. Parents who cope relatively well had a consistent philosophy throughout the course of the illness and a reliable support system. These parents also communicated well with their child throughout the illness and provided emotional support (McConville et al, 1990).

McConville and colleagues (1990) compared psychosocial distress in families whose children survived bone marrow transplantation and families whose children died or had many unexpected complications. They found that

> Fathers of the children who had more severe disorders showed greater distress, but the mothers were generally more supportive. Therefore, there seems to be a general pattern of cumulative stress responses and increased psychopathology associated with more severe clinical states. . . . Such stress disorders could well be associated with breakdowns in coping-defense mechanisms, as in the fathers' increased stress responses to more severely ill children. However, the more supportive responses of mothers to more severe illness in the children is interesting; perhaps the mothers used more adaptive emotive-based coping mechanisms than the fathers, who might have used less adaptive instrumental responses (McConville et al, 1990, p 773).

Liver Transplantation

General Considerations. The liver, the largest organ of the body, performs many complex functions. The first successful liver transplant was performed by Starzl in 1963. Once considered an experimental procedure, liver transplant has success rates as high as 80% in some centers (Sheets, 1989).

There are two types of liver transplant procedures—orthotopic and heterotopic. In orthotopic transplantation, the patient's liver is removed and replaced with a donor liver. In heterotopic transplantation, the recipient's liver remains intact and an extra liver is inserted. Patients are accepted on a waiting list if their liver disease will progress to death over the next 6 to 12 months; greatly impairs their quality of life; and cannot be treated by alternative therapy (Sheets, 1989).

As of September 1992, 2144 patients were registered on the national waiting list for liver transplantation. The length of time these candidates have been waiting for a donor liver is presented in Table 3–1. In 1990, the median waiting time to liver transplantation was 64 days. In 1992, 47 patients died while on the waiting list. Between 1987 and 1989 the 1-year graft survival rate among patients who underwent liver transplantation was 64.1%; the patient survival rate was 71.6%.

Stressors and Coping Strategies in the Adult Population

Patients Undergoing Transplants. In an attempt to decrease financial burden and increase the patient's sense of well-being, the preoperative evaluation is usually done in an outpatient setting. Patients and family members are encouraged to attend support group meetings to increase their support networks (Sheets, 1989).

The evaluation stage may be particularly stressful for patients with alcoholic liver disease. Some centers accept patients onto the waiting list only if they have abstained from alcohol for 6 months. Other centers evaluate both the patient and first-degree relatives because prolonged posttransplant abstinence is unlikely if the recipient's immediate family members are alcohol abusers (Neuberger, 1989).

Heyink and Tymstra (1990) found that patients may deliberately withhold information about family members during the evaluation process out of fear that an indiscretion on the spouse's part might disqualify them as transplant candidates.

Patients Rejected for Liver Transplantation. Heyink and associates (1989) and Heyink and Tymstra (1990) studied patients and families who were not accepted onto the waiting list, a stressor the patients and families conceptualized as a "death sentence." This rejection was a traumatic experience because hopes that were initially raised at the beginning of the evaluation process were permanently dashed. Ironically, patients often accepted this rejection more readily than did their relatives, perhaps because the patients had already resigned themselves to a premature death (Heyink & Tymstra, 1990).

Stressors encountered by these patients included the everpresent fear of fatal complications; fatigue, which limited both their employment and recreational options; and restrictions in mobility, which contributed to the loss of friends and acquaintances. Some patients coped with these losses by deepening their relationships

TABLE 3–1: WAITING TIME BY ORGAN, SEPTEMBER 1992

| | Organ | | | |
TIME WAITING	LIVER Number (Percent)	LUNG Number (Percent)	HEART Number (Percent)	TOTAL Number (Percent)
0–30 days	320 (14.9)	113 (12.4)	260 (10.1)	673 (12.0)
31–60 days	218 (10.2)	76 (8.4)	194 (7.6)	488 (8.7)
61–90 days	195 (9.1)	97 (10.7)	198 (7.7)	490 (8.8)
91–120 days	133 (6.2)	83 (9.1)	179 (7.0)	395 (7.1)
121–150 days	122 (5.7)	54 (5.9)	156 (6.1)	332 (5.9)
151–180 days	119 (5.6)	61 (6.7)	145 (5.6)	325 (5.8)
6 months to 1 year	465 (21.7)	272 (30.0)	638 (24.8)	1375 (24.5)
More than 1 year	572 (26.7)	152 (16.7)	799 (31.1)	1523 (27.2)
Total	2144	908	2569	5601

(From the Research Department, United Network for Organ Sharing, Richmond, VA.)

with their spouse, children, and parents. However, in two instances this increased interdependence led to divorce (Heyink et al, 1989).

Some patients coped by adjusting the psychological significance of the rejection. They reframed the rejection in positive terms by rationalizing that they were better off, even in the face of deteriorating physical status, because the "difficult transplant operation could have killed them" (Heyink et al, 1989, p 1069).

Young patients coped by trying to maintain a positive attitude. Others attempted to gain control of the situation by the use of astrology or magical stones (Heyink et al, 1989).

Stressors and Coping Strategies in the Pediatric Population. Gold and associates (1986) identified five major phases through which families progress during the pediatric organ transplantation process. These stages provide a convenient framework for categorizing the stressors associated with liver transplantation.

Stage 1. Preoperative Period. This phase extends from the initial evaluation through the waiting period. Stressors associated with this stage include raising funds for the transplant and arranging transportation to the medical center. Perhaps the two greatest stressors, however, are watching the child's condition become progressively worse and the fear of death. Parents are cognizant of the fact that the sickest children receive transplants first; therefore, their child must deteriorate to achieve priority status (Gold et al, 1986). Approximately 30% of children die while on the waiting list (Sheets, 1989). Parents have described this stage as "a helpless situation in which all feelings of control are lost" (Gold et al, 1986, p 740).

Stage 2. Intraoperative Period. This relatively brief phase begins with the location of a suitable donor organ and the arrival of the child at the hospital. Parents are stressed by the chaos of preoperative activity, by the long waiting time during the operation, and by the fear that their child might not be strong enough to survive the operation (Weichler, 1990). Parents describe themselves as numb and in shock during this stage (Gold et al, 1986).

Stage 3. Critical Care Period. This stage can be divided into two timeframes: the intensive care unit (ICU) period (generally 3 to 5 days) and the surgical ward period (approximately 2 weeks). The former period is one of great stress as parents see their child attached to a variety of tubes and monitors. Parents fear that their child might die. Some also have feelings of guilt about putting their child through so much suffering (Weichler, 1990). After the child leaves the ICU, stressors may temporarily decrease as parents experience feelings of exhilaration and a new beginning (Gold et al, 1986).

Stage 4. The Recovery Period. This period can last 4 weeks to 4 months depending on the number of complications that develop. It is a period of almost constant stress for both parents and children. Parents fear organ rejection and infection. Psychosocial stressors include feelings of isolation, vulnerability, lack of control, and marital discord. It is during this period that parents may acknowledge that they have traded liver disease for liver transplant disease (Gold et al, 1986). It is also during this stage that lack of support systems may surface as a stressor for families who have had to relocate to the transplant center (Williams & Rzucidlo, 1985).

Stage 5. Discharge Period. Stressors associated with this phase include continued fear of organ rejection and death, adaptation to a new parenting role (caring for a healthy, active child), readjustment of the family structure (Gold et al, 1986), and future growth, development and reproductive capability of the transplant recipient (Weichler, 1990).

Weichler (1990) identified several problem-focused coping mechanisms used by mothers of liver transplant recipients. These include talking to parents whose children had already gone through the liver transplant process; attending support group meetings; and obtaining information, especially during Stage 1 and Stage 4.

Lung Transplantation

General Considerations. The first successful lung transplant was performed in 1983. Common conditions that may necessitate a lung transplant include alpha-1 antitripsin deficiency, pulmonary fibrosis, chronic obstructive pulmonary disease, and cystic fibrosis. Typically, potential candidates must have end-stage lung disease, no other major organ disease, and a life expectancy of 18 months or less (Bright et al, 1990).

In 1991, 402 lung transplants were performed in the United States—399 cadaveric and 3 living donor. As of September 1992, 937 patients were registered on the national waiting list for lung transplantation. The length of time these candidates have been waiting for a donor lung is presented in Table 3–1. In 1990, the median waiting time for lung transplantation was 236 days. In 1992, 17 patients died while on the waiting list. Between 1987 and 1989 the 1-year graft survival rate among patients who underwent lung transplants was 52.3%; the patient survival rate was 53.8%.

Stressors and Coping Strategies. Bright and associates (1990) and Craven and co-authors (1990) studied the stressors encountered and coping strategies used by lung transplant candidates and their families throughout the transplantation process.

Stage 1. The Application and Assessment Period. Lung transplant candidates face serious financial stressors. Many third-party payors still classify the procedure as experimental. The potential candidate may be faced with making financial arrangements for the evaluation process, temporary living facilities, the surgical procedure, and postoperative medical and pharmaceutical care (Craven et al, 1990).

Few transplant centers perform lung transplantations. Therefore, many potential lung transplant candidates must relocate for an extended period of time. Some transplant centers mandate that a support person remain with the candidate throughout the entire transplant process. Relocation presents stressors to the support person in terms of prolonged absence from employment and other family members, especially children. The relationship between the candidate and the support person often becomes strained. These individuals may feel isolated and left out of events at home. In addition, they may experience guilt feelings about not being available to help family members at home (Bright et al, 1990).

During the assessment period, candidates fear that they may be found too ill to proceed with the operation or that a previously undiagnosed medical condition may eliminate them from further consideration (Bright et al, 1990). During the evaluation period, potential candidates may underreport emotional symptoms. This underreporting may be a coping mechanism, or it may indicate a belief that emotional problems will be deemed undesirable by the assessment team (Bright et al, 1990).

Stage 2. The Waiting Period. As with other transplant populations, candidates for lung transplants must cope with a disabling and life-threatening illness. Donor lungs are difficult to procure, and many patients die during the waiting period (Bright et al, 1990). Many candidates must be hospitalized for pulmonary insufficiency. Additional stressors are the need to restart steroid therapy or the development of a serious infection. Either of these complications can result in the removal of the candidate from the active waiting list (Craven et al, 1990).

As the waiting period lengthens, some candidates begin to wish for a donor lung. This wishing becomes a stressor when the candidate reinterprets it as "wishing for another person's death." Other candidates become preoccupied with their position on the waiting list and worry that other candidates have a higher priority. They may consider themselves in competition with other patients on the list who have a similar body size and blood type (Bright et al, 1990). Some candidates attempt to cope by using black humor. Bright and colleagues (1990, p 129) described a patient who remarked that he "would be waiting by the telephone for a drunk driver to have an accident." This coping mechanism, however, has the potential to become a stressor if it precipitates guilt and self-recrimination.

Some lung transplant centers mandate that candidates begin exercise training during the waiting period. This exercise regimen can serve as a coping mechanism in that it increases the candidate's exercise tolerance, functional capacity, and emotional well-being (Craven et al, 1990).

Candidates use both formal and informal support mechanisms during the waiting period. The formal support group, facilitated by members of the health care team, provides an environment of mutual support. It is particularly useful in helping candidates cope with a lack of control. Although individual candidates may lack control, the support group as a whole can exert control and express the needs of the group to the transplant team (Bright et al, 1990).

In the informal support network, candidates, support persons, and transplant recipients share information and resources. This coping mechanism is not always beneficial, however, and may itself become a stressor. Bright and colleagues (1990, p 129) explain:

> Patients who have relied primarily on denial to cope with their illness find their defense mechanism is challenged by daily contact with other candidates. Others have made close friends with patients who later died and found the grieving process a painful distraction from their own priorities.

Craven and colleagues (1990) note that candidates and family members may view use of these support networks as a sign of personal failure rather than an adaptive coping mechanism.

Stage 3. Postoperative Period. In their 1990 study, Craven and colleagues reported that major postoperative complications are stressors for family members. These complications may be doubly stressful. Not only are they stressful in their own right, but also they can precipitate guilt feelings in family members who encouraged the recipient to proceed with the lung transplant. Postoperative agitation, delirium, restlessness, disorientation, and combativeness are complications that have been noted in lung transplant recipients (Craven et al, 1990).

Lack of knowledge about the recipient's status is another postoperative stressor. Support persons and other family members report that frequent contact with the transplant surgeon and other members of the team is helpful in coping with this stressor (Craven et al, 1990).

Soon after the operation, lung transplant recipients resume a program of pulmonary rehabilitation. Most of these patients are pleased with their increased activity tolerance. However, staff expectations and performance anxiety may constitute stressors for some patients (Craven et al, 1990).

TABLE 3–2. LENGTH OF TIME 21,430 CANDIDATES HAVE BEEN WAITING FOR A DONOR KIDNEY, SEPTEMBER 1992

Length of Time	Number	Percent
0–6 months	6251	29.2
6–12 months	4522	21.1
1–2 years	5046	23.5
2–3 years	2397	11.2
3–5 years	2074	9.7
5–9 years	943	4.4
>9 years	197	0.9
TOTAL	21,430	100.0

(From the Research Department, United Network for Organ Sharing, Richmond, Va.)

Stage 4. Postdischarge Period. Some lung transplant recipients have difficulty leaving the transplant environment. This reluctance may be manifested in persistent somatic complaints. Prolonged pretransplant disability, childhood or adolescent disability, and an overprotective social network are but a few factors that may inhibit the recipient's autonomy (Craven et al, 1990).

Renal Transplantation

General Considerations. The Russian surgeon Voronoy performed the first documented human renal transplant in 1933. In 1954, the first renal transplant was performed in the United States. This initial transplant procedure involved an identical twin donor. It was not until the 1960s, however, that renal transplantation became common treatment of end-stage renal disease (Harasyko, 1989).

As of September 1992, 21,489 patients were registered on the national waiting list for renal transplants. The length of time these candidates have been waiting for a donor kidney is presented in Table 3–2. In 1992, 123 patients died while waiting for a kidney transplant (Wilson B., United Network for Organ Sharing, personal communication, November 1992).

Stressors and Coping Strategies in the Adult Population

Living-related Donors. Kidney transplantation is unique because of the availability of living-related donors. However, these donors must deal with potential stressors associated with the risks of an elective operation, rejection episodes, the failure of the donated kidney, and the death of the recipient (Harasyko, 1989; Holechek et al, 1991; Weizer, et al, 1989). Hirvas and associates (1976) reported that living-related donors with low self-esteem and limited inner resources experienced grief, anxiety, regression, and depression on the failure of the donated kidney. Weizer and colleagues (1989) documented the suicide of two living-related kidney donors upon graft rejection and the subsequent death of the recipients. These authors noted that supportive psychiatric treatment of the donor is usually not provided because of the lack of medical follow-up care of the donor after the death of the recipients. Furthermore, living-related donors who successfully complete the pretransplant evaluation are usually considered to be mentally stable. Therefore, health care providers may overlook symptoms of depression and the need for psychiatric intervention after the death of the recipient.

Soon after kidney transplantation became a common treatment of end-stage renal disease, Fellner and Marshall (1968) noted that kidney donors were often concerned about whether or not the recipient would truly appreciate the sacrifice and properly care for the donated organ. Kemph (1970) reported that kidney donors may actually "mourn" the loss of their kidney. Gardner and co-workers (1977, pp 630–631) compared these attitudes with those of bone marrow donors and theorized that

> These differences may be related to the fact that the kidney is conceptualized as a discrete organ which, once removed, does not regenerate. Thus the donor is aware not only of the temporary discomfort and disruption caused by hospitalization but also of the permanent sacrifice that increases his own risk of permanent disability or death, should the remaining kidney cease to function. By contrast, our bone marrow donors equate bone marrow with blood, saying they have plenty of both and can easily give some away, confident that it will soon regenerate.

Transplant Recipients: Preoperative. Candidates for renal transplantation face several unique stressors. Holechek and colleagues (1991) noted that candidates often must deal with the fear of organ rejection preoperatively as they watch fellow dialysis patients resume dialysis treatments after a failed transplant. Renal transplant candidates with certain systemic and renal diseases, such as malignant hypertension or antibiotic-resistant urinary tract infections, must undergo a pretransplant bilateral nephrectomy to prevent damage to the transplanted kidney. If there is concern about a patient's willingness to comply with the posttransplant regimen, some centers monitor and evaluate that patient's compliance with dialysis before accepting him or her as a candidate for renal transplantation (Harasyko, 1989). Renshaw (1987) noted that renal transplant candidates often have sexual concerns. Pain, fatigue, dyspnea, edema, and other symptoms are often countererotic. Decreased hormone levels or use of steroids may decrease libido. The risks associated with a pretransplant pregnancy are of concern to female renal transplant candidates.

Transplant Recipients: Postoperative. Hayward and associates (1989) asked 60 adult renal transplant recipients to rate potential stressors they experienced during the first 6 postoperative months on a four-point Likert scale ranging from "not stressful" to "very stressful." These patients identified the following items (listed in rank order; 44 possible stressors) as very stressful: (1) possibility of organ rejection; (2) possibility of infection; (3) uncertainty about the future; (4) cost of medications; and (5) side effects of immunosuppressive medications. The side effects of immunosuppressive agents include weight gain, acne, cataracts, hypertension, hair growth, gastrointestinal irritation, rash, bone marrow suppression, and increased risk of cancer.

It has been estimated that patients who receive immunosuppressants are 100 times more likely than the general population to have certain types of malignant tumors (Harasyko, 1989).

The patients in the study by Hayward and colleagues (1989) identified the following quality-of-life items as slightly stressful: (1) changes in family responsibility; (2) job opportunities; (3) time away from work; (4) changes in work; (5) changes in social activities; and (6) role reversal in family.

Using a similar approach, Sutton and Murphy (1989) asked 40 adult patients who had had renal transplants within the last 4 years to rate the severity of 35 potential stressors. The five most stressful items (in rank order) were (1) cost factors; (2) fear of organ rejection; (3) weight gain; (4) uncertainty concerning the future; and (5) limitation of physical activities. These investigators noted that although graft survival rates have improved, the potential for rejection remains an everpresent threat.

In this study, Sutton and Murphy (1989) also calculated each subject's total stress score. They found that subjects who received transplants 24 to 48 months before the study reported significantly more stress than subjects who received transplants 0 to 23 months before the study. The authors theorized that subjects in the 24-to-48-month posttransplant group might have reported more stress because graft survival rates decrease with time; patients tire of the side effects of medications; family members and friends expect more of the patient; and professional support declines with time. The lower stress scores of subjects in the 0-to-23-month posttransplant group may be reflective of the "honeymoon" phase during which renal transplant patients relish their newly found freedom from dialysis treatments and dietary restrictions.

Sutton and Murphy (1989) also studied the coping strategies used by these subjects. The five most frequently used coping strategies were (1) praying to or trusting in God; (2) looking at the problem objectively; (3) maintaining control over the situation; (4) obtaining more information about the situation; and (5) drawing on past experiences to help handle the present situation. Overall, the subjects used more problem-focused coping mechanisms than emotion-focused coping mechanisms. However, there were some differences in the coping mechanisms used by the two groups. Patients in the 24-to-48-month posttransplant group used significantly more emotion-focused coping mechanisms. The investigators noted that problem-focused coping mechanisms tend to be used in situations that are appraised as modifiable, whereas emotion-focused coping mechanisms tend to be used in situations that are viewed as less changeable. Sutton and Murphy (1989) theorized that subjects in the 0-to-23-months posttransplant group may have believed that they had more control over the situation than subjects in the 24-to-48-month posttransplant group.

Christensen and associates (1989) examined the role of family support in mediating psychological well-being among renal transplant recipients. Fifty-seven subjects completed questionnaires pertaining to family support, physical impairment, anxiety, and depression. These investigators found that family support mediated the physical impact of the illness on anxiety and depression. High levels of family support were associated with significantly lower levels of depression and anxiety. Christenson and co-authors (1989) theorized that a supportive family environment protects renal transplant recipients from potential psychological dysfunction. They noted that

"Higher levels of illness-related physical impairment were associated with more depression . . . and greater anxiety. Furthermore, patients incurring high levels of illness-related physical dysfunction reported significantly more psychological symptoms of depression and anxiety when they perceive a low rather than high degree of family support" (Christensen et al, 1989, p 261).

Using a prospective, cross-sectional design, Frey (1990) asked renal transplant recipients to rate the stressors they experienced during the first 6 weeks after the transplant. The following stressors (in rank order) were identified as most stressful: (1) possibility of repeated hospitalization; (2) possibility of organ rejection; (3) cost of medications; (4) uncertainty about the future; and (5) side effects of medications. Frey noted that it is important for health care professionals to discuss potential stressors with the patient and family when the patient is considering transplantation as an option. Postoperatively, it is important to remind the patient and family that these stressors are common and to suggest coping strategies that others have found useful.

White and associates (1990) also studied stress and coping in kidney transplant recipients during the first 6 months after the transplant. They found that even though renal transplantation is often equated with renewed health, the following health-related items were identified as most stressful: (1) uncertainty about the success of the transplant; (2) risk of infection; (3) side effects of medications; and (4) concern that changes in physical appearance will affect social life. These investigators noted that women were more concerned about their health than about family relationships or work and financial matters. With respect to coping, subjects in this study used positive attitudes (reframing) while maintaining a realistic outlook. The following strategies were reported most frequently: (1) staying cheerful and maintaining a positive attitude; (2) enjoying what life has to offer; (3) looking on the bright side of things; (4) remaining realistic; (5) making the best of it (White et al, 1990). The least-used coping strategies (escape or wishful thinking) were (1) making myself feel better by using drugs; (2) making myself feel better by smoking; (3) making myself feel better by drinking; (4) asking someone else to take care of me; (5) isolating myself (White et al, 1990). Female subjects reported using more outside resources in coping with their stressors than did male subjects.

With respect to nursing implications, White and colleagues (1990) noted that it is important to tell transplant candidates what to expect, so that they can identify coping resources. In addition, they should be encouraged to develop a wide range of coping mechanisms.

Renshaw (1987) reported that pregnancy is a potential stressor for both the renal transplant donor and the recipient. The donor's renal function should be evaluated before the pregnancy. Pregnancy in the recipient poses increased risk to both the mother and the fetus and requires multidisciplinary monitoring.

Voepel-Lewis and associates (1990) examined perceived stressors and coping strategies among family members of renal transplant recipients. Their findings were similar to those of White and colleagues (1990). During the first 6 months after the transplant, health-related items (such as side effects of immunosuppressive agents and medical complications) were identified as most stressful. The six most frequently used coping strategies were (1) remaining realistic; (2) trying to look on the bright side; (3) carrying on as I normally would; (4) trying to analyze the problem to better understand it; (5) drawing on past experiences; and (6) concentrating on what I have to do next. These investigators noted a positive correlation between the number of stressors reported and the number of coping strategies used. This correlation indicated that family members confronted with a large number of stressors tried a variety of coping strategies to deal with the stressors associated with the transplant experience.

Voepel-Lewis and colleagues (1990) also noted a difference in the way female and male family members coped. Women respondents sought significantly more social support and used significantly more positive reappraisal. One implication of this finding is that male family members should be encouraged to develop and use sources of informational, tangible, and emotional support. In addition, family members should be alerted to possible stressors before the transplant procedure. They also should be told which coping strategies have been successfully used by others.

Children and Adolescents. As the number of pediatric renal transplants increases, the age range of eligible candidates is widening; more infants and younger children are undergoing transplantation (Reynolds et al, 1991). Early studies of long-term adaptation to renal transplants among children and adolescents indicated a variety of stressors, including fear of rejection and damaged self-esteem (Korsch et al, 1973). Fine and associates (1978) noted decreased social adaptation among pediatric renal transplant recipients—a finding that suggested problems in peer relations.

The number of adolescents undergoing renal transplantation has increased because of advances in organ matching and immunosuppression. However, despite the success of the transplant procedure itself, teenagers may experience a number of social stressors stemming from growth retardation and pubertal delay related to the end-stage renal disease as well as the disfiguring cosmetic effects of immunosuppressive therapy (Melzer et al, 1989). Melzer and colleagues (1989) compared the social networks, self-esteem, and body image of adolescent renal transplant recipients with those of healthy teenagers. They found that the transplant recipients identified significantly fewer people in their total social networks and named significantly fewer opposite-sex peers. There were proportionally more family members in the social networks of the transplant recipients. The two groups were similar with respect to total self-esteem scores. However, the transplant recipients had significantly higher home self-esteem scores. This subscale reflects perceived acceptance by parents. Contrary to earlier findings, there were no significant differences between the two groups with respect to body image. This improved body image may be due to the recent trend toward early transplantation and the decreased used of steroids.

With respect to their findings, Melzer and associates (1989, p 311) wrote that the "high home self-esteem scores among the adolescents after transplantation suggests that parents and related peers may provide the needed social resources to help these adolescents maintain their self-esteem." The authors caution, however, that adolescents from stressed or dysfunctional families may be at risk for social isolation. To avoid future potential stressors, adolescent renal transplant recipients should be encouraged to participate in activities with their peers. Their families, in turn, may need help in dealing with the adolescent's increasing independence.

Regarding sexual stressors, Renshaw (1987) noted that social isolation before the transplant and countererotic symptoms may impede sociosexual learning and romantic exchange. As a result, adolescents may experience problems with dating and intimacy in the posttransplant period.

Allograft rejection is an overwhelming stressor for children and adolescents; it is a stressor that signals the return to pretransplant restrictions. Feelings of loss, denial, depression, anger, and guilt are common. Children and teenagers may equate their own self-esteem with the function of the kidney. When the kidney is rejected, these patients may reject themselves. Defense mechanisms such as denial, displacement, projection, rationalization, regression, and withdrawal may be used by children and adolescents in coping with graft rejection (Hudson & Hiott, 1986).

Heart Transplantation

General Considerations. As of September 1992, 2569 patients were registered on the national waiting list for heart transplantation. The length of time these candidates have been waiting for a donor heart is presented in Table 3–1.

In 1990, the median waiting time to heart transplantation was 186 days, In 1992, 71 patients died while waiting for a donor heart. Between 1987 and 1989 the 1-year graft survival rate among patients undergoing heart transplantation was 81.2%; the patient survival rate was 81.9% (Wilson B, United Network for Organ Sharing, personal communication, November 1992).

Stressors and Coping Strategies.

> *"I pray you to give me a heart, that I may be as other men."*
> L. Frank Baum, *The Wizard of Oz*

Many of the stressors associated with heart transplantation stem from the common perception that the heart is the center of emotions and personality. Stressors and coping strategies specific to each stage of the heart transplantation process are discussed in terms of the seven stages of emotional adjustment to cardiac transplantation developed by Kuhn and associates (1988).

Stage 1. Transplant Proposal. This stage extends from the first suggestion of transplantation until the patient and family decide to begin the evaluation process (Kuhn et al, 1990). In this stage, patients and families are confronted with the adaptive task of accepting heart transplantation as necessary for the preservation of life (Kuhn et al, 1988). The extent and duration of the patient's illness influence this adaptive process. In general, a patient whose physical condition has gradually deteriorated over time can more readily accept transplantation as a treatment option than can a patient with a sudden onset of cardiac disease. The latter patient, going suddenly from a healthy lifestyle to a catastrophic illness, has had little time to mentally adjust to the diagnosis. Neither the patient nor the family is accustomed to dealing with chronic illness.

Many are afraid that they may not "measure up" to all that will be expected of them (Hook et al, 1990; O'Brien, 1985).

During this stage, patients and family members often experience feelings of shock, disbelief ("a mistake has been made"), anger, and denial. Stressors confronting the patient may include the inability to work, loss of status, dependence, and role reversal, all of which may precipitate low self-esteem and social isolation. Family members may live with anticipatory grieving (O'Brien, 1985). To successfully pass through this stage and accept transplantation, a patient must reconcile intellectual acknowledgment of the heart as a circulatory pump with affective perception of the heart as the center of emotions and personality (Cardin & Clark, 1985).

Stage 2. Evaluation. This period extends from the time the patient accepts the need for transplantation to the time he or she is accepted as a candidate (Kuhn et al, 1990). The purpose of the evaluation is twofold: to determine if the patient can survive the transplant operation and achieve satisfactory rehabilitation and to provide the patient and family with information necessary for them to give informed consent (Christopherson, 1987).

Patients typically undergo rigorous physical and psychosocial assessments. In their recent review of this clinical assessment process, Kay and Bienenfeld (1991) noted that in addition to a battery of medical tests, potential candidates may be asked to complete as many as 12 psychological tests. During this stage, the adaptive task revolves around resolving any ambivalent feelings regarding transplantation and deciding whether or not to proceed with the operation (Kuhn et al, 1988). Zumbrunnen (1989, p 68) noted that the patient is faced with " . . . living two dramatically opposed, and equally possible, perspectives for his own future: either near death, or a quasi-miraculous revival through transplantation." One patient stated, "It seems to me that it is as if I was in a burning house, and asking myself whether I had to stay in the house or jump from the balcony" (Zumbrunnen, 1989, pp 68–69).

The evaluation phase is fraught with anxiety. The patient and family are given detailed information to meet informed consent requirements. This information, while necessary, highlights both the seriousness of the patient's condition and the specter of death (Porter et al, 1991). Patients may use denial to cope with mortality statistics, choosing to concentrate solely on survival rates (Cardin & Clark, 1985).

Once patients have opted for transplantation, fears that they may not be chosen as candidates may lead them to emphasize their physical suffering while presenting themselves in a psychologically "ideal" manner (Kuhn et al, 1988). Others may plead that they have "things left to do" and need "more time to spend with loved ones." Comments such as the following are common: "My first grandchild is due in August. I can't bear the thought of dying before I hold the baby" or "My children are two and three. If I die now, they'll never be able to remember that I was their mother. Please let me have just a few more years" (Christopherson, 1987, p 58). At the same time, equally fearful family members may try to please and convince the transplant evaluation team that the patient should be accepted as a candidate (Christopherson, 1987).

Zumbrunnen (1989) noted that the more coping mechanisms a patient has, the better the patient can adjust to this evaluation phase. Typical coping mechanisms associated with this stage include altruism; faith; seeking of attention, care, and information; social withdrawal; problem analysis; and passive cooperation.

Stage 3. The Waiting Period. This time period extends from the patient's acceptance as a candidate for a heart transplant until the actual operation (Kuhn et al, 1990). Once the initial euphoria associated with this acceptance fades, the patient is confronted with two adaptive tasks: accepting loss of control and dependency on health care providers while facing impending death. Anxiety levels increase as the waiting period is prolonged and the candidate's physical condition deteriorates (Kuhn et al, 1988). Patients strive to maintain a positive self-image and sense of self-worth in the face of a decreasing ability to perform their former roles (Cardin & Clark, 1985).

More than 80% of heart transplant candidates are unable to pursue gainful employment (Buse & Pieper, 1990). Grady and associates (1992) found that the most frequent and most distressing symptoms experienced by patients during the waiting period were fatigue, activity-related shortness of breath, difficulty sleeping, and weakness. Patients who did not work had significantly higher symptom distress levels than did patients who were employed. Higher symptom distress levels also correlated significantly with perceptions of higher stress levels, lower quality of life, less life satisfaction, and more functional disability.

Patients may be afraid to sleep at night, for fear of dying (Kuhn et al, 1988). As time goes by, they begin to doubt the decision to go ahead with the transplant. They may be plagued by questions such as, "Am I really on the waiting list?", "Did the consultant mean it or was he just saying it to keep me quiet?" and "Will I ever have the operation or will I die before a donor heart becomes available?" (O'Brien, 1985, p 230).

Several stressors are associated with the electronic pagers that patients are required to wear so they can be paged when a donor heart becomes available. Some patients believe they have been abandoned because they now have less contact with the transplant team. They may try to compensate by frequently calling or visiting the transplant center (Kuhn et al, 1988). On occasion, the patient's pager number is called by mistake. Extreme disappointment results when the patient is notified that a donor heart is available but, after closer scrutiny, is determined to be unsuitable (Muirhead, 1989).

Patients may fantasize about "donor weather," which increases accidents and therefore the availability of a donor heart. Others may pay close attention to ambulance sirens and news reports of accidents. Such activities usually precipitate severe guilt feelings (Christopherson, 1987; Kuhn et al, 1988).

In their recent study of coping among heart transplant candidates, Muirhead and associates (1992) found that most patients were dissatisfied with their quality of life because of such factors as physical symptoms and disabilities, sexual dysfunction, and psychological distress. However, despite these stressors, most patients were psychologically and socially well-adjusted. Frequently used coping mechanisms included maintaining a positive attitude and seeking social support. Negative coping mechanisms, such as confrontation, passive acceptance, and escapism, were uncommon.

Porter and colleagues (1994) studied perceived stressors and coping strategies among cardiac transplant candidates during the waiting period. The three stressors with the greatest intensity were "finding out that you need a heart transplant," "having terminal heart disease," and "having your family worry about you." The three most frequently used coping strategies were "thinking positively," "keeping a sense of humor," and "trying to keep life as normal as possible."

The waiting period is also stressful for family members. In their survey of 30 spouses, Buse and Pieper (1990) found that feelings of fear over the possible loss of one's spouse was the highest rated life-effect item. The uncertainty associated with this period becomes evident when spouses talk about funeral arrangements one minute and plan for a long-awaited family vacation the next minute (Christopherson, 1987). Support groups have been particularly effective in helping family members cope with this uncertainty (Buse & Pieper, 1990).

Nolan and associates (1992) examined perceived stressors and coping strategies among families of cardiac transplant patients during the organ waiting period. These researchers found that family members reported low to moderate degrees of stress. The three most frequently identified stressors were chores that don't get done, the illness of the family member, and medical expenses. The two most frequently used coping strategies were reframing (believing in family's problem-solving skills, facing problems head-on) and seeking social support.

In their landmark qualitative study of family adjustment to heart transplantation, Mishel and Murdaugh (1987) used the term *immersion* to characterize the waiting period. They defined immersion as " . . . a series of behaviors in which one family member, usually the partner, pledges self to the welfare of the patient" (Mishel & Murdaugh, 1987, pp 333–334). These researchers identified three concurrent categories of immersion: freeing self, symbiosis, and trading places.

1. Freeing self. The spouse frees the self from domestic, child-rearing, and social tasks and transfers all attention to the patient.
2. Symbiosis. In assuming the care-taker role, partners lose their self-identity. The personal pronoun "I" is replaced by "we" and "she" or "he" (referring to the patient). Energy previously spent on normal day-to-day activities is redirected at bonding with the patient. Patients are protected both psychologically and physiologically. By filtering information, partners shield the patient from any potentially upsetting news. All aspects of the patient's physical condition are monitored to make certain that the patient's condition remains stable.
3. Trading places. The partner "trades places" with the patient and assumes many of the patient's former roles and behaviors. "A major statement of [candidate's] partners was, 'Never say never', implying they were doing things they never thought they would do and they might take on other responsibilities in the future that they could not comprehend in the current situation" (Mishel & Murdaugh, 1987, p 335). This role disruption is a potential source of both marital and family stress (McAleer et al, 1985).

In general, patients' coping ability is a function of several factors, such as severity of illness, personality, previous illnesses, and amount of support available. Of these, severity of illness has the greatest impact on coping outcome (Zumbrunnen, 1989).

Symptoms that the patient's or family's coping skills are deteriorating include inability to identify and share feelings, inability to use support systems, self-deprecating statements, and feelings of powerlessness, hopelessness, withdrawal, and resignation. In facilitating effective coping strategies, it is essential to accept the patient and family's behavior rather than attempt to change it. Such attempts are likely to meet with resistance. Patients and family members are more willing to abandon negative coping behaviors if they first feel accepted as they are. A primary nursing model facilitates the development of a trusting environment in which patients and family members can try out more positive coping behaviors (Cardin & Clark, 1985).

Specific nursing interventions include encouraging patients and family members to express their feelings, encouraging hope, actively involving family members, and providing information (Cardin & Clark, 1985). Information and advice obtained from other patients and families is particularly helpful (O'Brien, 1985). A preoperative visit to the ICU, which prepares patients and family members for the actual operation through cognitive anticipation and role rehearsal, helps to prevent stress reactions in later stages of the transplantation process (Zumbrunnen, 1989).

Stage 4. The Perioperative Period. This relatively brief phase lasts from the actual operation until the patient is transferred out of the ICU (Kuhn et al, 1990). Because of the euphoria of this "honeymoon" period, relatively few stressors are associated with this stage. At this point, patients may naively hope that they will be one of the extremely rare recipients who never experience a rejection episode. Others may feel the need to fulfill a bargain they made with God during the waiting period (Christopherson, 1987).

Stage 5. In-hospital Convalescence. According to the stages described by Kuhn et al (1990), this period lasts from the time the patient is transferred out of the ICU until the patient is ready for discharge. Patients are confronted with the task of adjusting to the regimented structure of the convalescent period (Kuhn et al, 1990). Stressors reappear as the euphoria associated with the previous stage dissipates. The first endocardial biopsy, with its attendant possibility of rejection, reemphasizes the patient's vulnerability (Kuhn et al, 1988). Patients may begin to realize that they have substituted one disease for another (Christopherson, 1987). It is also during this stage that some patients may begin to wonder about the identity of the donor and how the donated heart may affect their personality (Kuhn et al, 1988; Rauch & Kneen, 1989).

As recovery continues, patients may be integrated into a network that includes other heart transplant recipients as well as candidates. Strong feelings of gratitude toward the transplant team may result in a desire to help patients who remain on the waiting list. The development of such close relationships, however, constitutes a double-edged sword. While recipients' self-esteem may be bolstered by their ability to help others, the death of a candidate or fellow recipient can be devastating. Patients may attempt to cope with such a loss by avoiding each other for awhile (Kuhn et al, 1988) or by differentiating themselves from the deceased, for example, "He died because he didn't have a good match but I have a good match and so I will live" (Rauch & Kneen, 1989, p 55).

Stage 6. Discharge. This period is the time immediately before and after discharge. Anticipating discharge, patients have the task of dealing with greater independence (Kuhn et al, 1990). This stage may be characterized by ambivalence and extreme anxiety as the patient contemplates a series of potential stressors, including transition from the patient role, leaving the safety net of the hospital, returning to work, or facing unemployment (O'Brien, 1985). Talking with others who have successfully made this transition is often a helpful coping mechanism (Kuhn et al, 1988). For exceptionally fearful patients, hospital passes of increasing duration can bolster patients' confidence in their ability to function outside the protective hospital environment. Such passes can also ease their reentry into the family unit (Christopherson, 1987).

Stage 7. After Discharge. This phase begins with the patient's return home and lasts until a perceived state of normalcy is achieved (Kuhn et al, 1990). The adaptive tasks associated with this phase include readjusting to the world outside the hospital, pursuing rehabilitation, and shedding the "transplant" identity. Psychological incorporation of the new heart occurs gradually. As patients become less conscious of having a donor heart, they begin to feel as though the new heart has always been theirs. The postdischarge phase may last at least several months. Kuhn and associates (1988, 1990) found that the first anniversary of the transplant is a major milestone. It is around this time that many patients report thinking of themselves as normal again.

Christopherson (1987) noted that two categories of stressors are likely to occur during the first 6 months after discharge. The first category consists of problems that are relatively common, such as side effects of medications and the responses of others to the transplant recipient. Solutions to these problems usually can be worked out through conversations with other transplant recipients or with the transplant team. The second category of stressors relates to family interactions and may center on control issues or feelings of family members who now are demanding attention. Such problems usually require professional counseling. It is important to note, however, that grievances that predated the transplant operation may be easier to resolve than before the transplant because of increased family caring and enhanced communication skills that developed during the transplant experience.

Several groups of researchers have examined psychosocial functioning and well-being in heart transplant recipients. Bohachick and associates (1992) measured the psychosocial functioning of heart transplant candidates before the operation and again 6 months after the operation. Patients reported a considerable amount of illness-related psychosocial distress immediately after being placed on the waiting list. However, most of these patients demonstrated a significant improvement in emotional state and psychosocial adjustment (domestic, sexual, social, and vocational functioning) 6 months after transplantation. Mai and associates (1990) reported similar findings 12 months after transplantation. Jones and colleagues (1988) examined psychological adjustment before transplantation, at discharge, and 4, 8, and 12 months after transplantation. They found significant postdischarge improvement in all parameters: depression, well-being, anxiety, body image, and quality of life. In a similar study, Jones and co-authors (1992) assessed psychological adjustment and well-being before transplantation, at discharge, 4, 8, and 12 months after transplantation, and again 3.5 to 5.2 years after transplantation. They reported significant improvement in anxiety, depression, and well-being scores over time. These findings, however, contradict those of Baumann and co-workers (1992), who found that 5 to 60 months after transplantation recipients reported stressors related to work problems, finances, role changes, lifestyle changes, and side effects of medications.

In regard to coping, Mai (1986) found that denial was a frequently used coping mechanism. He theorized that denial served as an intrapsychic adaptive mechanism that could be directed at the donated heart (graft denial), the donor, or both. Graft denial was expressed in statements such as "I try to forget about the new heart" or "I have no thoughts about my new heart" (Mai, 1986, p 1159). Donor denial was expressed in comments such as "I have not asked where it [the heart] came from" or "I never think about the donor" (Mai, 1986, p 1160).

With respect to stressors confronting spouses after the transplantation operation, Mishel and Murdaugh (1987) reported that as the patient regains strength, spouses begin to realize how drained *they* are, both emotionally and physically. As the patient becomes more independent, the previously symbiotic relationship between the patient and the partner begins to dissolve. Mishel and Murdaugh (1987) used the term "passage" to describe this phase—a phase characterized by catharsis, vacillation, and awareness.

Catharsis refers to the partner's emotional ventilation, a reliving and repeated sharing of the stressful events associated with the waiting period. This purging allows partners to express emotions that could not be expressed previously.

Vacillation refers to the ebb and flow in the spouse's belief that life will return to normal. It is caused by the unpredictable problems that arise during the first 6 weeks after the operation. Mishel and Murdaugh (1987) found that partners cope by buffering the growing realization that life will never return to normal. Two specific buffering mechanisms are unpredictability management and hope maintenance. Unpredictability management techniques attempt to bolster the belief that cues indicative of complications can be expected, prevented, or reversed. Hope maintenance is the positive reframing of transplant experiences. These mechanisms buffer the spouse's awareness that the patient's lifespan remains unpredictable by allowing aspects of this realization to be gradually integrated into his or her belief systems. Partners are thereby prevented from becoming overwhelmed by this unpredictability.

Mishel and Murdaugh (1987) used the term *awareness* to describe the process by which spouses come to acknowledge the necessity of redefining "normal." Confronted with a myriad of medications, diet restrictions, potential complications, such as an increased risk of malignant disease because of chronic immunosuppression, (Muirhead, 1989), and secondary illnesses, partners begin to realize that life will not return to normal.

Faced with this incessant unpredictability, spouses next attempt to negotiate a new lifestyle that takes this uncertainty into account. Mishel and Murdaugh (1987) identified several negotiation patterns—patterns that may lead to conflict between the partner and the patient. In one such pattern, the partners focused on obtaining security for themselves and their children by seeking or continuing employment, maintaining control over family finances, and retaining roles they had assumed during the transplant crisis. The patients, however, focused on enjoying the second chance they have been given by hedonistically pursuing lifelong dreams and desires. This and similar discrepancies regarding future goals and lifestyles can lead to conflict between patients and partners.

Stress Management Strategies. Members of transplant teams are in a unique position to help patients and families cope with the stressors associated with organ transplantation. Psychophysiologic self-regulation interventions such as guided imagery, along with music, humor, play, and relaxation therapies (including autogenic training, biofeedback, body scanning, progressive muscle relaxation, the relaxation response, and self-hypnosis) may be of considerable benefit to this population. The reader is referred to *Holistic Nursing: A Handbook for Practice* by Dossey and associates (1988) for additional information about each of these interventions.

In conclusion, this chapter reviews the literature with respect to stress and coping among transplant patients and their families. Such knowledge is essential if nurses are to anticipate problems and plan interventions to facilitate coping and long-term adjustment to transplantation.

REFERENCES

Baumann LJ, Young CJ, Egan JJ (1992). Living with a heart transplant: Long-term adjustment. *Transplant Int.* 5:1–8.

Bohachick P, Anton BB, Wooldridge P, et al (1992). Psychosocial outcome six months after heart transplant surgery: A preliminary report. *Res Nurs Health.* 15:165–173.

Brown H, Kelly M (1976). Stages of bone marrow transplantation: A psychiatric perspective. *Psychosom Med.* 38:439–446.

Bright JM, Craven JL, Kelly PJ (1990). Assessment and management of psychosocial stress in lung transplant candidates. *Health Soc Work.* 15:125–132.

Brown H, Kelly M (1984). Stages of bone marrow transplantation. In Moos RH, ed. *Coping with Physical Illness 2: New Perspectives* New York: Plenum, 241–252.

Buchsel PC, Kelleher J (1989). Bone marrow transplantation. *Nurs Clin North Am.* 24:907–938.

Buse S, Pieper B (1990). Impact of cardiac transplantation on the spouse's life. *Heart Lung.* 19:641–648.

Cardin S, Clark S (1985). A nursing diagnosis approach to the patient awaiting cardiac transplantation. *Heart Lung.* 14:499–504.

Christensen AJ, Turner CW, Slaughter JR, Holman HM Jr (1989). Perceived family support as a moderator: Psychological well-being in end-stage renal disease. *J Behav Med.* 12:249–265.

Christopherson LK (1987). Cardiac transplantation: A psychological perspective. *Circulation.* 75:57–62.

Collins C, Upright C, Aleksich J (1989). Reverse isolation: What patients perceive. *Oncol Nurs Forum.* 16:675–679.

Craven JL, Bright J, Dear CL (1990). Psychiatric, psychosocial, and rehabilitative aspects of lung transplantation. *Clin Chest Med.* 11:247–257.

Dossey BM, Keegan L, Guzzetta CE, Kolkmeier LG (1988). *Holistic Nursing: A Handbook for Practice.* Rockville, Md: Aspen.

Erikson EH (1950). *Childhood in Society.* New York: Norton.

Fellner CJ, Marshall JR (1968). Twelve kidney donors. *JAMA.* 203:2703.

Fine RN, Malekzadeh MH, Pennisi AJ, et al (1978). Long-term results of renal transplantation in children. *Pediatrics.* 61:641-650.

Freund BL, Siegel K (1986), Problems in transition following bone marrow transplantation: Psychosocial aspects. *Am J Orthopsychiatry.* 56:244-252.

Frey GM (1990). Stressors in renal transplant recipients at six weeks after transplant. *ANNA J.* 17:443-450.

Futterman AD, Wellisch DK, Bond G, Carr CR (1991). The psychosocial levels system: A new rating scale to identify and assess emotional difficulties during bone marrow transplantation. *Psychosomatics.* 32:177-186.

Gardner GG, August CS, Githens J (1977). Psychological issues in bone marrow transplantation. *Pediatrics,* 60:625-631.

George AL (1974). Adaptation to stress in political decision making: The individual, small group, and organizational contexts. In Coelho GV, et al, eds. *Coping and Adaptation.* New York: Basic Books, 176-245.

Gold LM, Kirkpatrick BS, Fricker FJ, Zitelli BJ (1986). Psychosocial issues in pediatric organ transplantation: The parents' perspectives. *Pediatrics.* 77:738-744.

Grady KL, Jalowiec A, Grusk BB, et al (1992). Symptom distress in cardiac transplant candidates. *Heart Lung.* 21:434-439.

Haberman M (1988). Psychosocial aspects of bone marrow transplantation. *Semin Oncol Nurs.* 4:55-59.

Hanigan MJ (1990). Complex problems of children following allogenic bone marrow transplantation. *J Pediatr Oncol Nurs.* 7:73-75.

Harasyko C (1989). Kidney transplantation. *Nurs Clin North Am.* 24:851-863.

Hayward MB, Kish JP, Frey GM, et al (1989). An instrument to identify stressors in renal transplant recipients. *ANNA J.* 16:81-85.

Hengeveld MW, Houtman RB, Zwann FE (1988). Psychological aspects of bone marrow transplantation: A retrospective study of 17 long-term survivors. *Bone Marrow Transplant.* 3:69-75.

Heyink J, Tymstra T (1990). Liver transplantation: The shadow side. *Fam Pract.* 7:233-237.

Heyink J, Tymstra T, Sloof MJH, Gips C (1989). Liver transplantation: The rejected patients. *Transplantation,* 47:1069-1071.

Hill R (1958). Generic features of families under stress. *Soc Casework,* 39:139-150.

Hirvas J, Enckell M, Kuhlback B, Pasternack A (1976). Psychological and social problems encountered in active treatment of chronic uraemia. II. The living donor. *Acta Med Scand.* 200:17-20.

Holechek MJ, Burrell-Diggs D, Navarro MO (1991). Renal transplantation: An option for end-stage renal disease patients. *Crit Care Nurs Q.* 13:62-71.

Holland J, Plumb M, Yates JM, et al (1977). Psychological response of patients with acute leukemia to germ-free environments. *Cancer.* 40:871-879.

Hook ML, Heyse TJ, Pawlak JC, Steckelberg JM (1990). Psychosocial care of the cardiac transplant patient: A nursing diagnosis approach. *Dimens Crit Care Nurs.* 9:301-309.

Hudson K, Hiott K (1986). Coping with pediatric renal transplant rejection. *ANNA J.* 13:261-263.

Jenkins PL, Linington A, Whittaker JA (1991). A retrospective study of psychosocial morbidity in bone marrow transplant recipients. *Psychosomatics.* 32:65-71.

Jones BM, Chang VP, Esmore D, et al (1988). Psychological adjustment after cardiac surgery. *Med J Aust.* 149:118-122.

Jones BM, Taylor F, Downs K, Spratt P (1992). Longitudinal study of quality of life and psychological adjustment after cardiac transplantation. *Med J Aust.* 157:24-26.

Kahn RL, Wolfe DM, Quinn RP, et al (1964). *Organizational Stress: Studies in Role Conflict and Ambiguity.* New York: Wiley.

Kay J, Bienenfeld D (1991). The clinical assessment of the cardiac transplant candidate. *Psychosomatics.* 32:78-87.

Kemph JP (1970). Observations of the effects of kidney transplant on donors and recipients. *Dis Nerv Syst.* 31:323.

Korsch BM, Negrete VF, Gardner JE, et al (1973). Kidney transplantation in children: Psychosocial follow-up study on child and family. *J Pediatr.* 83:399-408.

Kuhn WF, Brennan AF, Lacefield PK, et al (1990). Psychiatric distress during stages of the heart transplant protocol. *J Heart Transplant.* 9:25-29.

Kuhn WF, Davis MH, Lippmann SB (1988). Emotional adjustment to cardiac transplantation. *Gen Hosp Psychiatry.* 10:108-113.

Lazarus R (1966). *Psychological Stress and the Coping Process.* New York: McGraw-Hill.

Lazarus RS, Folkman S (1984). *Stress, Appraisal, and Coping.* New York: Springer.

Mai FM (1986). Graft and donor denial in heart transplant recipients. *Am J Psychiatry.* 143:1159-1161.

Mai FM, McKenzie FN, Kostuk WJ (1990). Psychosocial adjustment and quality of life following heart transplantation. *Can J Psychiatry.* 35:223-227.

McAleer MJ, Copeland J, Fuller J, Copeland JG (1985). Psychological aspects of heart transplantation. *J Heart Transplant.* 4:232-233.

McConville BJ, Steichen-Asch P, Harris R, et al (1990). Pediatric bone marrow transplants: Psychological aspects. *Can J Psychiatry.* 35:769-775.

McCubbin HI, Cauble AE, Patterson JM (1982). *Family Stress, Coping, and Social Support.* Springfield, Ill: Thomas.

McCubbin HI, Patterson JM (1982). Family adaptation to crises. In: McCubbin HI, et al, eds. *Family Stress, Coping, and Social Support.* Springfield, Ill: Thomas, 26-47.

Mechanic D (1962). *Students Under Stress: A Study in the Social Psychology of Adaptation.* New York: Free Press.

Mechanic D (1974). Social structure and personal adaptation: Some neglected dimensions. In: Coelho GV, et al, eds. *Coping and Adaptation.* New York: Basic Books, 32-44.

Melzer SM, Leadbeater B, Reisman L, et al (1989). Characteristics of social networks in adolescents with end-stage renal disease treated with renal transplantation. *J Adolescent Health Care.* 10:308-312.

Mishel MH, Murdaugh C (1987). Family adjustment to heart transplantation: Redesigning the dream. *Nursing Research* 36:332-338.

Muirhead J (1989). Heart and heart-lung transplantation. *Nurs Clin N Am.* 24:865-879.

Muirhead J, Meyerwitz BE, Leedham B, et al (1992). Quality of life and coping in patients awaiting heart transplantation. *J Heart Lung Transplant.* 11:265-271.

Murphy LB (1974). Coping, vulnerability and resilience in childhood. In: Coelho GV, et al, eds. *Coping and Adaptation.* New York: Basic Books, 69-100.

Neuberger JM (1989). Transplantation for alcoholic liver disease. *Brit Med J.* 299:693-694.

Nolan MT, Cupples SA, Brown MM, et al (1992). Perceived stress and coping strategies among families of heart transplant candidates during the organ waiting period. *Heart Lung.* 21:540-547.

O'Brien VC (1985). Psychological and social aspects of heart transplantation. *Heart Transplant.* 4:229-231.

Patenaude AF (1990). Psychological impact of bone marrow transplantation: Current perspectives. *Yale J Biol Med.* 63:515-519.

Pearlin LI, Schooler C (1978). The structure of coping. *J Health Soc Behav.* 19:2-21.

Pearlin LI, Schooler C (1982). The structure of coping. In: McCubbin HI, et al, eds. *Family Stress, Coping, and Social Support.* Springfield, Ill: Thomas, 109-135.

Pfefferbaum M, Lindamood MM, Wiley FM (1978). Stages in pediatric bone marrow transplantation. *Pediatrics.* 61:625-628.

Popkin MK, Moldow CF (1977). Stressors and responses during bone marrow transplantation. *Arch Intern Med* 137:725.

Porter RR, Bailey C, Bennett GM, et al (1991). Stress during the waiting period: A review of pretransplantation fears. *Critical Care Nurs Q.* 13:25-31.

Porter R, Krout L, Parks V, et al (1994). Perceived stress and coping strategies among cardiac transplant patients during the organ waiting period. *J Heart Lung Transplant.* 13:102-107.

Rauch JB, Kneen KK (1989). Accepting the gift of life: Heart transplant recipients' postoperative adaptive tasks. *Soc Work Health Care* 14:47-59.

Renshaw DC (1987). Sex and the renal transplant patient. *Clin Ther.* 10:2-7.

Reynolds JM, Garralda ME, Postlethwaite RJ, Goh D. (1991). Changes in psychosocial adjustment after renal transplantation. *Arch Dis Child.* 66:508-513.

Rodgers RH (1964). Toward a theory of family development. *J Marriage Fam.* 26:262-270.

Sheets L (1989). Liver transplantation. *Nurs Clin North Am.* 24:881-889.

Sutton TD, Murphy SP (1989). Stressors and patterns of coping in renal transplant patients. *Nurs Res.* 38:46-49.

Voepel-Lewis T, Ketefian S, Starr A, White MJ (1990). Stress, coping, and quality of life in family members of kidney transplant recipients. *ANNA J.* 17:427-431.

Weichler NK (1990). Information needs of mothers of children who have had liver transplants. *J Pediatr Nurs.* 5:88-96.

Weizer N, Weizman A, Shapira Z, et al (1989). Suicide by related kidney donors following the recipient's death. *Psychother Psychosom.* 51:216-219.

White MJ, Ketefian S, Starr AJ, Voepel-Lewis T. (1990). Stress, coping, and quality of life in adult kidney transplant recipients. *ANNA J.* 17:421-425.

Wikle T, Coyle K, Shapiro D (1990). Bone marrow transplant: Today and tomorrow. *Am J Nurs.* 90:48-56.

Williams L, Rzucidlo SE (1985). Care of the pediatric liver transplant patient in the ICU. *Crit Care Q.* 8:13-30.

Wolcott DL, Wellisch DK, Lawry FI, Landsverk J (1986). Adaptation of adult bone marrow transplant recipient long-term survivors. *Bone Marrow Transplant.* 41:478-484.

Zumbrunnen R (1989). Coping with heart transplantation: A challenge for liaison psychiatry. *Psychother Psychosom.* 52:66-73.

4

Organ and Tissue Donation

Julie Mull Strange
David C. Taylor

There is a critical need for suitable organs and tissues for transplant. The national list of patients waiting for a vital organ is constantly growing. Every 20 minutes a new name is added to the list (United Network for Organ Sharing [UNOS], personal communication, January 1994). During 1993, the list of patients waiting nationally for an organ transplant exceeded 32,000 (UNOS, 1993). The actual time a patient waits for a transplant depends in part on the type of organ required and the patient's geographic location. Many patients are listed at several transplant centers to increase their chance of receiving an organ. Estimates of the death rate among patients waiting for a transplant are as high as 20%, which means, on average, seven people die every day because an organ did not become available (UNOS, personal communication, January 1994).

According to a Gallup poll (1993), most Americans are aware of the benefits of transplantation and believe it is a necessary health care option. Similarly, many people have thought about organ and tissue donation and have even discussed it with their families (Gallup, 1993). Other studies show that health care professionals are equally knowledgeable and supportive regarding donation and transplantation (Bidigare & Oermann, 1991). In spite of public awareness of the need for organs, patients waiting for a transplant far outnumber the organs and tissues available.

This chapter presents an overview of the organ supply and demand crisis and reviews attempts being made to resolve it. It provides general information on donor recognition, referral, clinical management, surgical recovery, and the obstacles faced daily by procurement professionals in their attempts to recover organs and tissues for transplantation. And finally, this chapter touches on professional education efforts, hospital-wide donation systems, and public awareness programs that are all integral components in a successful donor campaign.

THE ORGAN DEMAND VERSUS SUPPLY CRISIS

Increased Demand for Organs for Transplantation

Scientific and medical advances made over the past decade have contributed to the long list of patients waiting to receive a transplant. Heart, lung, liver, pancreas, kidney, small intestine, stomach–intestine blocks, and a variety of tissues are all routinely and successfully transplanted (Table 4–1). Enhanced graft function and high patient and graft survival rates are now possible because of improved surgical and organ preservation techniques and decreased rejection rates associated with immunosuppressive agents. As function and survival rates continue to improve, more patients with end-stage organ failure are referred to transplant centers. In addition, previous restrictions on which patients could be considered for a transplant, including age and medical history, have been made more liberal than they once were (Siminoff et al, 1993; Evans et al, 1992). Improved technology, such as artificial cardiac devices that act as a bridge until a donor heart is available, has enabled more patients to survive while waiting for a transplant. Finally, the number of transplant centers across the United States has increased considerably, allowing greater numbers of patients to be listed for transplants.

Realities Regarding Donation

The reality of transplantation in the 1990s remains the inability to provide enough donor organs to treat the growing number of waiting recipients. Many organ procurement organizations (OPOs) have conducted death record reviews in their hospitals in an attempt to determine the potential number of donor organs. Unfortunately, the annual number of potential organ donors across the United States has not been well studied. Available data regarding potential donors indicate the range to be 12,000 to 20,000 donors (Caplan, 1991; Peters et al, 1989). Some reports indicate that as few as 26 to 42% of available donor organs are actually used (O'Connell et al, 1993). The one area of consensus is that more donors are available than are actually recognized and referred to certified OPOs. The number of donor organs recovered in the United States in 1991, 1992, and 1993 remained stable at approximately 4500, or 19 donors per 1 million population (Association of Organ Procurement Organizations [AOPO] data, 1993). This plateau in donor rates has been attributed to a variety of factors, the most important of which may be a decreasing incidence nationwide in deaths due to motor vehicle accidents (Evans et al, 1992). Safety campaigns to enforce speed limits, motorcycle helmet and seat belt laws, and air bag use, in addition to increased efforts to reduce drunken driving, have all contributed to a successful reduction in brain deaths due to blunt trauma. Sophisticated and effective emergency medical services systems have improved the response times and quality of care provided by prehospital personnel, leading to more lives saved. Although the number of patients who sustain penetrating

TABLE 4–1. TRANSPLANTABLE ORGANS AND TISSUES

ORGANS

Heart	Pancreas
Heart and lung	Pancreatic segment
Single or double lung	Pancreatic islet cells
Lung segment	Intestine
Liver	Stomach and intestine
Liver segment	Kidney

TISSUES

Skin	Saphenous veins
Bone (whole, crushed, segment)	Dura
Ligaments	Inner-ear bones
Soft tissues	Facial bones
Corneas	Vertebrae
Heart valves	

trauma may have remained constant or even increased in some geographic areas, many victims are either dead on arrival to the hospital or have such devastating multiorgan injuries that they are unsuitable candidates for organ donation. The acquired immunodeficiency syndrome (AIDS) epidemic also has decreased the number of potential donors (Caplan, 1991; Evans et al, 1992). These are all factors over which procurement and transplant professionals have little control. There are, however, a number of factors over which procurement personnel do have control. Table 4–2 lists some of these factors and several are discussed throughout this chapter. A number of these obstacles to donation and transplantation are inherent in the type of patient who becomes an organ donor. Organ and tissue donors are dead, and death is sensitive, personal, and often an uncomfortable experience for health care providers at all levels. Any misconception regarding brain death or the donation process can greatly interfere with the ability of a health care provider to participate and support the family of a potential donor. Conversely, a well-meaning, committed professional may unintentionally broach the subject of donation to a family prematurely, potentially causing a negative reaction and losing the organs for transplantation.

Efforts to Bridge the Donor–Recipient Gap

Although there are some legitimate and uncontrollable factors that have a negative impact on the number of potential donors, many professional and public policy issues may positively affect the number of potential donors.

Governmental Involvement. Federal laws have been enacted in an effort to improve donation rates and to ensure equitable allocation of transplantable organs. Many states have followed the federal lead and have also passed required request or routine referral legislation to ensure donors are recognized and referred and that

TABLE 4–2. OBSTACLES TO DONATION

Misconceptions in the health care community regarding brain death and difficulty discussing it with families

State laws proclaiming brain death as a legal definition or category of death but providing no specific criteria for the declaration process. Therefore, brain death criteria and the declaration process must be established by every individual hospital

Fear on the part of physicians and nurses that discussing donation may cause more pain for the grieving family

Treatment so aggressive that organs are rendered unsuitable for transplantation

Donor referrals to the recovery agency made too late in the process

Well-meaning personnel approaching the family prematurely or without the necessary information to appropriately offer the option of donation

Referrals not made because personnel believe a patient is not a suitable candidate for donation

Referrals not made because a patient was never identified as a potential donor

The complex critical care required by organ donors

Inability on the part of physicians and nurses to adjust to a patient's death and regard the patient as an organ donor

Concern regarding legal liability

Referrals not made because there is a general lack of understanding regarding how to make the referral and whom and when to call

Forgetting about organ donation in the midst of a crisis

families are given the option of donation. Although efforts by both state and federal lawmakers have made progress to protect the rights of donor families to make decisions regarding donation and to increase organ donation overall, they have not cured the organ shortage.

Joint Commission on the Accreditation of Healthcare Organizations. The Joint Commission on the Accreditation of Healthcare Organizations (JCAHO) provides oversight for donation programs. The JCAHO has begun monitoring hospitals' compliance with federal and state laws regarding donation. Hospitals must show evidence that they have established policies and procedures pertaining to donation; routinely offer the option of donation; refer potential donors to a certified OPO or tissue bank; and document outcomes in the patient's medical record (JCAHO, 1992). The anticipated outcome of increased organs and tissues for transplantation has not been achieved despite these efforts.

Presumed Consent. United States residents are encouraged to sign donor cards, designate themselves as donors on their driver's licenses, and discuss their wishes with their family. At the time of death, the patient's family is approached regarding donation, and consent is requested. Because this system of choosing to be a donor does not provide an adequate number of organs and tissues, many believe that the United States should adopt presumed consent. Several European countries have achieved higher numbers of donors per million population than in the United States by practicing presumed consent, but recipient waiting lists continue to grow (Stuart et al, 1981).

In presumed consent, a person is presumed to be a donor and organs are recovered unless a card denying donation is found or such wishes were made known by the patient's family. Proponents of this system believe that more transplantable organs and tissues would become available. Opponents, however, believe presumed consent would remove the family's right to be involved in the donation decision, a concept of which most Americans disapprove, as evidenced by a Gallup poll (Gallup, 1993). The poll indicated that the public did not support a physician's right to remove organs without consent from the next-of-kin. Even with presumed consent, organ recovery personnel would still have to speak with the donor's family to obtain a medical and behavioral history, thus affording the family the opportunity to oppose donation. OPOs would be reluctant, if not unwilling, to proceed with organ or tissue recovery under these circumstances. In addition, hospitals would look unfavorably on the negative publicity generated by organ recovery without family consent and in reality would most likely prohibit such activities.

Rewarded Gifting. Another controversial effort to improve donation rates is the concept of financial incentives, or "rewarded gifting." The current basis of the donation process is the donor family's altruistic capability to move beyond their own sense of profound sorrow and pain to think of the needs of others. Their gifts are made freely, and families often state that they view donation as an extension of the caring and giving nature of their loved one. Usually all they anticipate in return is a simple acknowledgment that the recipients are doing well and are appreciative. The notion of rewarded gifting implies that at some point the donor's family would receive financial compensation from the OPO in exchange for the donation. Whether a cash amount would be offered or a contribution made to defray funeral expenses, less than 20% of Americans polled by Gallup believed that financial incentives would influence their decision to donate (Gallup, 1993). Some proponents find a payment system acceptable (Peters, 1991). They believe that for many families receiving a reward might positively influence their decision to donate. Questions remain unanswered such as: Who will offer the money and when? Is the payment offer retracted if the organs are found to be unsuitable for transplantation? Who will safeguard the approach for donation to ensure no coercion takes place during donation discussions? Debate over financial incentives will surely continue in many arenas (Peters, 1991; Kuperberg, 1993; Price, 1993).

Expanded-criteria Donors. In the desperate search for ways to increase the number of organs and tissues available, many OPOs have expanded their previous donor criteria and are now evaluating and recovering organs from donors who would not have been considered suitable in the past. Satisfactory graft survival and function have been reported, even though these "marginal" or expanded-criteria donors may be older than the traditional age for donors, have long-standing medical problems, including hypertension and diabetes, have longer ischemic times, and have engaged in high-risk behavior (O'Connell et al, 1993; Siminoff et al, 1993; Alexander & Vaughn, 1991; Schuler et al, 1989; Sweeney et al, 1990; Mor et al, 1992; Sautner et al, 1991). Final donor suitability in such cases may not be confirmed until histologic information is received through biopsies of the liver and kidneys. Some transplant centers are now using both kidneys from an expanded-criteria donor with marginal biopsy results, for example, a biopsy indicative of existing glomerulonephritis, and transplanting them into a single recipient. The rationale is that despite compromised renal function individually, the kidneys together will provide adequate function and serve as a suitable graft (Ratner L, personal communication, January, 1993).

Nontraditional Transplants. In an effort to increase the number of organs available, some transplant centers are exploring the possibility of dividing a single kidney to transplant into two separate recipients (Ratner L, personal communication, 1993; UNOS, 1993). Success has been achieved in similar segmental transplants of the liver, pancreas, and lung. Data from the AOPO indicates that some transplant centers in the United States are reexploring the 1970s practice of recovering organs such as the liver and kidneys from donors without a heartbeat, specifically trauma patients who arrive at the hospital in cardiac arrest (AOPO, 1993; UNOS, 1993). Although there is interest in the possibility of such recoveries, public and professional debate continues surrounding the ethical and legal implications (Giordano, 1993). Organs from living-related donors, for example a kidney from one sibling to another, have had excellent graft survival rates (UNOS, 1993). Organs also are being transplanted from living-unrelated donors.

The donor shortage will not be resolved in the near future. Ideas and methods that seem quite controversial are being debated, researched, and tested. Before additional laws are drafted and enacted, before entire social and value systems are revised, before more experimental transplants are attempted, and before more lives are lost while waiting, society must take a closer look at what, if anything, is wrong with the donor system. The failings of the established system are not clear, but attempts are being made to design a new approach. Most available studies provide contradictory results and what remains is speculation. It would be more beneficial if health care professionals received the education and support they need to assist potential donors and their families. It also would be helpful if all physicians became comfortable with their knowledge of brain death and accepted the preestablished criteria for declaring death. All potential donors should be recognized and referred promptly to the appropriate recovery organization. Trained recovery professionals should be permitted to use their skills in determining donor suitability, in approaching all families for consent, and in managing the clinical needs of the donor. All Americans need to be cognizant of their option regarding donation and to discuss their wishes with their loved ones. While speculation continues, the present system should be perfected.

The National Donation System

The federal government oversees the Organ Procurement and Transplantation Network. It awards a contract to an organization to operate the network and to manage

TABLE 4–3. REGIONS OF THE UNITED NETWORK FOR ORGAN SHARING

Region 1
   Connecticut, Maine, Massachusetts, New Hampshire, Rhode Island, Vermont

Region 2
   Delaware, District of Columbia, Maryland, New Jersey, Pennsylvania
   Northern Virginia, West Virginia

Region 3
   Alabama, Arkansas, Florida, Georgia, Louisiana, Mississippi, Puerto Rico

Region 4
   Oklahoma, Texas

Region 5
   Arizona, California, Hawaii, Nevada, New Mexico, Utah

Region 6
   Alaska, Idaho, Montana, Oregon, Washington

Region 7
   Illinois, Minnesota, North Dakota, South Dakota, Wisconsin

Region 8
   Colorado, Iowa, Kansas, Missouri, Nebraska, Wyoming

Region 9
   New York

Region 10
   Indiana, Michigan, Ohio

Region 11
   Kentucky, North Carolina, South Carolina, Tennessee, Virginia

Source: UNOS Policy Manual. Policy 3.5.3.4. March 4, 1993

the national system for organ allocation and sharing. The UNOS has been awarded this contract since 1986. The UNOS is a voluntary, not-for-profit organization located in Richmond, Virginia. It is composed of a board of directors that represents 11 regions of the United States (Table 4–3) and various transplant professional organizations and the general public, including not-for-profit organizations, ethicists, and legal groups. The UNOS is responsible for (1) improving the effectiveness of cadaver organ procurement, distribution, and transplantation; (2) maximizing access to suitable organs for potential recipients; (3) systematically collecting donor and recipient data for quality analysis and control; and (4) maintaining the professional skills of those involved in the organ recovery and transplant process (O'Connell, 1993). The UNOS is responsible for maintaining the national list of all recipients awaiting organ transplants and for supervising organ distribution. Every organ donor and all waiting recipients must be listed on the UNOS computer, and all transplant centers, OPOs, and tissue typing laboratories must be members of UNOS. In addition, UNOS provides 24-hour access to its Organ Center to assist OPOs in local, regional, and national organ distribution.

Organ Procurement Organizations

There are approximately 68 OPOs in the United States. Although some are hospital-based and located within transplant facilities, most are independent, not-for-profit organizations. All OPOs are certified every 2 years by the Health Care Financing Administration. Although each OPO may carry out daily operations differently, all share the same mission: increasing the number of organs and tissues available for transplantation.

OPOs provide a variety of services to the hospitals and communities in their service areas. In addition to 24-hour, 7-day-a-week availability, a sampling of services is as follows:

- Receive, review, and process local donor referrals
- Evaluate patients to determine suitability for donation
- Assist in the medical care of the organ donor
- Obtain consent and provide grief counseling for donor families
- Share organs and assist with the surgical recovery process
- Provide public and professional education
- Assist hospitals in developing customized, realistic policies and procedures for a successful donation system.

THE DONATION PROCESS

Successful organ and tissue donation depends on the level of knowledge and personal and professional commitment to donation and transplantation of every person involved. Recognizing that a patient has the potential to become an organ or tissue donor and referring that patient to the appropriate procurement agency is the first step in the donation process.

Recognizing and Referring a Potential Donor

As many as 75% of the potential organ and tissue donors in Maryland in 1991 were never recognized and referred (Transplant Resource Center of Maryland [TRC], unpublished data, 1992). If a health care professional is unable to recognize a potential donor, the patient will not be referred to the appropriate agency; the patient's family will be denied their right to decide about donation; and valuable life-saving organs and life-enhancing tissues will be wasted. In this scenario, the hospital and the health care professionals have made the decision for the family that the patient will not become a donor; a decision that ethically, legally, and morally should be made by the family.

Hospital personnel in the TRC service area have been provided with broad criteria for organ and tissue donation. Any patient who meets these criteria are to be referred to the TRC. The difference between a potential organ donor and a potential tissue donor is that an organ donor's heart is still beating and is being mechanically supported with a ventilator. For example, any patient who has suffered a catastrophic brain injury or other cerebral event and who is at or near the point of brain death should be routinely referred to the procurement agency as a potential organ donor. Anyone who suffers a cardiac death in the hospital or who is dead on arrival is considered a potential tissue donor and should routinely be referred as such. Recent studies confirm that many health care professionals cannot differentiate between potential organ and potential tissue donors (Danneffel, 1992; Nelson, 1992; Caplan, 1991). Limitations due to age and medical history vary between potential organ and tissue donors and become even more specific depending on the individual organ or tissue being evaluated. This information is not necessary for hospital personnel to retain if a routine referral system is used. Although any health care provider should be able to recognize a potential donor, individual hospital policy often designates certain personnel as being responsible for making the actual referral call. The routine referral process at the TRC is as follows:

- A hospital staff member recognizes a potential organ or tissue donor
- A designated staff member refers the potential donor to the appropriate procurement agency
- An organ and tissue recovery coordinator performs an on-site evaluation to determine the suitability of the potential donor

This simple, routine referral procedure has been instituted in many hospitals throughout the United States for several reasons. First, the easier and quicker the referral system, the more likely are hospital personnel to remember how to access it and to refer patients promptly. Second, the routine referral of all potential donors eliminates the need for the staff to stay current on everchanging donor criteria, which, in some cases, may be recipient-dependent. In addition, the national shortage of available organs and tissues for transplant has led to the expansion of donor criteria previously mentioned (Alexander & Vaughn, 1991). Transplant surgeons are now more willing to accept organs from older donors and from donors who have medical conditions that previously were considered contraindications to donation. For example, in the past, a history of diabetes or hypertension or the need for more than 10 $\mu g/kg$ per minute of dopamine usually made the patient ineligible to donate any organs. No longer, however, do age, past medical history, or current hospital course, including the use of inotropic agents, automatically rule out the possibility that a patient can donate organs (Nygaard et al, 1990). Although the pancreas of a person with diabetes is not transplantable, the patient's heart, lungs, liver, and kidneys may be suitable for donation. It is unrealistic to expect health care personnel who are not directly involved with donation and transplantation on a regular basis to be qualified to determine medical suitability. The determination of donor suitability is the responsibility of the recovery coordinator in collaboration with transplant surgeons.

The routine referral procedure in most Maryland hospitals requires only one telephone call to alert the organ and tissue procurement agency about the potential donor. Although some patient information is needed (Table 4-4), this system is easy to use and takes little time on the part of the health care provider. If there are no obvious contraindications to organ donation, for example, the patient is known to be seropositive for human immunodeficiency virus (HIV) or to have an active malignant tumor (with the exception of a primary brain tumor or basal cell skin cancer), a recovery coordinator travels to the hospital to further evaluate the patient's suitability. In the unlikely event that the patient is deemed unsuitable for organ donation during the initial referral call, the recovery coordinator refers the potential donor on to the

TABLE 4–4. INITIAL REFERRAL INFORMATION

Essential Information

Name and status of referring person

Hospital and unit telephone numbers

Patient's name, age, race, sex

Diagnosis

Obvious track marks

Current neurologic status

Name of primary physician and nurse

Helpful Information if Time Permits

Current hemodynamic status (vital signs, urine output)

Past medical and social history

Family understanding and coping status

Patient's home address and date of birth[1]

Plan for declaration of brain death

Plan for further medical treatment

[1]This information enables an early call to the Motor Vehicle Administration/Maryland State Police to determine donor status.

appropriate tissue recovery team or eye bank agency. If the patient has an absolute contraindication to donation, the process ends and the caller is instructed to document this finding in the patient's medical record.

Donor Evaluation

Although the TRC provides liberal initial donor criteria to hospital staff, the actual evaluation process used by the recovery coordinator to screen potential donors is extensive and thorough. There are three distinct phases in the evaluation process:

1. Primary evaluation. The recovery coordinator performs an on-site assessment to determine general donor suitability.
2. Secondary evaluation. The recovery coordinator uses consultations with specialists and invasive diagnostic studies.
3. Tertiary evaluation. The recovery surgeons perform extensive organ visualization, palpation, and close inspection for any abnormalities (Transplant Resource Center of Maryland, 1993)

During the primary evaluation, the recovery coordinator uses information obtained from the following activities to determine the suitability of the potential organ and tissue donor. The recovery coordinator reviews the patient's medical record and documents the following pertinent information:

- Current hospital course
- Past medical and behavioral history
- Current neurologic status and plan for declaration of brain death

- Signs of any disease that would negate donation
- Trends in vital signs including blood pressure, heart rate, temperature, pulmonary artery pressures
- Trends in urine output, intake and output balance
- Intravenous fluids: type, rate, additives
- Vasopressor drips: type, rate, trends
- Trends in laboratory data

The recovery coordinator then performs a detailed total systems physical assessment, identifying signs of trauma, previous operations, and high-risk behaviors (track marks, tattoos, skin turgor), evaluating muscle tone, and documenting height and weight. After completing the review of the medical record and the physical examination, the recovery coordinator contacts the Maryland State Police to access the driver's license computer registry of all designated donors. Knowing that the patient is a designated donor usually enables the family to make the decision regarding donation without hesitation. During this initial evaluation phase the recovery coordinator also determines if the patient falls under the jurisdiction of the medical examiner. If so, the coordinator reviews the case and requests consent for donation from the medical examiner's office. Maryland law requires consent from the medical examiner's office in all homicides, suicides, accidental or suspicious deaths, and all deaths that occur in the hospital within 24 hours of admission (Maryland Post Mortem Examiners Commission, 1981). Finally, the recovery coordinator consults with the primary nurse and physician to discuss the patient's status, determine the plan for declaration of brain death if not yet completed, and to coordinate the effort for the timing and approach to the family for consent.

Brain Death

The understanding, recognition, acceptance and declaration of brain death remain critical obstacles to organ donation (Lucas et al, 1992; Baldwin et al, 1993; Vrtis & Nicely, 1993; Youngner, 1989). Although laws in every state consider brain death a legal form of death, developing a policy that directs the actual process to declare brain death remains the responsibility of individual hospitals with input from professionals such as neuroscientists, an ethics committee, and administration and nursing departments. Regardless of policies and procedures pertaining to brain death, there exists in many hospitals a reluctance to declare brain death. The experience of the staff at the TRC confirms that often potential organ donation falters at this point and fails to progress beyond it, and potential donor organs are lost.

Brain death may result from a number of injuries or cerebral events, the most common of which is spontaneous intercerebral hemorrhage and blunt or penetrating trauma. Other patients may become brain dead yet may go unrecognized as potential donors. For example, anoxic events caused by hanging, suffocation, overdose, drowning, and prolonged cardiac arrest may all lead to brain death. Primary brain tumors also may cause brain death. The recovery coordinator, although not permitted involvement in the declaration process, must ensure that proper methods have been used for declaring and documenting brain death because organ recovery may not take place until the declaration process is complete. Individual hospital policies may vary in the

TABLE 4–5. PROCEDURE FOR PERFORMING AN APNEA TEST

1. Preoxygenate the patient with 100% FiO_2 for 15 minutes. Before an apnea test is attempted, the patient's $PaCO_2$ should be normalized.

2. Disconnect the patient from ventilator and provide continuous oxygen at 8 to 12 L/min by inserting a catheter into the endotracheal tube (alternative method is to leave the patient connected to the ventilator in the continuous positive airway pressure mode).

3. Observe the patient for spontaneous respirations.[1]

4. Obtain an arterial blood gas sample after 10 minutes. Evaluate the $PaCO_2$ results. The $PaCO_2$ should rise to at least 60 mm Hg to ensure the test is accurate.

5. Reconnect the patient to the ventilator.

6. If there are no obvious respirations and the $PaCO_2$ is 60 mm Hg or higher, the patient is considered apneic.

[1]Note any desaturation or deterioration in cardiovascular status during the apnea test. If the patient becomes hypotensive, has dysrhythmias or clinically significant desaturation, abort the apnea test and place the patient back on mechanical ventilation. Other confirmatory studies may be required to confirm brain death.

process or type of examinations that must be performed. The most common method, however, is the clinical brain death evaluation. This assessment, which ensures that all brain and brain-stem function has ceased as required by law, includes the following criteria:

- No spontaneous movement (Spinal reflexes may still exist in the presence of brain death and should not interfere with the process)
- No response to painful stimuli
- No brain-stem reflexes
    No pupillary reflexes
    No corneal reflexes
    No doll's eye reflex
    No gag or cough reflex
    No oculovestibular response to caloric stimulation
- No spontaneous respiration in the presence of a $PaCO_2$ of 60 mm Hg or higher (Table 4–5) (Presidential Commission, 1981; Ad Hoc Com-mittee of the Harvard Medical School, 1968, 1984).

The clinical brain death examination is considered valid only in the absence of central nervous system depressants and in the presence of normotension, normothermia, normal metabolic balance and an established cause of the brain death (Presidential Commission, 1981; Kaufman & Lynn, 1986). Many hospitals require that two clinical examinations be performed by two different physicians with a predetermined interval of hours between examinations. Figure 4–1 shows a checklist used by some hospitals to document the clinical findings of the brain death examination. Table 4–6 presents the other physiologic changes that occur with brain death.

Diagnostic studies such as a negative cerebral blood flow study by use of arteriography or nucleotide scan and sequential isoelectric electroencephalograms (EEGs) may confirm the diagnosis of brain death (Mackersie, 1989). Although these studies may be helpful in selected patient situations, they are not required by Maryland law for the determination of brain death. The time the patient is declared brain dead is the actual time of death recorded in the medical record and on the death certificate. After the patient is declared brain dead, hemodynamic stability must be maintained until the patient's family has had the opportunity to consider organ and tissue donation.

Consent

Regardless of how knowledgeable, supportive, and committed health care personnel are on both a personal and professional level regarding donation, they usually identify the consent process as the most difficult and stressful part of donation (Lucas et al, 1992; Vrtis & Nicely, 1993; Danneffel, 1992). How and when a family is approached and by whom regarding the donation makes a great deal of difference in the outcome. For example, a family approached for consent before the declaration of death almost always says no to donation. Similarly, a requestor who says, "Even though I don't believe in this, the law says I still have to ask you," usually gets a negative response. A health care professional's feelings about donation have considerable impact on how an undecided family will respond (Vrtis & Nicely, 1993; Prottas & Batten, 1988). Although people should make the decision about donation for themselves, the reality is that most families must make the decision without knowing how their loved one felt about donation.

Data analysis from the TRC indicates that the consent process, often mismanaged or carried out by inexperienced or uncomfortable personnel, was responsible for 39% of all denials of donation in 1993 in the service area of the TRC. Figure 4–2 presents the reasons for lack of donation in 1993 in the TRC service area, including consent issues. Regardless of personal beliefs or feelings pertaining to donation, nurses should afford the family their legal right to donation. They should also be careful not to negatively influence a family's thinking (Vrtis & Nicely, 1993). Nurses and other health care professionals must be advocates for a patient's or family's values whether or not they agree and must support the family through the decision-making process (Corley et al, 1993; Martin, 1993).

Recovery coordinators are specially trained in the request process and because they are somewhat emotionally distanced from the family are more comfortable approaching a family regarding donation. The option of donation must be presented as a series of conversations, the staging of which represents a critical component for a successful donation. The option of donation should not be broached until after the family has had time to accept the finality of brain death and to say good-bye. Therefore, the first step in the consent process is a discussion among the family, physician, and nurse that describes the patient's prognosis and then centers on the declaration of brain death. The family must be afforded time to fully understand what brain death is and what it really means before they can accept that their loved one is legally dead, supported only artificially by machines and medications. The second step enables the family additional time to see the patient, say their good-byes, and begin grieving the loss of the loved one. The third and final step in the consent process is the discussion regarding organ and tissue donation. The family has now had time to accept the finality of brain death; they have had the opportunity to separate from their loved one; and now they must begin to make final arrangements to bring the experience to clo-

	First Exam	**Second Exam**
Date	_____	_____
Time	_____	_____
Body temperature	_____	_____
Electrolytes within normal limits? (yes or no)	_____	_____
Blood ethanol level? (If indicated)	_____	_____
Toxicology screen? (If indicated)	_____	_____
Confirmatory Tests Performed? (date/time) (EEG, cerebral arterial flow study)	_____	_____
Results of confirmatory test, if performed	_____	_____

Absence of Cerebral Functions

Is the patient completely unresponsive?	_____	_____
Any spontaneous movements?	_____	_____
Any movement to painful stimuli?	_____	_____

Spinal reflexes may be present in brain dead individuals.

Absence of Mid-Brain Functions

Pupillary reaction to light	_____	_____
Corneal reflexes	_____	_____
Oculocephalic response to head turning (doll's eyes)	_____	_____
Oculovestibular response (cold calorics)	_____	_____
Gag reflex or response to bronchial stimulation	_____	_____

Absence of Brain Stem Reflexes

Spontaneous respirations?	_____	
Apnea test in the presence of 100% O_2 (yes or no)	_____	
PCO_2 level at end of apnea test	_____	

Having considered the above findings, we hereby certify the death of:_____

Date:_____Time:_____AM/PM

A note certifying death has been placed in this patient's medical record along with a State of Maryland Death Certificate.

Physician's Signature: _____ MD _____ MD

Names Printed: _____ MD _____ MD

Figure 4–1. Checklist for determination of brain death.

TABLE 4–6. BRAIN DEATH: PHYSIOLOGIC CHANGES RELATED TO LOSS OF REGULATORY FUNCTIONS

Regulatory Mechanisms and Their Location in the Brain

Vasomotor regulatory center (medulla)

Respiratory regulatory center (medulla)

Cardiac regulatory center (medulla)

Water regulation (hypothalamic–pituitary loop)

Temperature regulation (hypothalamus)

Neuroendocrine regulatory mechanisms (hypothalamic–pituitary loop)

Physiologic Changes Due to Loss of Regulatory Mechanisms

Respiratory failure (hypoxemia, hypoxia)

Cardiovascular instability (changes in blood pressure, dysrhythmias, decreased cardiac output)

Hypovolemia

Metabolic derangements and fluid and electrolyte imbalances

Hypothermia or poikilothermy

Clotting disorders

---

sure. This step-by-step process, allowing sufficient time intervals between steps, was termed *decoupling* in a 1988 to 1990 collaborative study performed in Kentucky (Garrison et al, 1991). Decoupling is the temporal separation between conversations regarding brain death and donation. Most families cannot conceive of donating their loved one's organs and tissues until they are absolutely sure that death has occurred. The separation between conversations gives the family the time they need to accept the death. After they have separated for the last time, the family can begin to make the necessary decisions and arrangements.

The final phase in the consent process should be a collaborative approach with the patient's physician, nurse, social worker, and clergy, and the recovery coordinator. Whereas the hospital staff ideally conducts the brain-death conversations, the discussions regarding the option of donation should be led by the recovery coordinator. It was shown in the Kentucky study that when a hospital staff member approached a family alone, he or she obtained consent only 9% of the time. When the recovery coordinator approached the family, consent was given 67% of the time. When the recovery coordinator and a hospital staff member approached the family together consent was given 75% of the time (Garrison et al, 1991). The discussion should take place in a private setting away from the patient's bedside and be carried out in a caring and empathetic manner to enable the family to feel comfortable in asking questions. The recovery coordinator acknowledges the family's loss and ensures that they fully understand brain death before discussing donation. If the patient had never recorded or discussed his or her wishes, the family is offered the option of donation and is told of the benefits of transplantation. Questions families most often ask pertain to disfigurement, donation-related billing procedures, funeral arrangements, and the time required. Therefore, when appropriate in the conversation, the recovery coor-

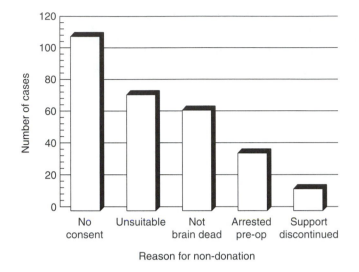

Figure 4–2. Non donation data. The total number of organ donor referrals in 1993 was 341. There were 68 organ donors, and 273 nondonations. Thirty-nine percent of the nondonations were due to lack of consent. In 50 cases the family was approached by a physician and a alone; in 4 cases by a physician and a nurse; in 3 by a physician and a donor advocate; in 7 by a physician and a Transplant Resource Center (TRC) staff member; in 12 by a nurse alone; in 9 by a TRC staff member alone; and in 10 by a donor advocate alone. In 3 cases the medical examiner refused consent. In 4 cases there was known prior patient objection. In 4 cases the physician refused the TRC access to the patient. Twenty-five percent of the Non-Donations were the result of the TRC's determining the patient was unsuitable for donation. In 53 cases the donor was ruled out because of history and age; in 14 cases because of high-risk social history; and in 1 case because of positive serologic results. In 22% of the nondonations (59 cases) the patient never met brain death criteria. In 11% (31 cases) the patient suffered a cardiac arrest prior to brain death declaration or time of surgery. Artificial support was withdrawn in 3% (9) of cases.

dinator explains the surgical procedure, including reconstruction and the length of time it will take to complete the donation. The coordinator reassures the family that they may have any type of funeral arrangements they desire and that the recovery team will work within any time restrictions necessary to comply with religious beliefs. The recovery coordinator also explains the billing procedure to the family so that they are aware that the recovery agency pays all costs associated with the donation.

If the family consents to donation, the recovery coordinator seeks comprehensive medical history information and elicits any medical or behavioral risk factors from the family. Personal questions regarding social behaviors including drug and alcohol use and sexual patterns must be asked at this time to evaluate the patient's suitability as a donor. The family is informed that all donors undergo blood testing for commu

TABLE 4–7 SEROLOGY TESTING

Human immunodeficiency virus 1 and 2

Human T-cell lymphotrophic virus

Hepatitis C virus (Non-A, non-B hepatitis)

Hepatitis B surface antigen (hepatitis B)

Cytomegalovirus

Rapid plasma reagin

Venereal Disease Research Laboratories test

nicable diseases such as HIV infection and hepatitis to prevent harm to the potential recipients of the organs. The legal next-of-kin, as prioritized by the law, then signs the donation consent form (Annotated Code of Maryland, 1974). A hospital staff member must witness and sign the consent as is done with other hospital informed consent procedures.

Secondary Evaluation

The secondary evaluation or screening phase takes place after consent for donation is obtained. It includes specific organ function and tissue assessment and consultation with specialists and possible diagnostic studies. The recovery coordinator ensures that ABO typing has been done and requests additional samples (approximately 60 mL) for serologic testing and preliminary tissue typing. Routine serologic tests required by UNOS policy for organ donors are listed in Table 4–7. Serologic samples are sent to the laboratory as soon after consent is obtained as possible because, on average, this panel of tests takes 4 to 6 hours to complete. Delays in receiving serologic results can delay transplantation because no organ can be transplanted until all serologic results are known. Blood samples for preliminary tissue typing are also sent to the laboratory as soon as possible because determination of the donor's human leukocyte antigen (HLA) status and then subsequent cross-matching with potential recipients can take as long as 10 hours to complete. Pancreas and kidney recipients are matched with the donor on the basis of the organ allocation criteria described later and the quality of HLA or antigen match. Ideally, the level of the antigen match and the results of the cross-match between the donor and recipient sera are completed before surgical recovery of the organ to minimize the time between recovery and transplantation. The recovery coordinator requests additional laboratory studies every 4 to 8 hours (Table 4–8) to monitor trends in organ function and to evaluate the effectiveness of management efforts.

Donor Management

Managing the clinical needs of a brain-dead organ donor can and often does become a complex struggle. Brain death, the irreversible loss of all regulatory functions previously performed by the brain, forces the rest of the body to fail as well. Ideally the patient should have a one-to-one nurse-to-patient assignment because his or her condition can change rapidly. A brain-dead patient is a challenge because high quality care must continue to ensure optimal organ function. The recovery coordinator

TABLE 4–8. ORGAN SPECIFIC LABORATORY DATA AND DIAGNOSTIC STUDIES

All organ donors	Liver
Electrolytes (including blood urea nitrogen, creatinine)	Total bilirubin
Complete blood count with differential	Direct and indirect bilirubin
Arterial blood gases	Alanine aminotransferase
Urinalysis	Aspartate aminotransferase
Blood culture	Alkaline phosphatase
Urine culture	Prothrombin time, partial thromboplastin time
Heart	**Lung**
Creatine phosphokinase with MB%	Stat sputum Gram stain
Chest radiograph	Sputum culture
Cardiac consultation	Chest measurements (by radiograph)
Electrocardiogram	Central venous pressure trends
Echocardiogram	100% FiO_2 challenge blood gas
Cardiac catheterization[1]	Bronchoscopy[2]
Pancreas	
Amylase	
Lipase	
Glucose	

[1]Cardiac catheterization may be requested when the donor exceeds local age and history criteria (if available in the donor facility)
[2]Bedside bronchoscopy may be necessary to determine if the lungs are suitable for transplantation.
MB, isoenzyme of creatine kinase that contains one M and one B subunit.

works in collaboration with the health care team to provide overall clinical management goals and offers guidance to prevent or minimize the complications associated with brain death. In addition, and often more important, the coordinator remains in the intensive care unit (ICU) throughout the process and lends personal as well as professional support to the personnel involved. The staff caring for this patient must make the transition from treating the patient as a survivor to accepting the fact that the patient is dead to treating the *organs* for optimal recipient outcome. All the while they must deal with their own emotions and reactions and with those of the donor family. The physiologic changes that take place with brain death are predictable and, in most cases, manageable with a planned, coordinated approach to care. The goals of donor management are: (1) correct, restore, and maintain the functions previously regulated by the brain; (2) modify clinical care to optimize organ function; (3) minimize the risk of contamination and infection; and (4) continue high quality critical care. Because a brain-dead patient has lost all vasomotor, cardiac, respiratory, and water-regulating functions, following the rule of 100's will assist the health-care team in providing basic donor management:

1. Maintain the blood pressure at greater than 100 mm Hg.
2. Maintain the PaO_2 at greater than 100 mm Hg.
3. Maintain the urine output at greater than 100 mL/hour.

How the team achieves these goals is different with each organ donor. How complex a patient's clinical needs become depends on many factors, including the cause of brain death, the presence of associated injuries or complicating factors, the patient's age and preexisting conditions, and the effects of the therapy previously provided in an attempt to treat the original cerebral event or injury. The average donor age and cause of brain death have changed over the recent past in the TRC service area; older patients who have extensive medical histories require different management techniques than young healthy donors. Table 4-9 provides the data on the changing TRC donor profile.   Additional goals and recommendations for clinical donor management are identified in the care plan found in Nursing Care Plan 4-1, p 103.

Organ Allocation and Placement

The donor's organs are allocated to recipients based on a point system established by UNOS policy. The recovery coordinator enters the patient into the national computer registry at UNOS as an organ donor by providing name, age, sex, weight, ABO type, available organs, and location of the donor hospital. From this information, the UNOS computer system generates a list of compatible potential recipients throughout the country. The factors used to determine the potential recipients for a given donor include the following:

- ABO type. The recipients must have identical or compatible blood types with the donor.
- Weight. Heart, lung, and liver recipients must be in the same weight range as the donor to ensure comparable organ size. (Height, although not currently recorded on the computer listing, is more helpful in matching lung recipients.)
- Status. Recipients awaiting a heart or liver are given a priority status based on their acuity. The more critical a waiting recipient's condition, the higher his or her name is on the waiting list. The accuracy of this listing is audited by UNOS to ensure compliance with established policies.
- Waiting time. Recipients accrue points based on the length of time they have been waiting for a transplant.
- Distance. The distance between the donor and the potential recipient is a factor for several organs because of time restrictions on how soon each organ should be transplanted after it is recovered. For example, the heart and lung teams in the TRC service area fly only 2000 miles to recover a heart because current practice indicates a heart should be transplanted within 4 to 6 hours after recovery to ensure optimal posttransplant function. The liver teams however, fly as far as 10,000 miles because a liver can tolerate a longer cold ischemic time.

When a potential recipient list is generated for a particular donor, the patient who matches the donor most closely by ABO and weight, who is the sickest, who is within acceptable proximity, and who has been waiting the longest has the highest score and is the first to be offered the available organ.

The organ allocation process begins when the list of potential recipients is generated. The TRC has found the most success in assigning the responsibility of placing

TABLE 4–9. SIX-YEAR ORGAN DONOR PROFILE FROM THE TRANSPLANT RESOURCE CENTER OF MARYLAND, INC, 1988–1993

Category	1988	1989	1990	1991	1992	1993
Number of Donors	47	45	52	62	65	68
Cause of Death %						
Motor vehicle accident	40	22	35	26	23	9
Cerebral event	30	40	25	44	35	60
Gunshot/stabbing	13	4	19	11	17	9
Head trauma	4	29	13	11	5	12
Cardiovascular	6	2	6	0	6	0
Asphyxiation	4	2	0	5	8	0
Drug overdose	2	0	0	2	5	2
Other	0	0	2	2	2	7
Age Range (%)						
0–10 years	9	15	8	10	11	9
11–20	36	13	31	24	23	9
21–40	36	40	35	34	25	23
41–50	11	15	19	16	17	21
51–60	6	9	0	13	15	19
61–70	2	7	8	3	8	16
>70	0	0	0	0	2	2
Gender (%)						
Male	51	58	77	60	63	60
Female	49	42	23	40	37	40
Race						
White	83	82	85	79	74	67
Black	13	11	13	18	25	33
Other	4	7	2	3	1	0

organs to an in-house coordinator while the recovery coordinator with critical care expertise remains in the ICU to oversee clinical donor management. Organs are offered to recipients on the local, regional, then the national waiting list. For example, an available liver is first offered to the recipients on the local waiting list of the OPO. If no local recipient is able to receive the liver, it is then offered to patients waiting within the UNOS region of the OPO. If no recipient is located within the region, the liver is offered to patients on the national waiting list.

The actual organ placement process includes contacting the surgeon or coordinator who is on-call for the respective recipient's transplant center and providing a detailed clinical report. All information regarding medical and behavioral history, current hospitalization, hemodynamic status, organ-specific laboratory data, results of serologic and diagnostic studies, and consultant recommendations are relayed to the recipient center. In addition, information regarding the tentative operating time and other organs that are to be recovered is shared to enable the receiving teams to estimate the probable length of the recovery. This information is essential for transplant personnel to accurately arrange transportation of their recovery team to and from the donor hospital and to schedule the transplant operation for the recipient. According to UNOS policy, once a full report is given to the recipient transplant center, they have 1 hour in which to make a decision to accept or decline the organ. If the transplant team for the first recipient on the waiting list declines the offered organ, the entire placement process begins again with the transplant center for the second patient on the waiting list. Organs are placed by the TRC in the UNOS-mandated order, which is as follows: heart; heart-lung; lung; liver; pancreas; pancreas-kidney; intestine; and kidney.

The organ placement phase, which takes the longest amount of time in the entire organ donation process, may last 12 or more hours. (Although TRC staff are committed to placing all organs available for transplantation, on occasion the instability of the donor's condition mandates that the placement process be terminated early and the patient be taken to the operating room as quickly as possible.) As the organs are being placed with the appropriate transplant centers, the recovery coordinator meets with the operating room charge nurse and anesthesiologist to schedule and discuss the organ recovery operation, review the plan for the surgical recovery, identify any specific equipment and medication needs, and report on the donor's current clinical status. Once all organs have been successfully placed with waiting recipients, the recovery coordinator finalizes the operating room time and then arranges for all recovery teams to arrive at the donor operating room at the scheduled time. Final serologic results have been received and reported to the recovery teams, and any updated patient information is provided as well. To ensure that all incoming recovery teams have adequate documentation regarding the organ donor, the recovery coordinator copies UNOS-required documents from the patient's medical record. A packet of information must accompany each organ. It includes items such as the OPO clinical donor evaluation forms (required by UNOS); ABO confirmation (required by UNOS); serologic results (required by UNOS); tissue typing results (if available) (required by UNOS); donation consent form; brain death declaration or death certificate; cardiology consult report; pertinent physician/nursing progress notes; and essential laboratory data.

Finally, the recovery coordinator activates the local recovery teams, packs and transports the necessary organ recovery equipment to the donor operating room, and ensures that all last-minute preoperative details have been addressed. Immediately before the donor is transferred to the operating room, a broad-spectrum antibiotic, usually cefazolin, is administered prophylactically.

Organ Recovery

Each transplant center that has accepted an organ sends a team to perform the recovery. If teams have traveled from outside the local OPO area, there are usually a recovery coordinator and at least two surgeons for each organ. Ideally, all participating team members discuss the case in advance to plan an efficient step-by-step recovery. This discussion is necessary because the teams are usually from different transplant centers and have never worked together before. In addition, because there may be more than 20 people including operating room staff, in the room, effective communication and interpersonal skills are essential for a successful operation. The recovery coordinator documents the names and medical license numbers of all participating surgeons. This information not only is required for the medical record but also is necessary to provide temporary surgical privileges to the visiting teams.

Once in the operating room, the donor is properly positioned on the table and all recovery equipment is arranged around the perimeter of the room. The recovery coordinator organizes the sterile table, where the organs are placed after removal for further inspection, measurement, and packing. During the operation, the recovery coordinator assists anesthesia personnel with donor management and guides the operating room staff through the procedure. Additional blood samples, lymph nodes, and spleen are obtained to accompany each organ so that potential recipients can be cross-matched with the donor. A cross-match tests the recipient's sera against the donor's to determine if the recipient will reject the transplanted organ.

As the time nears for the removal of the organs, the recovery coordinator ensures that medication is given to the donor at the appropriate time. Mannitol and furosemide, for example are administered no later than 15 minutes before the aorta is cross-clamped to promote renal vasodilatation and diuresis before a kidney is recovered. Heparin is given approximately 5 minutes before cross-clamping to prevent blood clots from forming before or during the time the heart is arrested and the organs are being flushed with preservation solution.

After all initial dissection is completed, the aorta is cross-clamped and the ventilator, cardiac monitor, and all intravenous lines are disconnected. The organs are cooled and preserved with an iced solution, usually University of Wisconsin (UW) solution and flushed rapidly through cannulae that have been placed in the aorta and portal vein. The UW solution is a high osmolar, potassium-rich solution that reduces cell degeneration during the ischemic time between recovery and transplantation. If the heart is being recovered, it is cannulated and flushed through the proximal aorta. The lungs are likewise cannulated and flushed through the pulmonary artery. In addition to the internal vascular cooling accomplished with the flushing process, topical organ cooling is performed by placing sterile saline slush in both the thoracic and abdominal cavities. The time at which the aorta is cross clamped, known as clamp time, is recorded as the beginning of the cold ischemic time. Tracking and minimizing the cold ischemic time is critical because the organs can be preserved on ice for only a limited period after recovery, ideally being transplanted as quickly after recovery as possible. For optimal organ function after transplantation, common practice is to transplant heart and lungs within 4 to 6 hours, liver and pancreas within 12 to 16 hours, and kidneys within 48 hours of recovery.

Once all organs are sufficiently flushed, final dissection is performed and the organs are removed from the body and taken to the back table, where they undergo the third or tertiary phase of the evaluation process. Organ appearance and anatomy are closely inspected, and the entire organ is palpated. If any abnormality is discovered, a biopsy is performed, and the transplant will not occur until the results of the biopsy are available. The recovery coordinator records the anatomy of the organ and any abnormalities identified. Recovery surgeons also record this information on standardized operative reports or directly in the donor's medical record. Additional information recorded in the medical record includes all surgical procedures performed and the planned disposition of the organs.

The recovery coordinator is responsible for ensuring that all organs and specimens are packed and labeled according to established policy and delivered safely to the appropriate institutions. Organs recovered by out-of-state teams or organs that will be transplanted immediately (heart and lungs) at a local facility, are delivered by the respective recovery teams. If an organ was recovered by a local team for an out-of-state transplant facility, transportation will involve either a commercial or private charter flight service. Other organs that are to be transplanted locally may be delivered by a ground courier service.

If consent for donation includes tissues, such as saphenous vein, fascia, bone, eyes/corneas, or skin, the tissue recovery team proceeds at the completion of the organ recovery process. Otherwise, the recovery coordinator assists the operating room staff with final care of the body and general cleaning of the surgical suite. All recovery supplies and equipment are cleaned and returned to the OPO office.

The average length of time required for the surgical recovery depends on the number of organs being recovered. For example, recovery of a kidney only takes $1^{1}/_{2}$ to 2 hours, whereas a multiple-organ recovery procedure may take as long as 4 to 5 hours. An additional 4 to 6 hours is needed if multiple tissues are also being recovered.

Activities After Organ Recovery

Donor-specific activities continue on for an additional 2 to 3 weeks after completion of the donation. These activities include documentation, staff debriefing, billing, and follow-up care of the recipient.

Billing. The finance office of the OPO requests a copy of the patient's itemized hospital bill on the first business day after the donation. The recovery coordinator for the case reviews the bill and identifies all charges related to the donation, including evaluation, critical care, and surgical recovery. The finance office of the OPO pays the donor hospital for these charges. The donor's family is not responsible for any costs associated with the donation. The hospital sends the revised bill to the donor's family or estate. Any costs incurred before the declaration of brain death remain the responsibility of family or estate.

Follow-up Care with the Donor Family and the Recipient and Documentation. After a donation, the recovery coordinator communicates with the transplant centers to obtain information about the recipients, including their posttransplant status and organ function. This information is used to provide follow-up care to the donor family and hospital personnel. A letter is sent to the donor family thanking them for their gift and to tell them briefly about the recipients. Although the names of the recipients remain confidential and are withheld, the donor family is told where the recipients are from; is given some personal information such as marital status, number of children, occupation or hobby; and is told how the recipient recovered since the transplant. The hospital staff are sent a similar letter, and an on-site visit is made to the hospital within a week after the recovery to review the case with the staff involved. This follow-up interview with the staff allows the recovery coordinator to answer any questions or concerns they may have and to educate the staff concerning any difficulties that may have occurred. It also enables the OPO team and the hospital staff to collaborate on and solve any problems to minimize recurrence. The recovery coordinator also obtains final culture results from the donor hospital and reports these findings to the transplant centers.

PUBLIC EDUCATION

The staff of an OPO spends a great deal of time and effort developing workable donor systems in hospitals. Establishing routine referral procedures, providing professional education, assisting with policy and procedure development, and performing regular quality improvement activities are all examples of how the OPO works collaboratively within the healthcare facility to promote donor awareness and enhance donation programs. An equally important focus, however, must be education and donor awareness efforts in communities surrounding the hospitals. The Gallup poll (1993) found that most Americans are aware of the many benefits of organ transplantation. Many have seen television reports and newspaper articles depicting the plight of a young child who awaits a vital liver or heart transplant in order to live. The media is also quick to cover a successful transplant story, especially when the recipient is a well-known community leader or public figure. The one angle that is often down-played in these stories however, is that organs from those who have died must first be made available before any of these stories can have happy endings.

The Transplant Resource Center is encountering an increased number of families who initiate the subject of organ donation. One can therefore assume that public awareness is improving regarding brain death and donation. Yet, ensuring that the public is informed and knowledgeable regarding their option of donation remains a priority in all procurement agencies. Efforts such as electronic media exposure, distribution of printed materials, collaborative activities with clergy, school systems, elected public officials, and community organizations, participation at health fairs, and targeted educational presentations all play integral roles in increasing community awareness. The key element, regardless of what avenue is used for promoting donor awareness, is that the special needs or concerns of the respective community be examined and addressed. For example, if a community is fearful or distrustful of the local hospital, donor awareness efforts will be in vain until the community's concerns are addressed and any misconceptions are dispelled.

While promoting donor awareness must be a year-round effort, national attention is raised annually during the third week of April, known as "National Organ and Tissue Donor Awareness Week." Procurement agencies nationwide go all out during April to celebrate the Gift of Life and to raise the consciousness and awareness of the citizens and communities they serve. Many of the agencies sponsor celebrations that are attended by donor families and recipients. These events publicly recognize the generosity of those who gave and the gratitude of those who received.

There are no easy answers or quick fixes for the on-going dilemma of the national organ shortage. There are, however, several key elements that must exist for the donor system to be successful. (1) The local procurement agency must be visible and viewed as a resource for all aspects of donation, in both the hospital and community settings. (2) Within the hospital, there must be an underlying philosophy that supports the family's right to decide about donation. Management and direct care providers alike must share this philosophy and truly be committed to the success of their donor program. While the procurement agency can help customize their system and provide the necessary education, it is only when the hospital staff assume ownership for their donation system that it will truly become effective and successful. (3) Within the community, the procurement agency can again provide the necessary education and materials needed for the public to become informed regarding their options. Yet, success in community efforts will not occur until each individual considers his or her own wishes and makes decisions regarding donation known to family members.

Increasing the number of organs and tissues available for the thousands of waiting recipients is a worthy yet monumental goal. This gap between donors and recipients, however, can be significantly narrowed with ongoing support from national organizations and the continued efforts of the local organ procurement organization working in collaboration with the public and healthcare professionals.

REFERENCES

Alexander JW, Vaughn WK (1991). The use of "marginal" donors for organ transplantation. *Transplantation* 51:135-141.

Ad Hoc Committee of the Harvard Medical School to Examine the Definition of Brain Death. (1968). A definition of irreversible coma. *JAMA.* 205:337-340.

Annotated Code of Maryland (1974). Anatomical Gift Act, Article 43. Annapolis.

Baldwin JC, Anderson JL, Boucek MM, et al (1993). Task Force 2: Donor guidelines. *J Am Coll Cardiol.* 22:15-20.

Bidigare SA, Oermann MH (1991). Attitudes and knowledge of nurses regarding organ procurement. *Heart Lung.* 20:20-24.

Caplan AL (1991). Assume nothing: The current state of cadaver organ and tissue donation in the United States. *J Transplant Coordination.* 1:78-83.

Corley MC, Selig P, Ferguson C (1993). Critical care nurse participation in ethical and work decisions. *Crit Care Nurse* 13:120-128.

Danneffel MB (1992). Knowledge and attitudes of healthcare professionals regarding organ and tissue donation. *J Transplant Coordination.* 2:127-135.

Evans RW, Orians CE, Ascher NL (1992). The potential supply of organ donors: An assessment of the efficiency of organ procurement efforts in the United States. *JAMA.* 267:239-246.

The Gallup Organization, Inc. (1993). The American public's attitudes toward organ donation and transplantation. Conducted for The Partnership for Organ Donation. Boston.

Garrison RN, Bentley FR, Raque GH, et al (1991). There is an answer to the shortage of organ donors. *Surg Gynecol Obstet.* 173:391-396.

Giordano BP (1993). You can have my organs, but please make sure I'm dead before you take them. *AORN J.* 58:202-204.

JCAHO Accreditation for Hospitals, MA 1.3.9, 1.3.10. (1992). Oak Brook Terrace, Ill: Joint Commission for the Accreditation of Healthcare Organizations.

Kaufman HH, Lun J (1986). Brain Death. *Neurosurgery* 19:850–856.

Kuperberg KG (1993). Will you soon become an organ broker? *Crit Care Nurs.* 13:124.

Lucas BA, Pitts LH, Keeter CS, et al (1992). The neurosurgeon's role in organ procurement. *Am Assoc. Neurol. Surg. Bull.*

Mackersie RC (1989). Organ procurement and brain death in trauma patients. *J Intensive Care Med.* 4:137–146.

Martin S (1993). Pediatric critical care nurses' perceptions and understanding of cadaver organ procurement. *Crit Care Nurse.* 13:74–81.

Maryland Post Mortem Examiners Commission (1981). *Maryland State Post Mortem Examiners Law and Regulations Governing Medical Examiners Cases.* Annapolis: State of Maryland Department of Post Mortem Examiners.

Mor E, Klintmalm GB, Gonwa TA et al (1992). The use of marginal donors for liver transplantation. *Transplantation.* 53:383–386.

Nelson, et al (1992). Evaluation of the impact of an organ procurement organization's educational efforts. *J Transplant Coordination* 2:117–121.

Nygaard CE, Townsend RN, Diamond DL (1990). Organ donor management and organ outcome: A 6-year review from a level I trauma center. *J Trauma.* 30:728–732.

O'Connell JB, Gunnar RM, Evans RW, et al (1993). Task Force 1: Organization of heart transplantation in the US. *J Am Coll Cardiol.* 22:8–14.

Peters TG (1991). Life or death: The issue of payment in cadaveric organ donation. *JAMA.* 265:1302–1305.

Peters TG, Vaughn WK, Spees EK (1989). The multiple organ donor: Prospective multicenter analysis of outcome in the United States of America. *Transplant Proc.* 21:1218–1220.

Presidential Commission for the Study of Ethical Problems in Medicine and Biomedical and Behavioral Research (1981). Guidelines for the determination of death. *JAMA.* 246:2184–2193.

Price CA (1993). How far should organ procurement go? *Dial Transplant.* 22:499.

Prottas J, Batten HL (1988). Health professionals and hospital administrators in organ procurement: Attitudes, reservations, and their resolutions. *Am J Public Health.* 78:642–645.

Sautner T, Gotzinger P, Wamser P, et al (1991). Impact of donor age on graft function in 1180 consecutive kidney recipients. *Transplant Proc.* 23:2598–2601.

Schuler S, Warnecke H, Loebe M, et al (1989). Extended donor age in cardiac transplantation. *Circulation* 80:133–139.

Siminoff LA, Arnold R, Virnig B, Caplan A (1993). Can we ever solve the shortage problem? *J Transplant Coordination.* 3:51–59.

Stuart FP, Veith FJ, Crawford RE (1981). Brain death laws and patterns of consent to remove organs for transplantation from cadavers in the United States and 28 other countries. *Transplantation.* 31:238–244.

Sweeney MS, Lammermeier DE, Frazier OH, et al (1990). Extension of donor criteria in cardiac transplantation: Surgical risk versus supply-side economics. *Ann Thorac Surg.* 50:1–2.

Transplant Resource Center of Maryland, Inc. (1993). *Clinical Standard Operating Procedures.* Baltimore: Transplant Resource Center of Maryland, Inc.

UNOS Update (1993). Number of patient registrations on the National Transplant Waiting List 9/30/93. 9:XXX.

Vrtis M, Nicely B (1993). Nursing knowledge and attitudes toward organ donation. *J Transplant Coordination.* 3:70–79.

Youngner SJ (1989). Brain death and organ retrieval. *JAMA.* 261:2205–2210.

NURSING CARE PLAN 4–1. THE POTENTIAL ORGAN DONOR

Nursing Diagnosis or Collaborative Problem	Expected Outcomes	Nursing Interventions
Impaired Gas Exchange *Related to* • Inadequate ventilatory support (hypoventilation) • Acute obstructive problems (faulty endotracheal tube placement, intubation of right main stem bronchus) • Extrapulmonary restrictive problems (obesity, abdominal distention, pleural disease/effusion, pneumo/hemothorax) • Pulmonary restrictive problems (atelectasis, pneumonia, ARDS, neurogenic pulmonary edema, cardiogenic pulmonary edema) • Hypoxia (anemia, decreased blood supply, smoke inhalation, banked blood)	• Adequate gas exchange is established. Stable ABG results (PaO$_2$ > 100 mm Hg) • Adequate ventilation is established, evidenced by normal breath sounds, chest wall symmetry	• Check placement of endotracheal tube and cuff integrity. • Chest radiograph results q 6 hr. • Monitor breath sounds. • Monitor chest wall movement. • Never clamp chest tubes. • Aggressive pulmonary hygiene. (Chest PT & suction q 1–2 hours. Turn patient q 2 hours.) • Sputum culture and stat gram stain. • Lasix for infiltrates, pulmonary edema. • Transfuse fresh banked CMV negative blood (<72 hours old) • Ventilator settings 　Tidal volume: 10–15 mL/kg (max = 22 mL/kg) 　Respiratory rate: 10–12 breaths/minute 　FiO$_2$%: keep PaO$_2$ > 100 mm Hg 　PEEP: 5 cm if on > 40% FiO$_2$ (hydrate first) 　Humidification and warming *(continued)*

103

NURSING CARE PLAN 4–1. THE POTENTIAL ORGAN DONOR (*continued*)

Nursing Diagnosis or Collaborative Problem	Expected Outcomes	Nursing Interventions

Decreased Cardiac Output and Tissue Perfussion
 	
Related to
 	
• Hypovolemic shock state (internal hemorrhage/3rd spacing; external hemorrhage; therapeutically-induced dehydration; insensible losses)
 	
• Neurogenic shock state (destruction of the sympathetic nervous system)
 	
• Cardiogenic shock state (ischemic heart disease, dysrhythmias, pneumo/hemothorax, direct cardiac injury, ruptured diaphragm)
 	
• Acute DIC (trauma, transfusion of mismatched blood, drowning, cardiogenic shock due to acute MI, obstetrical complications)
	• Normal CO.
	• HR/BP WNL for age/size of donor (> 100 mm Hg)
	
	• Adequate tissue perfusion—stable VS, normal CRTs and peripheral pulses; normal color; normal arterial blood pH and adequate U/O
		• Monitor heart rate and BP at least once per hour.
		• Continuous ECG monitoring.
		• Monitor skin color/temperature, CRTs, peripheral pulses.
		• Two large-bore peripheral IV lines started.
		• Radial A-line and central/PA line started.
		• Monitor CVP/PA pressures hourly.
		• Hourly input/output records.
		• Resuscitate with
		    Colloids—Albumin, plasmanate, Hetastarch
		    Crystalloids—LR, 45% sodium chloride, D51/2NSS, D51/4NSS
		    No NSS or Plasmalyte for volume resuscitation
		• Component therapy (PRCs, platelets, FFP, cryoprecipitate).
		• Vasopressor agents (hypovolemia +/−)
		    Dopamine
		    Neosynephrine

No Aramine, Levophed or epinephrine–severe vasoconstriction

- Monitor serum electrolytes, BUN, creatinine, osmo, cardiac enzymes; CBC and clotting profile every 4 to 6 hours.
- Monitor O_2 challenge ABG's every 2 to 4 hours.
- Monitor intake/output balance at least once an hour.
- Monitor vital signs hourly.
- Maintenance IV fluids (usually D51/2NSS or D51/4NSS) given to replace U/O cc/cc + 50–100 cc/hr).
  After initial fluid resuscitation
- Monitor urine specific gravity q 2 hours.
- Monitor serum and urine electrolytes and osmolality q 4 hours.
- Administer electrolyte alloquots as indicated
- Titrated continuous Pitressin drip (usually start—0.5 units/hr)
  No SQ/IM injections

- Monitor serum/urine glucose levels q 4 hours.
- Avoid fluid resuscitation with D5W solution.

(continued)

- Adequate fluid balance—stable vital signs, adequate/controlled urine output
- Balanced electrolyte status—stable/normal serum/urine electrolyte levels

- Adequate circulating glucose—serum glucose levels 120–200

Fluid Volume Deficit and Electrolyte Imbalance

Related to

- Diabetes insipidus (decrease in synthesis and release of ADH secretion)
- Hypovolemia (previously discussed)
- Hyperkalemia (acidosis, oliguria, banked blood, supplemental potassium, tissue necrosis, hemolysis
- Hypokalemia (↑ excretion, polyuria, gastric suctioning)
- Hypernatremia (inadequate replacement of water, excessive infusion of sodium chloride IV solutions, metabolic acidosis)

Hyperglycemia

Related to

- Excess administration of dextrose solutions

105

NURSING CARE PLAN 4–1. THE POTENTIAL ORGAN DONOR (continued)

Nursing Diagnosis or Collaborative Problem	Expected Outcomes	Nursing Interventions

• Altered glucose uptake by cells (lack of insulin stress response)
 	
• Acidosis
		• Adjust maintenance IV fluids based on results of glucose level results.
		
		• Insulin to maintain glucose level at 120–200:
		
		1 unit/hr via drip, plus ++
		  2 units IV push if glucose is 200.
		  3 units IV push if glucose is 300.
		  4 units IV push if glucose is 400, and so on.
		
		Monitor q 1 hr glucose by fingerstick method
		Hold IV infusion for 1 hour, if glucose is <120; then reevaluate.

Hypothermia *Related to* • Hypothalamic destruction • Altered metabolic rate • Direct heat loss • Cold or room temperature IV solutions	• Adequate body temperature is maintained. Normal core temperature readings are obtained.	• Monitor core temperature q 1 hour, if no continuous method is available. • Apply warming device on ventilator is activated. • Use thermia blanket. • Infuse warmed IV fluids (PRCs can be mixed with warm NSS or Plasmalyte). • Use warming lamps.

Potential for Infection

Related to

- Artificial airway
- Indwelling urinary catheter
- Multiple intravenous sites
- Immobility

- Absence of infection evidenced by afebrile state, clear urine, absence of purulent secretions/wound drainage

- Use proper handwashing technique.
- Use aseptic/sterile techniques—foley care, suctioning, wound care, dressing changes, IV catheter insertion.
- Observe all wounds, catheter insertion sites, incisions for redness, drainage, skin integrity.
- Obtain blood, urine, sputum cultures.
- Perform wound, catheter tip cultures as indicated
- Send for serial CBCs with differentials.
- Perform aggressive pulmonary hygiene.
- Give antibiotics as indicated.

5

Heart Transplantation

Sharon M. Augustine
Maryhelen Masiello-Miller

Cardiac transplantation, once considered a bold new experiment, has become almost routine in the 1990s. Almost a full century has passed since Carrel and Guthrie reported the experimental transplantation of the heart of a puppy into the neck of an adult dog (Carrel & Guthrie, 1905; Carrel, 1907). Animal research continued sporadically over the next 60 years. The first successful canine heart transplant was performed in 1960 by Lower and Shumway (1960). Reemtsma and associates (1962) reported the first use of immunosuppression in canine heart transplants in 1962. Soon thereafter, James Hardy was planning to perform the first human heart transplant at the University of Mississippi. The patient's condition, however, became very unstable and with no appropriate heart donor available, a chimpanzee heart was transplanted. Although the transplant was a success, the primate heart was too small to support the circulation and failed 2 hours after transplantation (Hardy et al, 1964). This procedure awakened the scientific community to the feasibility of heart transplantation.

The first successful human heart allograft procedure was performed in Cape Town, South Africa, in 1967 by Christiaan Barnard (1967). Enthusiasm rose sharply during the next year, but it quickly dampened because of complications of rejection and infection. Only a small number of centers, most notably Stanford University, but also the University of Cape Town, South Africa, the Medical College of Virginia, and Hopital de la Pitie, Paris (Firth, 1987) continued their efforts. One of the most important clinical advances of the 1970s was the development of the endomyocardial biopsy by Philip Caves and associates (Caves et al, 1973). It was not until cyclosporine was introduced in 1981 that cardiothoracic transplantation met with routine success at a number of centers around the world (Reitz, 1990). Table 5–1 outlines the highlights of advances during this century. Readers interested in a more in-depth history of heart transplantation are encouraged to read *The History of Heart and Heart-Lung Transplantation* by Reitz (1990).

According to the International Society of Heart and Lung Transplantation (Kaye, 1993), as of April 1992, 21,664 transplants had been performed worldwide. The 10-year actuarial survival rate for patients who underwent heart transplantation from 1967 through 1992 is shown in Figure 5–1. The survival rate is 79% for 1 year, 68% for 5 years, and 56% for 10 years.

INDICATIONS FOR HEART TRANSPLANTATION

The primary indications for heart transplantation are cardiomyopathy (50%) and coronary artery disease (43%) (Kaye, 1993). Valvular heart disease and congenital heart disease are less common indications. As time passes, the need for retransplantation due to accelerated coronary artery disease increases. Thus far, 577 retransplant procedures have been performed worldwide for the following reasons (Kaye MP, personal communication, April 1994).

60%	Coronary artery disease
17%	Nonspecific graft failure
10%	Other (wide variety)
9%	Acute rejection
3%	Hyperacute rejection
1%	Restrictive or constrictive disease

Patients who require heart transplantation for ischemic heart disease may have had several myocardial infarctions (MIs) over a period of years or may have experienced a severe MI that produced massive injury to the left ventricle that could not be repaired by revascularization.

Patients with cardiomyopathy are often young and have been generally healthy before the disease developed. Cardiomyopathies can be characterized as dilated, hypertrophic, or restrictive (Bulkley, 1984; Miller & Borer, 1983). Dilated cardiomyopathy is characterized by severe thinning and dilatation of the ventricles. The cause is usually unknown, although cases with documented viral causes have been recognized. Postpartum cardiomyopathy, a form of dilated cardiomyopathy, remains obscure in terms of causation (Julian & Szekely, 1985).

Hypertrophic cardiomyopathy, also referred to as idiopathic hypertrophic subaortic stenosis, hypertrophic obstructive cardiomyopathy, or asymmetric septal hypertrophy, results when the myocardium becomes hypertrophied and hyperdynamic. Restrictive cardiomyopathy is characterized by a normal left ventricular cavity but thickened ventricular walls. The thickening is caused by infiltration rather than hypertrophy and usually reflects systemic disease, thus it is rarely an indication for transplantation.

TABLE 5–1. ADVANCES IN HEART TRANSPLANTATION DURING THE TWENTIETH CENTURY

1905	First canine heart transplant Carrel and Guthrie
1960	First successful canine heart transplant Lower and Shumway
1962	First use of immunosuppression in canine model James Hardy
1964	First chimpanzee–to–human heart xenograft James Hardy
1967	First successful human heart transplant Christiaan Barnard
1973	First endomyocardial biopsy Philip Caves
1977	Distant organ procurement Donald Watson
1981	Cyclosporine used in clinical trials

PRETRANSPLANT EVALUATION

Recipient Selection

One of the most important factors in ensuring a good outcome of the transplant procedure has been adherence to strict selection criteria. In recent years, however, there has been a tendency to relax criteria to include previously marginal candidates. In this

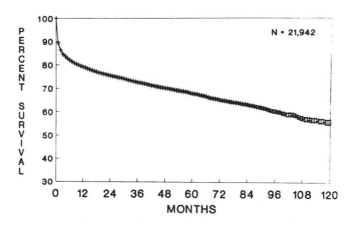

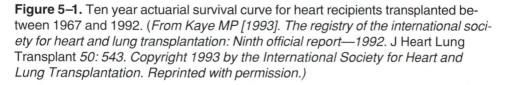

Figure 5–1. Ten year actuarial survival curve for heart recipients transplanted between 1967 and 1992. (*From Kaye MP [1993]. The registry of the international society for heart and lung transplantation: Ninth official report—1992.* J Heart Lung Transplant *50: 543. Copyright 1993 by the International Society for Heart and Lung Transplantation. Reprinted with permission.*)

TABLE 5–2. INDICATIONS FOR CARDIAC TRANSPLANTATION

End/stage heart disease not amenable to any medical or surgical therapy

Patient New York Heart Association Class III or IV with ≤ 50% chance of surviving 1 year

Physiologic age of ≤ 60 years

Absence of systemic illness or other organ system disease that limits long-term survival

Psychosocial stability

Family support

day of profound donor scarcity, it is important to evaluate all referrals in light of the need to allocate organs to those most likely to have successful long-term outcomes.

Table 5-2 lists the generally accepted criteria for heart transplantation. Candidates for a transplant must have end-stage heart disease for which every other medical or surgical therapy has been tried or considered. It is incumbent on the transplant center to carefully evaluate all prior test results and perhaps repeat certain diagnostic tests, including catheterization, if there is any possibility that more conventional therapy may be used. For example, patients with life-threatening arrhythmias may be referred for transplantation when another procedure may be more appropriate, such as endocardial stripping, surgical implantation of an automatic defibrillator, or electrophysiologic testing as a guide to new drug therapy.

An endomyocardial biopsy is often performed on patients with nonischemic cardiomyopathy to rule out sarcoidosis or myocarditis, both conditions that might respond to medical therapy. In addition, the diagnosis of a systemic disease such as amyloidosis or lupus erythematosus may be identified, in which case transplantation is usually contraindicated (Achuff, 1990). A report summarizing the results of heart transplantation in patients with myocarditis concluded that these patients were subject to a higher incidence of rejection and lower survival rates (O'Connell et al, 1990).

Although it is difficult to predict survival objectively, it is an important factor that must be considered carefully. It is desirable to reserve transplantation until absolutely necessary but not beyond the point at which clinical deterioration would make transplantation an unacceptable risk. As stated earlier, the 1-year survival rate after transplantation has been reported to be 79% (Kaye, 1993). Therefore, any patient with a lower survival rate because of cardiac disease could potentially benefit from transplantation.

Patients with severely impaired left ventricular function (ejection fraction less than 20%) are reported to be at higher risk than patients whose ejection fraction is 20% or greater (Keogh et al, 1990; DiBianco et al, 1989). In controlled and uncontrolled clinical trials involving patients with New York Heart Association (NYHA) Class IV symptoms of congestive heart failure, survival rates were 50–60% (Consensus Trial Study Group, 1987; Wilson et al, 1983; Franciosa et al, 1983; Cohn et al, 1984; Keogh et al, 1988). Table 5-3 reviews NYHA functional class.

Results of uncontrolled studies involving NYHA Class III patients suggest the survival rate to be 40 to 70% (Wilson et al, 1983; Franciosa et al, 1983; Cohn et al, 1984; Keogh et al, 1988). The Studies of Left Ventricular Dysfunction (SOLVD) trial, which

TABLE 5–3. THE FUNCTIONAL CLASSIFICATIONS OF PATIENTS WITH DISEASES OF THE HEART

Class I	Patients with cardiac diseases but without resulting limitations of physical activity. Ordinary physical activity does not cause undue fatigue, palpitation, dyspnea, or anginal pain.
Class II	Patients with cardiac disease resulting in slight limitation of physical activity. They are comfortable at rest. Ordinary physical activity results in fatigue, palpitation, dyspnea, or anginal pain.
Class III	Patients with cardiac disease resulting in marked limitation of physical activity. They are comfortable at rest. Less than ordinary physical activity causes fatigue, palpitation, dyspnea, or anginal pain.
Class IV	Patients with cardiac disease resulting in inability to carry on any physical activity without discomfort. Symptoms of cardiac insufficiency or of the anginal syndrome may be present even at rest. If any physical activity is undertaken, discomfort is increased.

Note: The classification of patients according to their cardiac functional capacity gives only a part of the information needed to plan the management of the patient's activities. A recommendation or prescription regarding physical activity should be based on information derived from many sources. The functional classification is an estimate of what the patient's heart will allow and should not be influenced by the character of the structured lesion or by an opinion as to treatment prognosis.

Excerpted from *Diseases of the Heart and Blood Vessels-Nomenclature and Criteria for Diagnosis.*, 6th Edition, Boston, Little Brown and Company, copyright 1964 by the New York Heart Association, Inc. The classifications are not included in the 7th edition, revised 1973.

evaluated a cohort of Class II and Class III patients treated with enalapril, suggested a better prognosis than previously reported (SOLVD Investigators, 1991). In ambulatory NYHA Class III patients, impairment of exercise tolerance, defined as a $\dot{V}O_2$ max of less than 14 ml/kg per minute, was reported to be a poor prognostic sign (Mancini et al, 1991). The American Heart Association position statement (O'Connell et al, 1990) provides an excellent review of these studies.

Some patients may be in NYHA Class I or Class II but have life-threatening symptoms. They should be considered for a transplant. Measurements of hemodynamic values and oxygen consumption, histopathologic findings, neuroendocrine status, and electrophysiologic results were studied and reviewed by Levine and Levine (1991) and may provide a general guideline for the timing of activation. All of these objective criteria must be considered in concert with the patient's course and rate of progress of the disease.

The upper age limit for patients who undergo heart transplantation is a controversial issue. Most centers agree that physiologic age rather than chronologic age is a more appropriate criterion (Carrier et al, 1986; Olivari et al, 1986). Patients who undergo heart transplantation should be free of systemic illnesses or diseases of other organ systems that would limit their likelihood of long-term survival.

Psychosocial stability cannot be overemphasized. It includes the patient's emotional status, history of compliance, and strong evidence of family or friends who have the ability and motivation to support the patient in the long term if complications arise. This is a difficult area to assess because the patient and family are often less than

TABLE 5-4. CONTRAINDICATIONS TO CARDIAC TRANSPLANTATION

Advanced age
Severe pulmonary hypertension
Irreversible organ failure
Peripheral or cerebrovascular disease
Chronic lung disease
Recent pulmonary infarction
Active peptic ulcer disease or diverticulitis
Active infection
Insulin-dependent diabetes mellitus
Malignant neoplasms
Alcohol or drug abuse
Some psychiatric illnesses

totally truthful in order to make a good impression. It is for this reason that referrals from the family physician should include a frank and comprehensive overview of the patient's past behavior. Thorough evaluation by the social worker or psychologist is important, not to eliminate candidacy, but to predict possible problem areas so that the transplant team is prepared to identify and assist with these problems should they arise after transplantation.

Contraindications to Cardiac Transplantation

Table 5-4 shows the generally accepted contraindications to heart transplantation. Experience has shown that there are few absolute contraindications to transplantation. However, several relative contraindications combined can decrease the potential for long-term survival. Advanced age, generally more than 60 years, has been shown to effect long-term outcome. Patients should be judged by all subjective and objective means to be physiologically 60 years of age or younger to withstand the rigors of transplantation (Loebe et al, 1989; Achuff, 1990).

Severe pulmonary hypertension is one of the few absolute contraindications. A fixed pulmonary vascular resistance (PVR) of 6 Wood units or more at rest is traditionally considered unacceptable because the donor heart is incapable of maintaining adequate right ventricular stroke work against the elevated resistance (Shinn, 1985; Funk, 1986; Augustine, 1990; Addonizio et al, 1987; Costard-Jackle et al, 1991). PVR is defined as mean pulmonary artery pressure minus pulmonary capillary wedge pressure divided by cardiac output. A PVR of more than 3 Wood units necessitates pharmacologic intervention to determine the reversibility of pulmonary hypertension. Pharmacologic interventions expected to produce a similar decrease in PVR postoperatively must be identified (Bolman & Saffitz, 1990). Vasodilating agents such as nitroprusside, nitroglycerine, prostacyclin, or oxygen may be used to reduce PVR in some patients (Costard et al, 1989). Transplanting a larger heart or heterotopic transplantation may be considered for patients with borderline PVR.

Irreversible organ failure as is seen in hepatic or renal disease (not secondary to decreased cardiac output) is an adverse factor for transplantation (Shroeder & Hunt 1987; Myerwitz, 1987, Levine & Levine, 1991). Severe cerebrovascular or peripheral vascular disease is usually a solid contraindication to cardiac transplantation, unless surgical correction is feasible, because of the potential for exacerbation of the disease by steroids. The likelihood of increased risk of hepatotoxicity and nephrotoxicity from cyclosporine alone or in combination with antibiotics should be considered (Achuff, 1990). Immunosuppression increases the risk of recurrent pulmonary infections in patients with chronic obstructive pulmonary disease (COPD) or chronic bronchitis. A recent pulmonary infarction or pulmonary embolism increases the risk for pulmonary infection and must be totally resolved before transplantation and immunosuppression (Levine & Levine, 1991; Copeland, 1988; Rogers et al, 1989; Young et al, 1986). Patients with active peptic ulcer disease or diverticulitis face a serious risk for bleeding and perforation and may have fungal or viral superinfections of the ulcer with catastrophic sequelae. Patients should be treated with H2 inhibitors, and the ulcers must be completely healed before transplantation (Levine & Levine, 1991; Copeland et al, 1987; Augustine et al, 1991). Patients with active infections are temporarily excluded from transplantation because of the need for immunosuppression. Many of these problems can be treated and present only temporary lack of acceptance as a heart transplant candidate.

Insulin-dependent diabetes mellitus once was considered an absolute contraindication to heart transplantation because of the almost certain steroid-induced exacerbation and the potential for widespread vasculopathies. These patients are also believed to be at increased risk for infection and poor healing, accelerated end-organ damage including nephropathy and retinopathy, and premature coronary graft atherosclerosis (Levine & Levine, 1991). Many centers have transplanted hearts into patients with diabetes with satisfactory results, but they still consider insulin-dependent diabetes mellitus a relative contraindication and judge each patient independently, looking carefully for evidence of preexisting end-organ damage (Badellino et al, 1988; Gradinec et al, 1988; Rhenman et al, 1988).

Malignant neoplasms other than primary brain tumors are almost always considered an absolute contraindication to heart transplantation. Again, some centers have transplanted hearts into patients who had convincing evidence of a remote cancer considered cured (Armitage et al, 1989).

The importance of a thorough psychosocial evaluation has already been discussed. Active or recent drug or alcohol abuse is considered a serious threat to long-term survival, and patients professing to be totally free of drugs should be thoroughly evaluated by a professional experienced in treating people with problems related to drug and alcohol abuse.

An approach used by some centers in an attempt to give patients with marginal psychosocial criteria the benefit of the doubt is to enroll these patients in clinical end-stage heart disease research protocols. This provides an opportunity for longitudinal assessment of the patient's compliance, motivation, and ability to cope with stress (Achuff, 1990; Herrick et al, 1987). Some psychiatric diagnoses that render a patient unable to or unmotivated to comply with prescribed medical therapy and procedure should be considered contraindications.

TABLE 5–5. CARDIAC TRANSPLANT EVALUATION

Complete history and physical examination

Laboratory studies
  Serum electrolytes, liver function tests,
  cholesterol, triglycerides, complete blood count,
  prothrombin time, partial thromboplastin time,
  creatinine clearance

ABO type, human leukocyte antigens, preformed antibody screen

Cultures
  Viral for cytomegalovirus (CMV)

Serologic Testing
  CMV, Epstein-Barr virus (EBV), herpes simplex
  virus (HSV), varicella-zoster virus, toxoplasmosis,
  hepatitis B surface antigen (HBsAg), anti-hepatitis C virus (HCV),
  human immunodeficiency virus (HIV)

Chest radiograph

Right heart catheterization

Left heart catheterization[1]

Endomyocardial biopsy[1]

Electrocardiogram

Pulmonary function tests[1]

MUGA scan[1]

Exercise testing with oxygen consumption[1]

Abdominal ultrasonography[1]

Carotid and peripheral Doppler flow studies[1]

---

[1]If indicated.
Abbreviation: MUGA, multigated blood panel imaging.

Evaluation Process

The evaluation may be performed in the hospital or on an outpatient basis at the transplant center. The patient and family members are usually seen by various members of the transplant team, which usually includes a cardiologist, a cardiac surgeon, a social worker and psychologist, and a nurse coordinator. People in other disciplines may see the patient in consultation as needed, for example a nutritionist, gastroenterologist, oral surgeon, gynecologist, and dentist. Table 5-5 lists typical evaluation procedures.

The widely acceptable ischemic time for donor hearts is 4 hours. It is, therefore, impractical to specifically crossmatch all donors with recipients before transplantation. For this reason the prospective recipient's sera are tested against a panel of random donors to screen for preexisting human leukocyte antigen (HLA) antibodies. This procedure is called an antibody screen and the results are described as a panel reactive antibody (PRA). The PRA describes the level of sensitization of the recipient to the panel of cells. A positive PRA warrants a specific donor–recipient crossmatch before transplantation. The patients most likely to have high PRAs are women who have been pregnant and patients who have received blood transfusions. This can possibly mean a longer waiting time for a suitable, crossmatch-negative donor. With the advent of typing and crossmatching of cadaveric donors prospectively or before organ retrieval, much of the ischemic time can be reduced.

Once a patient has been accepted as a transplant candidate, he or she is listed through the transplant center's organ procurement organization (OPO) with the United Network for Organ Sharing (UNOS) and placed on a computerized list. Unfortunately, many more patients are listed for transplants than actually receive hearts because of the scarcity of donor organs. The median waiting time for Status 2 patients (patients not in an intensive care unit [ICU] or using assist devices or inotropic support) is 426 days (UNOS Organ Procurement Transplant Network, 1994). As the recipient pool expands and the donor pool remains unchanged or shrinks, more patients die while waiting for a donor heart.

Matching requirements for heart transplantation include only ABO blood type and body weight and size. HLA testing is usually done for retrospective study only.

SURGICAL PROCEDURES

Orthotopic Cardiac Transplantation

Orthotopic transplantation is the excision of the native heart and replacement with a donor heart in the normal anatomic position, as first described by Lower and Shumway (1960). This simplified technique has remained the technique of choice of virtually every transplant center for more than 20 years (Baumgartner, 1990).

On arrival in the operating room, the recipient undergoes placement of intravenous lines, anesthesia, intubation, and standard preparation and draping. A median sternotomy is made and cannulation for cardiopulmonary bypass performed by standard techniques with minor variation. The aorta and pulmonary artery are divided at the level of the commissures of the semilunar valves. The atria are transected at the level of atrioventricular grooves, leaving the posterior right and left atrial walls and their venous connections intact (Fig. 5–2). Similar excision of the donor heart leaves the sinus node and blood supply intact. Atrial remnants are trimmed to fit those of the recipient.

Implantation of the graft begins with anastomosis of the left atrium, followed by the right atrium, pulmonary artery, and then the aorta. Two temporary pacing wires are secured on the donor right atrium. Chest tubes are inserted and the chest is closed (Baumgartner, 1990).

Heterotopic Cardiac Transplantation

Heterotopic transplantation is the placement of a donor heart in the right chest cavity ("piggyback" to the recipient's heart) followed by end-to-side anastomosis of the donor superior vena cava and aorta to the recipient vessels. The pulmonary artery also is anastomosed end to side but may require a small Dacron polyester graft if the donor pulmonary artery is not long enough to reach the recipient pulmonary artery (Baumgartner, 1990).

The indications for heterotopic transplantation are irreversibly elevated PVR or a small donor heart. Both situations represent instances in which a normal donor heart

Figure 5–2. Four anastomoses are required, starting with the left atrium, followed by the right atrium, pulmonary artery and aorta. *(Reprinted with permission from Augustine SM et al [1994]. The Johns Hopkins Manual of Cardiac Surgical Care. St. Louis: Mosby.)*

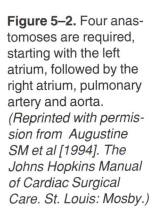
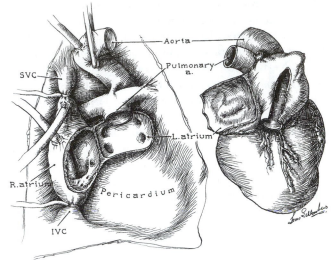

alone would be incapable of maintaining adequate right ventricular function. The donor heart then acts as an auxiliary pump to the native heart. Limitations include potential thromboembolism from the native heart, which necessitates anticoagulation for all heterotopic transplant recipients; continued angina in patients with ischemic heart disease; and the use of prosthetic graft material if needed for pulmonary anastomosis (Baumgartner, 1990; Copeland et al, 1988; Macdonald & Naucke, 1990).

POSTOPERATIVE CARE

The postoperative care of transplant recipients is similar to that of other patients who undergo open heart operations and intensive nursing care. Special considerations are given to the effects of denervation, the effects of ischemia, and immunosuppressive therapy. An example of a nursing care plan is provided at the end of this chapter (Nursing Care Plan 5–1).

Immediately Postoperative Phase
Patients are transported immediately to the ICU after heart transplantation. Operating room personnel provide information concerning the operative procedure, complications, current status, and pertinent medical history. Patients are intubated and receive full ventilator support. Arterial blood gases are measured frequently, and pulse oximetry is used to monitor continually arterial blood oxygen saturation. Invasive lines and drains are similar to those used in any patient who undergoes an open heart operation. A double-lumen internal jugular line is used to measure central venous pressure (CVP) and to administer vasoactive drugs, antibiotics, and immunosuppressant agents.

There is often an immediate depression of left ventricular function postoperatively. This effect has been attributed to ischemia during removal of the donor heart and implantation. Marti et al (1992) demonstrated that a total ischemic time of more than 150 minutes was related to an increased incidence of graft dysfunction and to increased mortality.

In the early postoperative period there are elevations in both right and left-sided filling pressures that gradually recede (Uretsky, 1990). The donor cardiac output is depressed because of limitation of the stroke volume. Cardiac output and stroke volume spontaneously return to normal or nearly normal levels over the first 4 postoperative days (Stinson et al, 1975).

Right ventricular failure can result from a primary decrease in right ventricular contractility due to an increase in PVR because of long-term pretransplant left ventricular failure or poor preservation. The donor right ventricle has difficulty pumping against this increased resistance, which leads to ventricular dilatation and failure. Therefore, it is important to frequently monitor CVP and to observe for signs and symptoms of right ventricular failure (Funk, 1986).

The resting heart rate is usually 70 to 90 beats per minute. Many patients have bradyarrhythmias secondary to sinus node dysfunction possibly related to ischemia or surgical trauma. Isoproterenol is used initially to augment heart rate and to improve ventricular function. A temporary pacemaker may be required to maintain heart rate at 100 beats per minute if isoproterenol is not successful. However, most patients' heart rates increase spontaneously to 100 to 120 beats per minute by the third to fifth postoperative day (Miyamoto et al, 1990). The denervated transplanted heart has a generally increased heart rate because of the absence of parasympathetic influence. Miyamoto and associates (1990) demonstrated that immediately after orthotopic heart transplantation, 65% of recipients maintained normal sinus rhythm. Bradyarrthymias occurred in 18% of the patients and other arrhythmias (junctional, atrial fibrillation, and atrial flutter) occurred in 17% of the patients. The use of amiodarone before the transplant may cause temporary bradyarrhythmia. Patients with sinus node dysfunction who do not recover within 2 weeks may require permanent pacemaker implantation. Redmond and associates (1993) demonstrated the effectiveness of theophylline in the treatment of posttransplant bradyarrhythmia. A large percentage of patients achieved sinus rhythm with a rate of more than 90 beats per minute. The need for permanent pacing was greatly reduced. The dose of theophylline ranged from 150 mg to 300 mg orally every 8 to 12 hours. Indications for permanent pacemaker insertion include sinus bradycardia, complete heart block, or a slow junctional rhythm accompanied by symptoms of dizziness, light-headedness, and syncope. The development of severe dysrhythmias in the early and late posttransplant period may be an indication of rejection (Blanche et al, 1992).

Measures to improve cardiac output are instituted immediately and may be initiated when the patient is separated from coronary pulmonary bypass. Isoproterenol is routinely administered to all transplant recipients because of its chronotropic and inotropic effects on the myocardium. Isoproterenol is a potent β_1 and β_2 agonist and has direct effects on the pulmonary vasculature resulting in vasodilation (Bolman & Saffitz, 1990). Other inotropic agents that may be used are dobutamine, low-dose dopamine, and amrinone. Temporary pacing of the heart may be used to maintain a heart rate of 100 beats per minute if isoproterenol is ineffective.

Vasodilating agents (sodium nitroprusside and nitroglycerin) are required to maintain a mean arterial pressure of 65 to 75 mm Hg and to improve right ventricular function. Infusion of prostaglandin E, another vasodilating agent with effects on the lung vasculature, is useful in the care of patients with pulmonary hypertension after cardiac transplantation (Vincent et al, 1992). If arterial hypotension occurs, norepinephrine, infused through a left atrial catheter, minimizes the vasoconstricting effects on the pulmonary circulation (Vincent et al, 1992).

Careful assessment of cardiac status and patient response to measures to improve cardiac output is important. Vital signs and hemodynamic values are monitored continuously. In the absence of a pulmonary artery catheter, cardiac output should be assessed by peripheral pulses, neurologic status, color, temperature, capillary refill, and urinary output. Volume status and filling pressures are evaluated by CVP and urinary output. The heart rate and rhythm as well as atrial and ventricular ectopy are documented and treated if necessary. A 12-lead electrocardiogram (ECG) is obtained on admission, 8 hours after admission, and every day thereafter.

Mediastinal and pleural tubes are usually removed 24 hours postoperatively or when the drainage is less than 25 mL/hour. These tubes should be removed only when drainage is considerably reduced because pleural and pericardial effusions frequently develop in the early postoperative phase. Preoperative fluid overload and renal dysfunction may contribute to the formation of pleural effusions. Pericardial effusions may result when a large pericardial space is made by removal of a heart with dilated cardiomyopathy (Borkon & Augustine, 1990). A full nursing assessment is performed and documented at the time of admission and updated frequently. Hourly intake and output is strictly recorded. The admission laboratory evaluation includes a chemistry panel, liver function tests, complete blood count (CBC) with differential, and coagulation studies. Daily chemistry and hematology panels are obtained and recorded on a flowsheet for easy access by the many health care professionals involved in the care of these patients.

Immunosuppressive Considerations

Some centers advocate the use of induction therapy. Muromonab-CD_3 or antithymocyte preparations are given immediately postoperatively for 7 to 14 days to lower the incidence of rejection. Triple-drug maintenance therapy, consisting of prednisone, azathioprine, and cyclosporine is used for immunosuppression of heart transplant recipients (Table 5–6). Cyclosporine blood levels are obtained daily and should be obtained approximately 12 hours after administration of the drug to provide accurate trough levels. Dosage is adjusted according to cyclosporine and serum creatinine levels. Cyclosporine can be administered orally (liquid or gelatin capsule form) or intravenously. Intravenous doses are first given at approximately one-fourth to one-third the oral dose and may need to be adjusted further. When using intravenous infusion of cyclosporine, blood samples for drug levels may be obtained at any time because the drug is administered as a constant infusion. Nephrotoxicity is an adverse effect of cyclosporine and is reported in one-third of transplant patients (Shannon & Wilson,

TABLE 5–6. IMMUNOSUPPRESSION

Timing	Cyclosporine	Methylprednisolone	Prednisone	Azathioprine
Preoperative	10 mg/kg orally	—	—	—
Intraoperative	—	500 mg IV in one dose	—	—
Postoperative	10 mg/kg a day orally or 0.5–1.0 mg/kg a day IV	125 mg IV every 8 hours for 3 doses	1 mg/kg a day (divided doses) tapered to 0.4 mg/kg by 14 days	2 mg/kg a day

1992). Strict intake and output, as well as daily BUN and creatinine, must be monitored. After the initiation of intravenous cyclosporine, patients should be observed continuously for at least 30 minutes and at frequent intervals thereafter to detect allergic or other adverse reactions (Shannon & Wilson, 1992). After discharge, to appropriately compare levels if patients have their cyclosporine levels processed at a laboratory different from the one used while they were in the hospital, it is important to determine the laboratory procedure used and whether the second laboratory uses whole blood or serum in samples.

Azathioprine is administered in the immediately postoperative phase at a dose of approximately 2 mg/kg through oral gastric tube or by mouth. This dose is adjusted to maintain a white blood cell (WBC) count of 4500 cells/mm³ or more (Bolman & Saffitz, 1990). Azathioprine may cause bone marrow suppression and leukopenia, resulting in an increased risk for infection. Concomitant use of allopurinol increases azathioprine activity considerably (McGoon & Frantz, 1992).

Methylprednisolone 500 mg is administered intraoperatively and in the immediately postoperative phase at 125 mg every 8 hours for three doses. Prednisone is then started at 1 mg/kg and tapered daily to achieve a dose of approximately 0.4 mg/kg. Transient hyperglycemia may be seen during this period of administration of high doses of corticosteroids.

Rejection

The accurate diagnosis and effective treatment of allograft rejection remains one of the crucial factors in both short-term and long-term survival (Miller, 1992). Rejection can be divided into three categories: hyperacute, acute, and chronic on the basis of immunologic mechanisms and rate (Murdock et al, 1987). Hyperacute rejection may result from ABO blood group incompatibility and the presence of preformed cytotoxic antibodies (Murdock et al, 1987). This type of rejection may be prevented by ensuring ABO blood group compatibility and establishing a negative lymphocyte cytoxic antibody screen against a panel of donor antigens obtained from a pool of random blood donors. If this random screening test is positive, a donor-specific crossmatch must be performed before transplantation. Hyperacute rejection develops almost immediately after transplantation, frequently in the operating room. It can cause diffuse interstitial edema and plugging of small arteries, arterioles, capillaries, and venuoles by platelet aggregation as well as fibrin deposition. Damage to the coronary arteries accompanied by hypotension and cardiogenic shock is the end result (Weil et al, 1981; Shumway, 1990). Hyperacute rejection is usually fatal; retransplantation may be the only possible treatment (Shinn, 1989).

Acute rejection is most common in the first few weeks after transplantation, the incidence progressively decreasing by 3 months after transplantation (Bolman & Saffitz, 1990). Acute rejection begins when the surface cell antigens of the transplanted heart are recognized as foreign bodies (Murdock et al, 1987). It is characterized histologically by interstitial and perivascular mononuclear cell infiltration. The usual criterion for treatment is the presence of diffuse myocytic necrosis.

Chronic rejection may represent a low-grade immunologic response (Murdock et al, 1987), the exact cause of which is unclear. It is exhibited as cardiac allograft vasculopathy (transplant coronary artery disease). Humoral and cell-mediated injury to the donor endothelium appear to be the primary events (Eich et al, 1991).

Cyclosporine has changed the pattern of acute rejection. There are often no clinical signs or symptoms unless rejection is severe (Shinn, 1989). Some symptoms that may indicate rejection are fatigue, malaise, and shortness of breath (Bolman & Saffitz, 1990). The signs of severe rejection may include peripheral edema, pulmonary crackles, jugular venous distention, S_3 gallop, pericardial friction rub, dysrhythmia (primarily atrial), decreased ECG voltage, decreased cardiac output, hypotension, and cardiac enlargement on radiographs (Macdonald & Naucke, 1990).

Histologic rejection can take place without hemodynamic changes. Routine endomyocardial biopsies remain the standard of reference for detection of rejection in a transplanted heart (Bolling et al, 1991). At our institution, cardiac biopsies are performed every 10 days during the first month after transplantation, every 2 weeks during the second month, once a month for the next 4 months and then every 3 months. This protocol varies widely among transplant centers.

An endomyocardial biopsy is an invasive procedure in which percutaneous and transvenous technique is used; it is usually well-tolerated. Complications are rare. They include pneumothorax and transient rhythm disturbances. Local anesthetic is used, and the procedure takes approximately 15 minutes. A bioptome is introduced through the right internal jugular vein and is advanced into the right ventricle with the use of echocardiography or fluoroscopy (Caves et al, 1973; Reitz, 1992).

The biopsy procedure and possible complications should be explained to patients; informed consent is required. Adequate time for questions and for expression of anxieties should be provided. Patients should receive nothing by mouth after midnight the night before a biopsy.

Treatment of Rejection

Table 5–7 shows the protocol used at our institution for the treatment of acute rejection. The traditional sequence of treatment options used in the treatment of moderate rejection usually begins with an increased dose (100 mg) of oral prednisone for 3 days. Some centers then taper the daily dose each day until that patient's baseline is reached. Other centers revert promptly to the maintenance dose. The next step, if oral prednisone proves to be insufficient, is intravenous administration of methylprednisolone in 1-g doses each day for 3 days. If the rejection episode is unusually severe

TABLE 5–7. TREATMENT OF REJECTION

Prednisone taper
    100 mg/day (divided doses) $\times$ 3 days followed by taper of 5 mg/day (total dose) until baseline
    is reached

Methylprednisolone
    1 g/day for 3 days followed by maintenance dosage of prednisone

Antithymocyte Globulin (ATGAM)
    15 mg/kg IV for 14 days

Skin test is administered and read before first dose is administered

T cells checked 3 times per week

Normal saline solution is used to prepare ATGAM

Administered over 4 to 6 hours

Patient monitored for signs of reaction, including fever, chills, rash, urticaria, diaphoresis, dyspnea,
    and headache

Muromonab-CD3 (OKT3)
    5 mg/day (1 vial) IV push for 10 to 14 days

    T cells checked 3 times per week

    Complete blood count with differential every day

PREMEDICATION FOR OKT3
Methylprednisolone
    1 mg/kg 1 hour before administration of OKT3 for the first 3 doses then as needed.

Hydrocortisone
    100 mg 30 min after OKT3 for the first 3 doses then as needed

Diphenhydramine and acetaminophen
    1 hr and 4 hours after OKT3 for the first 3 doses then as needed

Rabbit Anti-Thymocyte Serum
    0.2 to 0.5 ml/kg of body weight

Currently in clinical trial, not FDA approved

CD3 lymphocyte count should be reduced to below 150 cells per mm^3

Skin test should be performed before treatment

If the desired response is not observed, the dosage may be increased by 0.1 to 0.2 ml/kg with reeval-
    uation of CD3 2 to 3 days after the dosage change

---

or early in the posttransplant period, the oral dosing may be skipped. The third step is usually administration of an intravenous antithymocyte or antilymphocyte preparation to decrease circulating T_3 cells to less than 150 per mm^3 for 10 to 14 days or treatment with monoclonal antibodies (muromonab-CD3).

It is important that nurses who care for cardiac transplant patients be familiar with maintenance schedules and treatment protocols. Nurses also should be familiar with the major actions and side effects of each drug. The initial administration of antithymocyte products or muromonab-CD3 is often accompanied by systemic release of lymphokines, which may result in fever, chills, diarrhea, nausea, wheezing, and peripheral vasodilatation (McGoon & Frantz, 1992). Acetaminophen can be administered before treatment to control fever and chills. Patients must be carefully assessed before, during, and after administration of muromonab-CD3. If weight gain occurs, or if there is any evidence of pulmonary interstitial fluid, the patient should undergo diuresis to avoid pulmonary edema during muromonab-CD3 therapy (Rogers et al, 1989).

Infection Control

Infection resulting from immunosuppressive therapy is one of the major causes of mortality and morbidity among transplant recipients (Heck et al, 1989). In the early postoperative phase, nosocomial organisms such as *Pseudomonas aeruginosa, Proteus, Klebsiella,* and *Escherichia coli* are frequently encountered in transplant patients (Reitz, 1992). Heart transplant recipients are more susceptible to these infections than are other patients because of their reduced immune status.

There is a wide diversity of infection control practices among centers; they range from no special precautions to strict reverse isolation. Lange and associates (1992) surveyed several heart transplant programs in the United States to identify infection control practices used in the care of heart transplant recipients. They determined that there was no significant correlation between the number of infection control measures used and survival rates.

Nystatin suppositories are administered orally four times a day after extubation to prevent oral candidiasis. Prophylactic cephazolin 1 g is administered intravenously upon closure of the chest and every 8 hours until the central line is removed. Vancomycin 1 g every 12 hours is used in patients with penicillin or cephalosporin allergies.

Strict hand-washing is the most effective measure in preventing infections. Other measures to prevent infection include strict sterile technique with dressing changes and line care. Invasive-line dressing changes are performed every 24 hours with careful inspection of insertion sites for any signs of redness, swelling, or drainage. The patient's temperature is monitored carefully. Temperatures higher than 38°C necessitate collection of urine, sputum, and blood specimens by sterile technique for culture and sensitivity. A chest radiograph is obtained to detect pulmonary infiltrates. Broad-spectrum antibiotic coverage should be started immediately after the appropriate culture specimens have been obtained (Reitz, 1992).

Recovery

Once the effects of anesthesia and sedation have waned and the patient begins to take spontaneous respirations, extubation should occur as soon as blood-gas and respiratory values are within normal limits. Immediately after extubation, aggressive pulmonary toilet is instituted; this includes coughing and deep breathing and the use of an incentive spirometer.

Once hemodynamic stability and normotension are achieved, inotropic support may be discontinued and invasive lines may be removed. At this point, the patient can begin mobilization. Activity is gradually increased, and physical therapy should begin as soon as mobilization begins. Ambulation usually begins in the room and progresses to longer distances. Patients are usually riding a stationary bicycle 3 to 5 days after transplantation.

The sympathetic nervous system does not stimulate the denervated heart, but β-adrenergic receptors are intact. Changes in heart rate, conduction, and contractility occur only in response to circulating catecholamines released from the adrenal gland (Muirhead, 1992). Therefore, this response is slower than in a normal heart. When patients start to exercise, there is no immediate increase in stroke volume, heart rate, or contractility, as in an innervated heart, because those increases are the result of the sympathetic stimuli (Roos, 1986). Therefore, prolonged warm-ups and cool-downs are required to allow the heart compensatory time for catecholamine stimulation. Orthostatic hypotension may occur because of the lack of compensatory tachycardia when venous pooling decreases preload. This should be considered when the patient sits upright or when vasodilation occurs; adequate preload must be maintained (Augustine, 1994).

Patients initially eat a high-calorie and high-protein diet to promote wound healing and help replenish protein stores. Many patients experience altered nutrition related to their debilitated preoperative state, in which they were receiving less than their body's nutritional requirements (Shinn, 1989). Patients also are restricted to 1200 to 1500 mL of fluid on each of the first 3 postoperative days. All stool and gastric secretions should be tested for occult blood.

Family members need to be constantly informed of the patient's progress. Family members are often excited after a prolonged wait for a donor heart. They often experience anxiety related to restrictive visiting hours while the patient is in the ICU. They also may experience anxiety regarding their future. Nurses have the opportunity to assist the family in maintaining emotional stability so that they can provide emotional, social, and physical support.

Standardized teaching-learning flow sheets are helpful to outline and document patient and family education. Key aspects include the physiologic properties of the denervated heart, diet, activity, pulmonary toilet, rejection, infection, and medications. Teaching should be performed consistently throughout the postoperative period when the patient is well rested and comfortable.

Late Postoperative Care

Patients are transferred out of the ICU when their hemodynamic condition is stable and when their arterial blood-gases on low-flow oxygen are normal without ventilatory support. Patients are usually transferred with only one peripheral intravenous line and continue to undergo cardiac monitoring or telemetry. Preparation for discharge is the main focus of nursing care.

Discharge Instructions

The patient and at least one family member should be given thorough instructions about each medication and its action. Dosage, frequency, administration guidelines, side effects, and strict compliance with the regimen should be emphasized. The patient should be provided with written instructions about diet, activity, medications, and follow-up visits. Table 5–8 lists self-care behaviors that should be reviewed. A rationale should be given for each behavior.

Recipients were often found to have a high rate of compliance with medications. In a study by Baumann and associates (1992), 100% of the recipients interviewed

TABLE 5–8. SELF-CARE BEHAVIORS FOR ALL HEART TRANSPLANT RECIPIENTS

Adherence to scheduled follow-up appointments with cardiologist or nurse transplant coordinator

Adherence to regular appointment with dentist and ophthalmologist

Adherence to regular exercise program

Adherence to low-fat and low-sodium diet

Adherence to proper personal hygiene with particular attention to meticulous skin, mouth, and foot care.

Participation in support-group activities.

Reporting temperatures >38°C or infection to physician or transplant coordinator immediately

Reporting chest pain to physician or transplant coordinator immediately

Avoidance of alcohol, tobacco, and illicit drugs

Avoidance of direct sun exposure. Use of sunscreen and sunglasses when exposed to sunlight

Avoidance of people with obvious infections

Consulting with physician or transplant coordinator before using over-the-counter medications

6 months after transplantation reported taking three immunosuppressive medications all the time. Both recipients and family perceived more difficulty in managing mood swings than in following a low-fat diet, exercising regularly, or taking medications.

Recipients and their family members may be encouraged to join a support group with other transplant recipients to provide a social and emotional outlet that extends beyond immediate family. Groups serve as sources of social support for their members, and vital information is shared among members; they often contribute greatly to an individual's well-being (Sampson & Marthas, 1990).

LONG-TERM FOLLOW-UP CARE

A schedule of follow-up tests and procedures is provided in Table 5-9. The goals of long-term care are to detect rejection, infection, and coronary artery disease; to monitor therapeutic drug levels and assess for long-term complications of immunosuppressive therapy; and to provide proper management of these complications.

Coronary Artery Disease

Accelerated coronary artery disease (also referred to as transplant coronary disease and cardiac allograft vasculopathy) is present in a large number of recipients. At 2 years and 5 years the occurrence rate has been reported at 20 to 30% and 40%, respectively (Gao et al, 1988; Uretsky et al, 1987). Heart transplant recipients with cytomegalovirus infections had more frequent and severe graft atherosclerosis (Grattan et al, 1989). The pathogenic mechanisms involved in the development of accelerated coronary artery disease are unknown (Hosenpud et al, 1992).

More cardiac lesions developed in patients who received hearts that were older than 35 years than in patients who received younger donor hearts in a study conducted by Bieber and associates (1981). It was also demonstrated that serum triglyc-

TABLE 5–9. SCHEDULE OF FOLLOW-UP VISITS

Procedure	Timing
Endomyocardial biopsy	Every 10 days for 3 procedures
	Every 2 weeks for 2 procedures
	Every month for 4 months
	Every 3 months thereafter
Electrolyte, blood urea nitrogen, creatinine, glucose, magnesium levels	Every visit (with biopsy) and as needed
Complete blood count	Every visit (with biopsy) and every 2 weeks
Cyclosporine levels (troughs)	Every visit (with biopsy) and as needed
Lipid profile	Every 6 months
Chemistry profile	Every visit (with biopsy) and as needed
Chest radiographs in posteroanterior and lateral projections	Every 6 months and as needed
Echocardiogram	Every visit (with biopsy) and as needed
Electrocardiogram	Once a year and as needed
Coronary angiogram	Once a year

eride levels greater than 280 mg/dL were found to be associated with arteriosclerosis. A study by Carrier and associates (1991) demonstrated that older donor age and higher pretransplant triglyceride levels in the recipient were predictors of the development of accelerated coronary atherosclerosis. The data from this study also suggest that the recipient's initial cardiac disease may be related to this development.

Cardiac allograft vasculopathy has been attributed to chronic rejection. In most cases, allograft vasculopathy is different from coronary artery disease, as demonstrated in Table 5–10. It is of a diffuse nature with concentric narrowing of the vessels. The vasculopathic process is limited to the allograft and involves the great arteries and venous structures up to the suture line (Hosenpud et al, 1992). Figure 5–3 shows a cross section of a coronary artery with accelerated arteriosclerosis. The intima is diffusely and concentrically thickened by the accumulation of lymphocytes, macrophages, and smooth-muscle cells. Annual coronary angiograms are obtained to evaluate transplant coronary disease. Small distal penetrating arteries may be affected before the large epicardial vessels, which can make angiographic diagnosis difficult (Neish et al, 1992).

Several theoretic mechanisms have been suggested relating to the development of cardiac allograft vasculopathy. There is evidence to suggest that this disease is primarily immune-mediated and that the cellular and humoral systems play an important role (Miller, 1992). Endothelial injury, CMV, and hyperlipidemia may also be involved.

The diffuse distribution of lesions and rapid progression of transplant coronary disease limit the use of coronary bypass operations or percutaneous angioplasty for these patients. Elective retransplantation is the only recognized treatment (Gao et al, 1988). Patients are instructed to modify cardiac risk factors by eating a low-fat diet, exercising, and avoiding tobacco.

TABLE 5–10. HISTOLOGIC COMPARISON BETWEEN CARDIAC ALLOGRAFT VASCULOPATHY (CAV) AND CORONARY ARTERY DISEASE (CAD)

Histologic attribute	CAV	CAD
Angiographic localization	Diffuse, distal	Focal, proximal
Intimal proliferation	Concentric	Usually eccentric
Calcium deposition	Absent	Frequently present
Internal elastic lamina	Intact	Disrupted
Inflammation, vasculitis	Infrequent	Never
Rate of development	Months	Years

(From Hosenpud J, Shipley G, and Wagner C (1992). Cardiac allograft vasculopathy: Current concepts, recent developments, and future directions. J Heart Lung Transplant. 11:10. Copyright 1992 by The Journal of Heart and Lung Transplantation. Reprinted by permission.)

Studies demonstrating sensory reinnervation in humans after cardiac transplantation suggest that chest pain should not be dismissed as noncardiac in origin (Stark et al, 1991). Patients should report symptoms of chest pain to the physician or nurse coordinator immediately. The clinician should take chest pain seriously in transplant recipients, even if recent angiograms are normal, because of the rapidly progressive nature of transplant coronary disease (Uretsky, 1992).

Complications of the Long-Term Use of Immunosuppressive Agents

Almost all organs in the body can be affected by long-term triple-drug immunosuppressive therapy. Patients require special instructions to minimize side effects and routine physical examinations to detect complications of immunosuppression.

Heart transplant patients have a high incidence of malignant disease related to immunosuppressive therapy (Sklarin et al, 1991). Non-Hodgkin lymphomas make up a high percentage of the neoplasms and are not uncommon in heart transplant recipients (Penn & Brunson, 1988). Before the use of cyclosporine, most non-Hodgkin lymphomas were extranodal (Penn, 1983). With cyclosporine it has been observed that 48% of non-Hodgkin lymphomas are nodal and 52% are extranodal (Penn & Brunson, 1988). The degree of immunosuppression appears to be related to the subsequent development of lymphoma (Weintraub & Warnke, 1982).

Heart transplant recipients are at risk for a variety of side effects associated with the long-term use of steroids. The effects include hyperglycemia, fat deposition in the trunk and face, muscle wasting, peptic ulcers, pancreatitis, severe mood changes, osteoporosis, and an increased susceptibility to infection (Shannon & Wilson, 1992). Patients are also at risk for cataracts and glaucoma (Schaefer & Williams, 1991).

To minimize gastric irritation, prednisone should be given with food and antacids. H2 inhibitors are often used if the patient has a history of peptic ulcer disease. Patients need to be instructed to report low-grade fevers with mild abdominal discomfort to the physician or nurse coordinator immediately. These may be the only symptoms of severe abdominal problems in long-term users of steroids (Augustine

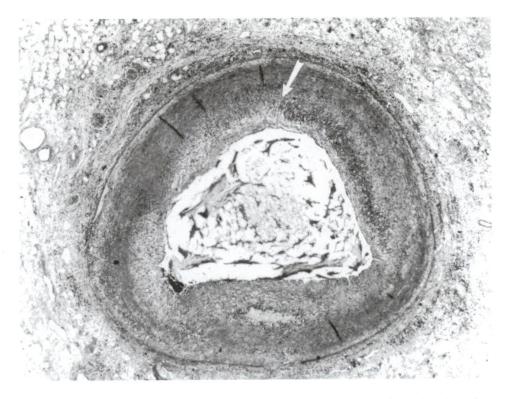

Figure 5–3. Cross section of a coronary artery with accelerated arteriosclerosis. The intima (*arrow*) is diffusely and concentrically thickened by the accumulation of lymphocytes, macrophages, and smooth muscle cells.

et al, 1991). The gastrointestinal (GI) tract is the site of a large number of complications after cardiac transplantation. In one study, diarrhea was the most frequent GI complication in heart and heart-lung transplant patients (Augustine et al, 1991). The other types of complications were perforated viscera, gastrocutaneous fistulas, perforated gastric ulcers and retroperitoneal abscesses, cholecystitis, gastric atony, perianal abscesses, GI bleeding and ulcers, esophageal reflux or spasm, pancreatitis, pancreatic abscesses, hepatitis, and CMV infection. Fifty percent of all complications occurred in the first 6 months after transplantation, corresponding to the period of highest immunosuppression. The remaining 50% were distributed over the seventh to 61st months after transplantation.

The use of steroids may cause solar sensitivity and an increased susceptibility to some skin cancers. Transplant recipients should be encouraged to limit sun exposure, wear sun block and a hat while exposed to the sun, and to avoid tanning beds (Schaefer & Williams, 1991). Thorough skin assessments are necessary on a routine basis, and patients should be encouraged to report skin lesions.

Weight gain is common; it may be related to an increase in appetite and a change in metabolism with steroid use. Obesity was cited as a chronic postoperative problem at 1, 2, and 3 years after heart transplantation (Grady et al, 1991). In this study, 1 year postoperatively the patient's body weight was 117% of ideal body weight and 106% of usual body weight. Patients need to be encouraged to adhere to a low-fat diet and exercise routine. Obese heart transplant recipients have an increased cardiac output and left ventricular dilatation and a lower ejection fraction (Ventura et al, 1992).

To reduce the risks of long-term steroid use, corticosteroid-free immunosuppression has been studied (Lee et al, 1991; Ratkovec et al, 1990; Renlund et al, 1987). Double-drug protocols were instituted. In the study by Lee and associates (1991), when a patient exhibited more than two episodes of rejection, the double-drug protocol was considered to have failed, and therapy was converted to the triple-drug regimen. One-third of the patients had such a change. Steroids were successfully tapered and eventually discontinued for 50% of these patients. Patients who survived 6 months observing the double-drug protocol had a low incidence (5%) of requiring steroids because of rejection. Furthermore, they had an excellent chance of remaining on the same regimen in the long term without a high risk of late graft rejection.

Renlund and associates (1987) demonstrated that patients who were successfully withdrawn from maintenance corticosteroids had fewer cushingoid characteristics and fewer infections and exceeded ideal body weight to a lesser extent. According to Ratkovec and colleagues (1990), corticosteroid minimization or withdrawal did not adversely affect the prevalence or the progression of transplant coronary disease during the first 2 years after transplantation.

Long-term use of cyclosporine causes at least a 20% reduction in renal function in almost all patients; however, the clinical course is generally benign (Kahan, 1989). Most of the renal damage occurs in the first 6 months after transplantation with an increase in serum creatinine level. Creatinine levels increase progressively over the following 3 years (Costanzo-Nordin et al, 1990).

Hypertension is a serious complication of the use of cyclosporine; the incidence is 40 to 90% among transplant recipients (Costanzo-Nordin et al, 1990). This hypertension is characterized by an expansion of plasma volume and the absence of major abnormalities of the renin-angiotensin-aldosterone system (Bellet et al, 1985).

It has been demonstrated that treatment with cyclosporine alone causes an increase in the total cholesterol level from the baseline measurement; thus change is related to an increase in low density lipoprotein (LDL) levels (Ballantyne & Podet, 1989). In a study by Ballantyne and associates (1992), total cholesterol and triglyceride levels increased between the first and the third month after transplantation. LDL levels also increased. High density lipoprotein (HDL) cholesterol levels showed an increase from baseline 1 month after transplantation but declined slightly 3 months after the transplant. Lovastatin 20 mg a day was effective when total cholesterol levels were greater than 240 mg/dL on two or more consecutive measurements taken after 6 months of dietary therapy. Lovastatin 20 mg daily was also shown effectively to lower cholesterol levels after cardiac transplantation in a study by Kobashigawa and associates (1990). Ballantyne and associates (1992), however, observed that when lovastatin was administered at 40 mg twice daily, there was an unacceptably high incidence of myositis.

Heart transplant recipients present unique physical and psychosocial challenges to nurses. These challenges range from the acute care to out-patient follow-up care. The well-being of heart transplant patients can be influenced greatly by the knowledge and commitment of nurses. Nurses, in turn, receive abundant rewards seeing these patients leave the hospital and return to physically active and satisfying lives.

REFERENCES

Achuff SC (1990). Clinical evaluation of potential heart transplant recipients. In: Baumgartner WA, et al, eds. *Heart and Heart-Lung Transplantation.* Philadelphia: Saunders, 51–57.

Addonizio LJ, Gersony WM, Robbins RC, et al (1987). Elevated pulmonary vascular resistance and cardiac transplantation. *Circulation.* 76 (Suppl V):V52–V55.

Armitage JM, Griffith BP, Kormos RL, et al (1989). Cardiac transplantation in patients with malignancy. *J Heart Transplant.* 8:89 (Abstract 24).

Augustine SM (1990). Nursing care of the heart and heart-lung transplant patient. In: Baumgartner WA, et al eds. *Heart and Heart-Lung Transplantation.* Philadelphia: Saunders, 139–156.

Augustine SM, Baumgartner WA, Stuart RS, Acker MA (1994). Heart and lung transplantation and cardiomyoplasty for end-stage cardiopulmonary disease. In: Baumgartner WA, Owens S eds. *The Johns Hopkins Manual of Cardiac Surgical Care,* St. Louis: Mosby, 461–484.

Augustine SM, Yeo CJ, Buchman TG, Achuff SC (1991). Gastrointestinal complications in heart and in heart-lung transplant patients. *J Heart Lung Transplant.* 10:547–556.

Badellino M, Nairns B, Fucci P, et al (1988). Influence of diabetes mellitus on the course of cardiac transplantation. *J Am Coll Cardiol* 11:103A [Abstract].

Ballantyne C, Podet E (1989). Effects of cyclosporine on plasma lipoprotein levels. *JAMA.* 262:53–56.

Ballantyne C, Radovancevic V, Farmer A, et al (1992). Hyperlipidemia after heart transplantation: Report of a six year experience, with treatment recommendations. *J Coll Cardiol.* 19(6):1315–1321.

Barnard CN (1967). The Operation. A human cardiac transplant: An interim report of a successful operation performed at Groote Schuur Hospital, Cape Town. *S Afr Med J* 41:1271–1274.

Baumann L, Young C, Egan J (1992). Living with a heart transplant: Long term adjustment. *Transplant Int.* 5:1–8.

Baumgartner WA (1990). Operative techniques utilized in heart transplantation. In: Baumgartner WA, et al, eds. *Heart and Heart-Lung Transplantation.* Philadelphia: Saunders, 113–133.

Bellet M, Cabrol C, Sassano P, et al (1985). Systemic hypertension after cardiac transplantation: Effect of cyclosporine on the renin-angiotension-aldosterone system. *Am J Cardiol.* 56:927–931.

Bieber C, Hunt SA, Schwinn S, et al (1981). Complications in long term survivors of cardiac transplantation. *Transplant Proc.* 13:207–211.

Blanche C, Czer L, Trento A, et al (1992). Bradyarrhythmias requiring pacemaker implantation after orthotopic heart transplantation: Association with rejection. *J Heart Lung Transplant.* 11:446–452.

Bolling S, Putman J, Abrams G, Deeb G (1991). Hemodynamics versus biopsy findings during transplant rejection. *Am Thorac Surg.* 51:52–55.

Bolman RM, Saffitz J (1990). Early postoperative care of the cardiac transplantation patient: Routine considerations and immunosuppressive therapy. *Prog Cardiovasc Dis.* 33:137-148.

Borkon AM, Augustine SM (1990). Immediate postoperative management of the heart transplant recipient. In: Baumgartner WA, et al, eds. *Heart and Heart-Lung Transplantation.* Philadelphia: Saunders, 134-138.

Bulkley BH (1984). The cardiomyopathies. *Hosp Pract.* 19:59-73.

Carrel A (1907). The surgery of blood vessels, etc. *Johns Hopkins Hosp Bull.* January, 18:18-28.

Carrel A, Guthrie CC (1905). Functions of a transplanted kidney. *Science.* 22:473.

Carrier M, Emery RW, Riley JE, et al (1986). Cardiac transplantation in patients over 50 years of age. *J Am Coll Cardiol* 8:285-288.

Carrier M, Pelletier G, LeClerc Y, et al (1991). Accelerated coronary atherosclerosis after cardiac transplantation: Major threat to long-term survival. *Can J Surg.* 34:133-136.

Caves PK, Stinson EB, Billingham M, Shumway NE (1973). Percutaneous transverse endomyocardial biopsy in human heart recipients. *Ann Thorac Surg.* 16:325-336.

Cohn JN, Levine TB, Olivari MT, et al (1984). Plasma norepinephrine as a guide to prognosis in patients with chronic congestive heart failure. *N Engl J Med.* 311:819-823.

Consensus Trial Study Group (1987). Effects of Enalapril on mortality in severe congestive heart failure: Results of the cooperative North Scandinavian Enalapril survival study (CONSENSUS). *N Engl J Med.* 316:1429-1435.

Copeland JG (1988). Cardiac transplantation. *Current Probl Cardiol.* 13:157-224.

Copeland JG, Emery RW, Levinson MM, et al (1987). Selection of patients for cardiac transplantation. *Circulation.* 75:2-9.

Costanzo-Nordin M, Grady K, Johnson M, et al (1990). Long-term effects of cyclosporin in cardiac transplantation: The Loyola experience. *Transplant Proc.* 22:6-11.

Costard A, Hill I, Schroeder J, Fowler M (1989). Response to nitroprusside: Predictor of early posttransplant mortality. *J Am Coll Cardiol.* 13:62A [Abstract].

Costard-Jackle A, Hill I, Schroeder JS, Fowler MB (1991). The influence of preoperative patient characteristics on early and late survival following cardiac transplantation. *Circulation.* 84(Suppl III): III-329–III-337.

DiBianco R, Shabetai R, Kostuk W, et al (1989). A comparison of oral milrinone, digoxin, and their combination in the treatment of patients with chronic heart failure. *N Engl J Med.* 320:677-683.

Eich D, Thompson J, Daijin K, et al (1991). Hypercholesterolemia in long-term survivors of heart transplantation: An early marker of accelerated coronary artery disease. *J Heart Lung Transplant.* 10:45-49.

Firth BG (1987). Southwestern internal medicine conference: Replacement of the failing heart. *Am J Med Sci.* 293:50-63.

Franciosa JA, Wilen M, Ziesche S, Cohn JN (1983). Survival in men with severe chronic left ventricular failure due to either coronary heart disease or idiopathic dilated cardiomyopathy. *Am J Cardiol.* 51:831-836.

Funk M (1986). Heart transplantation: Postoperative care during the acute period. *Crit Care Nurse.* 6:27-45.

Gao S, Alderman E, Schroeder J, et al (1988). Accelerated coronary vascular disease in the heart transplant patient: Coronary arteriographic findings. *J Am Coll Cardiol.* 12:334-340.

Gradinac S, Frazier OH, VanBuren CT, Radovancevic B (1988). Heart transplants in diabetic patients. *Circulation.* 78(Suppl II):II-252 (Abstract 1003).

Grady K, Costanzo-Nordin M, Herold L, Shoda R (1991). Obesity and hyperlipidemia after heart transplantation. *J Heart Lung Transplant.* 10:449-459.

Grattan M, Moreno-Cabral C, Starnes V, et al (1989). Cytomegalovirus infection is associated with cardiac allograft rejection-atherosclerosis. *JAMA.* 261:3561–3566.

Hardy JD, Chavez CM, Kurrus FD, et al (1964). Heart transplantation in man. *JAMA.* 188: 1132–1140.

Heck C, Shumway S, Kaye M (1989). The registry of the international society for heart transplantation: Sixth official report. *J Heart Lung Transplant.* 8:271–276.

Herrick CM, Mealey PC, Tischner CS, Holland CS (1987). Combined heart failure transplant program: Advantages in assessing medical compliance. *J Heart Transplant.* 6:141–146.

Hosenpud J, Shipley G, Wagner C (1992). Cardiac allograft vasculopathy: Current concepts, recent developments and future directions. *J Heart Lung Transplant.* 11:9–29.

Julian DG, Szekely P (1985). Peripartum cardiomyopathy. *Prog Cardiovasc Dis.* 27:223–240.

Kahan B (1989). Cyclosporine. *N Engl J Med.* 321:1725–1738.

Kaye MP (1993). The registry of the international society for heart and lung transplantation: Ninth official report-1992. *J Heart Lung Transplant.* 12:541–548.

Keogh AM, Baron DW, Hickie JB (1990). Prognostic guides in patients with idiopathic or ischemic dilated cardiomyopathy assessed for cardiac transplantation. *Am J Cardiol.* 65:903–908.

Keogh AM, Freund J, Baron DW, Hickie JB (1988). Timing of cardiac transplantation in idiopathic dilated cardiomyopathy. *Am J Cardiol.* 61:418–422.

Kobashigawa J, Murphy F, Stevenson L, et al (1990). Low-dose lovastatin safely lowers cholesterol after cardiac transplantation. *Circulation.* 82(Suppl IV):281–283.

Lange S, Prevost S, Lewis P, Fadol A (1992). Infection control practices in cardiac transplant recipients. *Heart Lung.* 21:101–105.

Lee K, Pierce J, Hess M, et al (1991). Cardiac transplantation with corticosteroid-free immunosuppression: Long-term results. *Ann Thorac Surg.* 52:211–218.

Levine AB, Levine TB (1991). Patient evaluation for cardiac transplantation. *Prog Cardiovasc Dis.* 33:219–228.

Loebe M, Schuler S, Warnecke H, Hetzer R (1989). The effect of older age on the outcome of heart transplantation. *J Heart Transplant.* 8:307 (Abstract 96).

Lower RR, Shumway NE (1960). Studies on orthotopic homotransplantation of the canine heart. *Surg Forum.* 11:18–19.

Macdonald S, Naucke N (1990). Heart transplantation. In: Smith S, ed. *Tissue and Organ Transplantation.* St. Louis: Mosby, 210–244.

Mancini DM, Eisen H, Kussmaul W, et al (1991). Value of peak exercise oxygen consumption for optimal timing of cardiac transplantation in ambulatory patients with heart failure. *Circulation.* 83:778–786.

Marti V, Ballester M, Auge J, et al (1992). Donor and recipient determinants of fatal and nonfatal cardiac dysfunction during the first week after orthotopic heart transplantation. *Transplant Proc.* 24:16–19.

McGoon M, Frantz R (1992). Techniques of immunosuppression after cardiac transplantation. *Mayo Clinic Proc.* 67:585–595.

Miller DH, Borer JS (1983). The cardiomyopathies: A pathophysiologic approach to therapeutic management. *Arch Intern Med.* 143:2157–2162.

Miller L (1992). Cardiac allograft vasculopathy disease. *Literature Scan: Transplantation.* 8: cover.

Miyamoto Y, Curtiss E, Kormos R, et al (1990). Bradyarrhythmias after heart transplantation. *Circulation* 82(Suppl IV):313–317.

Muirhead J (1992). Heart and heart-lung transplantation. *Crit Care Nurs Clin North Am.* 4:97–109.

Murdock D, Collins E, Lawless C, et al (1987). Rejection of the transplanted heart. *Heart Lung.* 16:237–245.

Myerowitz PD (1987). Donor selection and organ procurement for heart transplantation. In: Myerwitz PD, ed. *Heart Transplantation.* Mount Kisco: Futura, 89–111.

Neish A, Loh E, Schoen F (1992). Myocardial changes in cardiac transplant-associated coronary arteriosclerosis: Potential for timely diagnosis. *J Am Coll Cardiol.* 19:586–592.

O'Connell JB, Dec GW, Goldenberg IF (1990). Results of heart transplantation for active lymphocytic myocarditis. *J Heart Transplant.* 9:351–356.

O'Connell JB, Bourge RC, Costanzo-Nordin MR, et al (1992). Cardiac transplantation: Recipient selection, donor procurement, and medical follow-up. *Circulation* 86:1061–1079.

Olivari MT, Antolick A, Kaye M, et al (1986). Heart transplantation in the elderly. *J Heart Transplant.* 5:366 (Abstract 14).

Penn I (1983). Lymphomas complicating organ transplantation. *Transplant Proc.* 15:2790–2797.

Penn I, Brunson ME (1988). Cancers after cyclosporine therapy. *Transplant Proc.* 20:885–892.

Ratkovec R, Wray R, Renlund D, et al (1990). Influence of corticosteroid-free maintenance immunosuppression on allograft coronary artery disease after cardiac transplantation. *J Thorac Cardiovasc Surg.* 100:6–12.

Redmond J, Zehr K, Gillinov M, et al (1993). Use of theophylline for treatment of prolonged sinus node dysfunction in human orthotopic heart transplantation. *J Heart Lung Transplant.* 12:113–139.

Reemtsma K, Williamson WH, Iglesias F, et al (1962). Studies in homologous canine heart transplantation: Prolongation of survival with a folic acid antagonist. *Surgery.* 52:127–133.

Reitz BA (1990). The history of heart and heart-lung transplantation. In: Baumgartner WA, et al, eds. *Heart and Heart-Lung Transplantation.* Philadelphia: Saunders, 1–13.

Reitz BA (1992). Heart and heart-lung transplantation. In: Braunwald E, ed. *Heart Disease.* Philadelphia: Saunders, 520–534.

Renlund D, O'Connell J, Gilbert E, et al (1987). Feasibility of discontinuation of corticosteroid maintenance therapy in heart transplantation. *J Heart Transplant.* 6:71–78.

Rhenman MJ, Rhenman B, Icenogle T, et al (1988). Diabetes and heart transplantation. *J Heart Transplant* 7:356–358.

Rogers K, Sinnott J, Ferguson J (1989). Using OKT3 to reverse cardiac allograft rejection. *Heart Lung.* 18:490–496.

Roos R (1986). Exercise training for heart transplant patients. *Physician Sports Med.* 14:165–174.

Sampson E, Marthas M (1990). *Group Process for the Health Professions,* 3rd ed. Albany: Delmar.

Schaefer M, Williams L (1991). Nursing implications of immunosuppression in transplantation. *Nurs Clin North Am.* 26:291–313.

Schroeder JS, Hunt S (1987). Cardiac transplantation: Update 1987. *JAMA.* 258:3142–3145.

Shannon M, Wilson B (1992). Prototype drugs. In: *Govoni & Hayes Drugs and Nursing Implications.* 7th ed. Norwalk: Appleton & Lange, 45–264.

Shinn JA (1985). New issues in cardiac transplantation. In: Douglas MK, Shinn JA, eds. *Advances in Cardiovascular Nursing.* Rockville, Md: Aspen Systems, 185–195.

Shinn J (1989). Cardiac transplantation. In: Underhill S, et al, eds. *Cardiac Nursing.* Philadelphia: Lippincott, 585–600.

Shumway S (1990). Basic immunologic concepts involved in organ transplantation. In: Baumgartner WA, et al, eds. *Heart and Heart-Lung Transplantation.* Philadelphia: Saunders, 15–24.

Sklarin N, Dutcher J, Wiernik P (1991). Lymphomas following cardiac transplantation. *Am J Hematol.* 37:105–111.

SOLVD Investigators (1991). Effect of enalapril on survival in patients with reduced left ventricular ejection fractions and congestive heart failure. *N Engl J Med.* 325:293-302.

Stark R, McGinn A, Wilson R (1991). Chest pain in cardiac-transplant recipients. *N Engl J Med.* 324:1791-1794.

Stinson E, Caves P, Griepps R, et al (1975). Hemodynamic observation in the early period after human heart transplantation. *J Thorac Cardiovasc Surg.* 69:264-270.

UNOS Organ Procurement Transplant Network (1994). Database.

Uretsky B (1990). Physiology of the transplanted heart. *Cardiovasc Clin.* 20:22-85.

Uretsky B (1992). Sensory reinnervation of the heart after cardiac transplantation. *N Engl J Med.* 326:66-67.

Uretsky B, Murali S, Reddy S, et al (1987). Development of coronary artery disease in cardiac transplant patients receiving immunosuppressive therapy with cyclosporine and prednisone. *Circulation.* 76:827-834.

Ventura H, Johnson M, Grusk B, et al (1992). Cardiac adaptation to obesity and hypertension after heart transplantation. *J Am Coll Cardiol.* 19:55-59.

Vincent J, Carlier E, Pinsky R, et al (1992). Prostaglandin E infusion for right ventricular failure after cardiac transplantation. *J Thorac Cardiovasc Surg.* 103:33-39.

Weil R, Clarke D, Iwaki Y, et al (1981). Hyperacute rejection of a transplanted human heart. *Transplantation.* 32:71-72.

Weintraub J, Warnke R (1982). Lymphoma in cardiac allotransplant recipients. *Transplantation.* 33:348-356.

Wilson JR, Schwartz JS, Sutton MS, et al (1983). Prognosis in severe heart failure: Relation to hemodynamic measurements and ventricular ectopic activity. *J Am Coll Cardiol* 2:403-410.

Young JN, Yazbeck J, Esposito G, et al (1986). The influence of acute preoperative pulmonary infarction on the results of heart transplantation. *J Heart Transplantat.* 5:20-22.

NURSING CARE PLAN 5–1. CARDIAC TRANSPLANTATION

Nursing Diagnosis Collaborative Problem	Expected Outcomes	Nursing Interventions
Ineffective Breathing Pattern	• Patient is weaned from ventilator in first 24 hours after operation	• Assess breath sounds every 4 hours as needed according to the patient's condition. Document abnormal breath sounds.
Related to	• Respiratory rate effort remains normal	
• Effects of anesthesia and sedation	• Breath sounds clear and chest radiograph normal	• Assess respiratory rate, rhythm, and effort every hour as needed according to the patient's condition
• Incisional pain	• Patient is able to participate in pulmonary exercises on extubation	
• Prolonged intubation	• Patient is given an explanation of respiratory physiology and understands interventions used to improve pulmonary status	• Consult with physician concerning chest radiographic findings
• Ventricular dependency		
• Pulmonary effusions		• Provide continuous pulse oximetry during ICU stay
• Infiltrates		
Defining Characteristics		• Wean patient from ventilator according to unit protocol
• Mechanical ventilation requirement for the initial 8 to 16 hours postoperatively		
• Abnormal chest radiographic finding		• Upon extubation, encourage aggressive toilet, coughing, and the use of the incentive spirometer
• Failure to wean from ventilator		
• Inability to participate in pulmonary exercise coughing, deep breathing, and the use of incentive spirometer		

Altered Health Maintenance Knowledge Deficit

- Immunosuppressive therapy
- Diet
- Exercise
- Follow-up appointments, examination, tests

- Before discharge from hospital patient and at least one family member verbalize an understanding of triple immunosuppressive regime, other discharge medications, diet, exercise, and follow-up appointments, examinations, and tests.
- Patient demonstrates compliance with medication regime
- Patient complies with diet and exercise regime
- Patient attends scheduled examinations and tests

- Assess patient's and family members' level of understanding concerning transplant needs
- Educate patient and at least one family member about medication, diet, exercise, follow-up appointments

  Use teaching, learning, flow sheet to document instruction and patient feedback

  Assure that environment promotes learning and facilitates teaching

  Allow ample time for questions

  Use creative techniques such as pictures, role-playing, and games

- Supply patient with telephone numbers of resource people (primary nurse, social worker, physician, cardiologist, nurse coordinator)

(continued)

NURSING CARE PLAN 5–1. CARDIAC TRANSPLANTATION (*continued*)

Nursing Diagnosis Collaborative Problem	Expected Outcomes	Nursing Interventions

Decreased Cardiac Output
 	
Related to
• Effects of graft ischemia
• Conduction disturbances
• Fluid shifting
• Right-sided heart failure (in recipients whose preoperative intrapulmonary pressures were high)
• Effects of rejection
 	
Defining Characteristics
• Bradycardia
• Diminished peripheral pulses
• Cool, clammy, extremities
• Decreased urinary output
• Altered mental status
	• Cardiac output remains adequate as demonstrated by palpable peripheral pulses, warm extremities, and urinary output >30 ml/hour
	• Heart rate for first 3 to 5 days is 100 to 110 beats per minute
	• Patient has explanation of effects of decreased cardiac output and understands cardiac failure and interventions used to improve cardiac output
		• Monitor cardiac rhythm and rate and obtain 12-lead ECG once a day
		• Obtain vital signs according to unit protocol.
		• Assess peripheral pulses, capillary refill, neurologic status every 4 hours as needed
		• Monitor central venous pressure
		• Strictly record intake and output
		• Weigh patient every day
		• Monitor for signs of heart failure
		   Check skin turgor for edema
		   Note jugular venous distention
		   Auscultate lung sounds for crackles
		   Auscultate heart for S_3
		• Assess chest radiographs for cardiac enlargement
		• Initiate atrial pacing if needed to maintain heart rate between 100 and 110 beats per minute
		• Administer isoproterenol at 0.1 to 0.2 mg (titrate) according to physician orders; Assure heart rate does not exceed 110 beats per minute

138

- Administer vasoactive drips, IV sodium nitroprusside, nitroglycerine to maintain mean arterial pressure at 75 to 85 mm Hg.
- Administer inotropic agents such as dobutamine and amrinone according to physician order
- Administer fluid colloids and chrystalloids according to physician order
- Administer diuretics according to physician order
- Describe at patient's and family members' level of understanding the importance of maintaining heart rate between 100 and 110 beats per minute and the importance of other interventions to promote adequate cardiac output

(continued)

(continued)
NURSING CARE PLAN 5–1. CARDIAC TRANSPLANTATION

Nursing Diagnosis Collaborative Problem	Expected Outcomes	Nursing Interventions
High Risk for Infection *Related to* • Immunosuppressed state • Invasive lines *Defining Characteristics* • Temperature >38.0C • WBC >10,000 or <5000 • Reddened or tender wounds • Drainage from wounds or insertion sites of invasive lines • Infiltrates on chest radiograph • Change in sputum • Urinary tract infection • Positive culture results	• Patient remains free of signs and symptoms of infection • Patient demonstrates and verbalizes measures to reduce risk for infections	• Assess for signs and symptoms of infection Obtain complete blood count once a day Observe and document status of incisional wounds and insertion sites of invasive lines Obtain temperature every 4 hours as needed according to unit protocol • Observe strict hand-washing techniques • Observe isolation techniques according to unit protocol • Maintain strict aseptic technique during dressing changes and endotracheal suctioning • Cap all stopcocks • Administer prophylactic antibiotics according to unit protocol • Describe to patient and family prevention, transmission, signs and symptoms of infection

6

Heart-Lung and Lung Transplantation

Sharon G. Owens
Janice M. Wallop

The idea for heart-lung transplantation was first suggested in the early 1900s. Alexis Carrel proposed the notion of replacing the heart and lungs as a method of treating patients with severe abnormalities and physical limitations (Reitz, 1990a). Experimental replacements were performed on animals as early as the 1950s. Although dogs were initially used in these studies, abnormal breathing patterns resulted from the denervation of their lungs. Primates did not experience these respiratory complications and therefore emerged as the model for human heart-lung transplantation. Between 1969 and 1971 attempts at transplantation in humans were not successful because of allograft rejection, severe infection, and failure of the anastasmoses to heal. With the advent of cyclosporine, rejection became easier to treat without large doses of steroids and their attendant complications. The first successful heart-lung transplant in a human was performed in 1981 at Stanford University by B.A. Reitz and his colleagues (Reitz et al, 1982).

Lung transplantation had been considered in the laboratory since the 1940s, when Demikhov, a Russian physiologist, performed hemografts of individual canine lobes in 1947 (Kirklin & Barratt-Boyes, 1993). The first lung transplant in a human was performed by James Hardy at the University of Mississippi in 1963 (McCarthy et al, 1992). This field of transplantation was plagued by obstacles similar to those in heart-lung transplantation. Other problems for lung transplantation included an extremely limited donor pool and the technical difficulties associated with the double-lung procedure. In the 1980s, with the advent of new methods to prevent, detect, and treat rejection, as well as technical advances in the operating room, the field of cardiopulmonary transplantation began to flourish. Despite the problems of rejection and infection, transplantation continues to offer patients with a limited life expectancy the chance for increased survival. Figure 6–1 depicts the current survival statistics for patients who undergo heart-lung, double-lung, and single-lung transplantation (Kaye, 1993). This chapter focuses on the diseases that necessitate transplantation; donor and recipient selection; and operative and postoperative care.

DISEASES THAT NECESSITATE TRANSPLANTATION

Various diseases may necessitate either heart-lung or lung transplantation. Table 6–1 list conditions commonly treated by each operation.

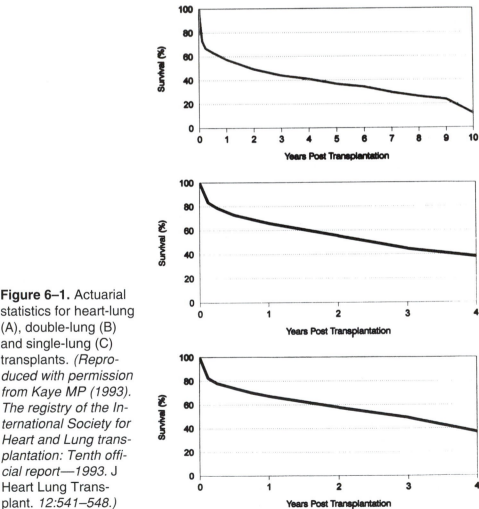

Figure 6–1. Actuarial statistics for heart-lung (A), double-lung (B) and single-lung (C) transplants. *(Reproduced with permission from Kaye MP (1993). The registry of the International Society for Heart and Lung transplantation: Tenth official report—1993.* J Heart Lung Transplant. *12:541–548.)*

TABLE 6–1. DIAGNOSES

Diagnoses Leading to Heart and Lung Transplantation
Eisenmenger syndrome
Cystic fibrosis
Primary pulmonary hypertension

Diagnoses Leading to Lung Transplantation
Chronic obstructive pulmonary disease (bronchiectasis, emphysema)
α-1-antitrypsin deficiency
Primary pulmonary fibrosis
Cystic fibrosis
Primary pulmonary hypertension

Cystic Fibrosis

Cystic fibrosis is a lethal, autosomal recessive disorder of infants, children, and young adults with widespread dysfunction of the exocrine glands. Abnormally thick mucus obstructs organ passages and leads to respiratory, digestive, integumentary, and reproductive impairment and damage. Progressive pulmonary obstructive disease, multiple acute and chronic pulmonary infections, and malnutrition secondary to malabsorption characterize the clinical situation. With current medical therapies and nutritional support, most patients survive into the third decade of life. Pulmonary disease continues to be the most common cause of death. The primary pulmonary abnormality of cystic fibrosis is thick secretions that cause obstruction of the small and large airways. Atelectasis secondary to mucous plugging promotes bacterial infection by *Pseudomonas aeruginosa, Staphylococcus aureus,* and *Haemophilus influenzae* which leads to ventilation and perfusion abnormalities. The cycle of repeated infections and chronic irritation results in progressive airway and parenchymal fibrosis and respiratory insufficiency. Hypoxia and pulmonary vascular changes often progress to pulmonary hypertension and cor pulmonale. With the final appearance of spontaneous pneumothorax and congestive heart failure, chances for recovery are limited (Scott Hutter et al, 1988; Shennib et al, 1992; Smyth et al, 1990).

Eisenmenger Syndrome

Eisenmenger syndrome involves congenital cardiac lesions such as ventricular septal defect and transposition of the great vessels, which result in an abnormal communication between the systemic and pulmonary circulations. Such communications reverse the normal blood-flow patterns within the heart. In the case of a ventricular septal defect, blood from the left ventricle flows into the right ventricle, leading to increased pressure. If the underlying cardiac defect remains uncorrected, changes in the pulmonary vasculature occur and lead to pulmonary hypertension. The term *Eisenmenger syndrome* also has been used to describe any anomaly that leads to obliterative pulmonary vascular disease, including pretricuspid and postricuspid shunts (Friedman, 1988; Kloner, 1984). Patients with Eisenmenger syndrome may experience dyspnea, fatigue, syncope, hemoptysis, atypical chest pain, and grossly elevated hematocrits to compensate for low arterial oxygen saturation levels. Pulmonary vascular resistance is elevated to 75% of systemic vascular resistance (SVR). Initial treatment includes diuretics, sodium restriction, treatment of right ventricular failure, phlebotomy, and chronic oxygen therapy. The prognosis is poor once this syndrome develops; patients rarely live past the age of 30 years. Although the largest group of recipients of heart-lung transplants are those with an underlying anomaly and associated pulmonary hypertension, many with congenital heart defects may not be acceptable transplant candidates. Those who have undergone surgical correction of these anomalies are prone to extensive intrathoracic adhesions. These adhesions can cause excessive surgical bleeding, increasing the patient's risk for complications and death (Reitz, 1990b).

Primary Pulmonary Hypertension

Primary pulmonary hypertension is increased pulmonary vascular resistance and pulmonary hypertension usually of unknown origin. Several theories have been investigated regarding the cause of this disease. They include the possibility of recurrent pulmonary emboli, thrombus formation in small pulmonary arteries, and autoimmune phenomenon vasculitis. Internal thickening occurs in the small pulmonary arteries, producing an onion-skin appearance. Eventually necrotizing arteritis with thrombosis and atherosclerosis occurs. Patients experience dyspnea, fatigue, dizziness, syncope, weakness, and atypical chest pain (Renfroe, 1992; Rubin, 1993). Pulmonary artery and right ventricular pressures are elevated and sometimes equal systemic pressures. Treatment may include pulmonary vasodilators such as isoproterenal, prostaglandins, or hydralazine, and oxygen administration. The outcome for this disease is generally poor; the life expectancy is often less than 2 years after the initial diagnosis.

Chronic Obstructive Pulmonary Disease

Chronic obstructive pulmonary disease (COPD) affects approximately 10 million people in the United States. The term actually relates to a group of diseases that includes asthma, bronchitis, emphysema, bronchiectasis, and α-1-antitrypsin deficiency (Wilson & Thompson, 1990). Not all of these diseases inevitably progress to end-stage lung disease. Emphysema, α-1-antitrypsin deficiency, and bronchiectasis are the most common disorders that necessitate an evaluation for lung transplantation.

Emphysema. Approximately 2.5 million people in the United States have anatomic changes within the air spaces of the lung known as emphysema. Primarily affected are the areas distal to the terminal bronchioles. Destruction of the lung wall occurs, resulting in increased compliance, decreased capacity for diffusion of oxygen and carbon dioxide, and air trapping with a decreased ability to expire carbon dioxide (Higgins, 1984). Most patients also suffer from chronic bronchitis characterized by hypertrophy and hyperplasia of the submucosal glands that lead to increased production of mucus. Most instances of emphysema are caused by cigarette smoking (Snider, 1988). The remainder, 1 to 2% of cases, can be attributed to α-1-antitrypsin deficiency (Fishman, 1992).

Most patients experience the onset of symptoms in the sixth or seventh decade of life. The overall course of the illness varies with the individual and with how effectively complications are managed. One indicator believed to be valuable in relation to outcomes, is the forced expiratory volume in 1 second (FEV_1). Patients who have an FEV_1 of less than 0.75 L are known to have a mortality of 30% in the first year of illness and 95% at 10 years (Snider, 1988).

α-1-antitrypsin Deficiency. The deterioration seen in α-1-antitrypsin deficiency is similar to that of emphysema. The difference lies in the mechanism that causes the pathologic condition. This deficiency can result from any number of different mutations of the same gene. These mutations cause a deficiency in the production of the antiprotease known as α-1-antitrypsin. This substance has a protective effect on the lung by inhibiting the potential proteolytic actions of certain enzymes. Insufficient levels of α-1-antitrypsin allow these proteases to destroy lung tissue, causing the same airway problems as described for emphysema. Most patients are affected in the third or fourth decade of life, resulting in a 10-year decrease in life expectancy. Smoking is believed to accelerate the disease process by at least 10% (Fishman, 1992). Therapies under investigation for the treatment of this disorder may hold promise for the future. However, the only known cure for the illness at present is lung transplantation.

Bronchiectasis. Bronchiectasis is irreversible dilatation and eventual destruction of the elastic and muscular components of the bronchi and bronchioles. Chronic infections and inflammation of the bronchial tree are often present. Patients experience a loose, productive cough, often with purulent secretions. Treatment is essentially palliative with postural drainage and percussion along with the use of expectorants. Prognosis for this condition is poor (Baum & Hershko, 1989).

Idiopathic Pulmonary Fibrosis. Idiopathic pulmonary fibrosis is a thickening of the alveolar interstitium. Eventually, alveoli are destroyed and adjacent capillaries are obliterated. Pulmonary fibrosis usually affects people in the fourth or fifth decade of life and has a fairly aggressive course. Patients usually have a life expectancy of 3 to 6 years after diagnosis (Crystal et al, 1984). The presenting clinical manifestations are dyspnea on exertion, cough, rales, and nail clubbing. As the disease progresses, the lungs become stiff, shrunken, and noncompliant. Treatment usually involves the use of steroids but is ineffective in preventing progression of the disease.

RECIPIENT SELECTION

Since the early years of transplantation, much has changed in relation to recipient selection. Patients once thought to benefit only from double-lung procedures are now being successfully treated with single-lung transplantation. Single-lung procedures have been shown to be successful for patients with primary pulmonary hypertension. In the past, these patients were believed only to be candidates for heart-lung transplantation. Figure 6–2 demonstrates the process of matching the appropriate recipi-

Candidate with end-stage pulmonary disease

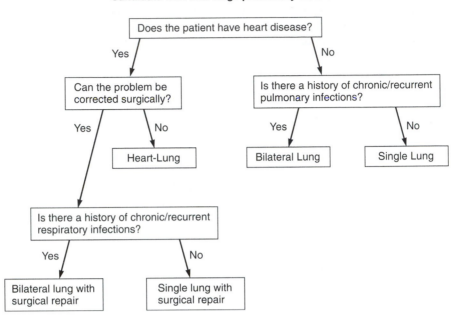

Figure 6–2. Decision tree. Matching the recipient to the appropriate procedure.

ent to the appropriate procedure. These findings are encouraging in light of the limited donor pool. The need for one lung as opposed to two or for one lung or two lungs as opposed to a heart and a lung could greatly increase the number of people who might benefit from one donor.

Essential to the success of transplantation is careful screening and evaluation of potential candidates. A complete history and physical examination and extensive testing are warranted to determine the suitability of the patient for transplantation. The components of the evaluation process are listed in Table 6–2.

Upon referral, patients undergo evaluation of their current medical condition and their ability to undergo the difficult operation and postoperative follow-up therapy. The family accompanies the patient for this evaluation. General recipient selection guidelines are shown in Table 6–3.

The patient should be motivated for recovery, be able to follow a complex medical regimen, and have a strong support system. In general, patients should have end stage disease not amenable to any other medical or surgical intervention and have a life expectancy less than 18 to 24 months (Onofrio & Emory, 1992). They should have demonstrated compliance to medical regimens in the past and be free of any major systemic illness (Bolman et al, 1991). It is recommended that patients not take steroids for at least 1 month before the procedure because of potential complications to healing. Patients who have had a previous thoracic operation are considered by most centers not to be good candidates for heart-lung transplantation or double-lung pro-

TABLE 6–2. EVALUATION PROCESS FOR RECIPIENT SELECTION

Medical history and physical examination

Routine laboratory tests

ABO blood type

Serologic tests for hepatitis, HIV antibody, and cytomegalovirus antibodies

Pulmonary studies:
    Chest roentgenogram
    Pulmonary function tests
    Arterial blood gas measurements
    Ventilation–perfusion scan

Cardiovascular studies
    Electrocardiogram
    Multiple gated (image) acquisition (MUGA) scan
    Right heart catheterization
    Left heart catheterization (heart and lung candidates and all patients older than 40 years)

Rehabilitation assessment
    Six-minute walk test (distance walked and supplemental O_2 requirements)

Psychosocial assessment

cedures (Hardesty & Griffith, 1987; Wallwork, 1989). The presence of adhesions may lead to excessive postoperative bleeding that necessitates massive volume resuscitation; the outcome is generally poor (Baumgartner, 1990). Lung transplant recipients should have adequate cardiac function as demonstrated by a multiple gated (image) acquisition (MUGA) scan (Boychuck & Malen, 1990). If the person does have impaired function, the question of reversibility becomes an issue. If the cardiac problem is believed to be secondary to the pulmonary problems, there is potential for improvement once the lung or lungs have been replaced.

TABLE 6–3. HEART AND LUNG RECIPIENT SELECTION

Presence of

End-stage pulmonary or cardiopulmonary disease

Life expectancy < 1 year

Age no more than 50–55 years (heart and lung, bilateral lung) 60–65 years (single lung)

Strong family support

Absence of

Systemic illness, malignant neoplasm

Previous, major thoracic operation

Irreversible liver impairment

Renal impairment

Lack of compliance with supportive medical regimens

Potential recipients therefore undergo a very thorough evaluation. The purpose is not only to ensure that the patient is qualified as a candidate but also to plan a pretransplant program. This program involves a combination of medical therapies, physical therapy, and a comprehensive nutritional plan. The goal is to optimize the recipient's overall state of health before transplantation. The main focus should be in the areas of nutrition and physical rehabilitation. By enhancing these areas the patient will be in a better position to withstand rigorous medication and treatment protocols postoperatively. If the patient does not have sufficient caloric intake, intravenous therapy may be necessary. A physical therapist sees these patients and develops a program focused on cardiovascular and pulmonary endurance, mobility, cardiopulmonary hygiene, and postural assessment and exercise. A major component of the program includes patient and family education. *All* patients, including those not accepted as candidates, are provided a comprehensive health plan.

DONOR SELECTION

Cadaveric Donors

The single most limiting factor for these procedures involves the scant donor pool. The lack of available donors and organs poses a problem for all types of transplantation and is particularly problematic with lung procedures. The reasons for this are varied. The first involves the nature of the lung itself, which is in constant contact with the environment. This results in an increased susceptibility to infection and injury, potentially limiting the use of certain lungs. The second problem relates to the nature of the donors themselves, who are often victims of motor vehicle accidents and require mechanical ventilation. Motor vehicle accidents are often associated with chest trauma and can result in damage to one or both lungs. Intubation increases the potential for infection and, if done in an emergency, may be associated with aspiration. As a result, even when a donor becomes available, the lung or lungs may not be suitable for transplantation.

Any possibility of infection before transplantation may lead to a life-threatening problem after the transplant because of immunosuppression and mechanical ventilation. In general, the donor must have a Po_2 greater than 100 mm Hg on a Fio_2 of 40% (Table 6–4). Size matching is important because use of donor lungs larger than the recipient's lungs may lead to compression, causing atelectasis and shunting. Matching is achieved by comparing the chest sizes according to chest radiographic measurements (Shennib et al, 1992).

TABLE 6–4. HEART AND LUNG DONOR CRITERIA

Size compatibility
$Po_2 > 100$ mm Hg on 40% Fio_2
Normal lung compliance
Absence of pulmonary infection or gross infiltrate as demonstrated by a chest radiograph
Absence of infectious disease such as HIV infection or hepatitis B

Living-Related Donors

Living-related lung donations are a recent occurrence. The first lung transplant of this type took place in October of 1990 at Stanford University. A 12-year-old patient with bronchopulmonary dysplasia received a right upper lobe from her mother (Goldsmith, 1990). Later, at the same institution, a 1-year-old child received a lobe of a lung from an unrelated donor (McCarthy et al, 1992). Although there are ethical implications of allowing healthy people to donate organs or portions of organs, this type of donation does offer hope to people with end-stage lung disease. A special type of living donor situation existed with the "domino donor" transplant. In the late 1980s a patient with cystic fibrosis required a transplant. His heart function was normal, but at that time very few isolated lung procedures were being performed. Most centers treated these patients as heart-lung candidates. When the organs became available the patient with cystic fibrosis donated his heart to a recipient who required a heart transplant alone. The two transplants were performed simultaneously. This practice has been abandoned because cystic fibrosis is now treated with bilateral lung transplantation.

SURGICAL MANAGEMENT

During the surgical procedure, the operating room nurse has responsibility for the donor organs and for the recipient. Heart-lung procedures are performed with the patient use of cardiopulmonary bypass. First the heart is removed and the phrenic nerves are isolated. The lungs are removed individually by dividing the inferior pulmonary ligaments and transecting the pulmonary hilar structures. Sufficient left atrium is removed to allow the donor's right lung to fit into the right pleural space. The donor heart and lung bloc is placed into the recipient's chest, and the tracheal anastamosis is completed (Ahrens & Powers, 1990; Novitzky & Cooper, 1990) (Fig 6–3).

Single-lung transplants are performed through an anterolateral thoracotomy (Fig 6–4 and 6–6a). Some patients may require cardiopulmonary bypass such as those with primary pulmonary hypertension or Eisenmenger syndrome (Bolman et al, 1991). The double-lung transplant procedure has been modified to a bilateral single lung transplant procedure with the individual bronchial anastamoses (Fig 6–5 and 6–6b). The double-lung procedure had been associated with increased complications and mortality perioperatively because of the requirement for cardiopulmonary bypass.

POSTOPERATIVE MANAGEMENT

The postoperative condition of patients who undergo heart-lung transplantation depends on preoperative status, the length of cardiopulmonary bypass, and recovery from the operation. Prevention of infection and rejection and complications related to preoperative disease, such as cystic fibrosis, is vital. A plan of care should address the most important nursing diagnoses (see Nursing Care Plan 6–1, pp 161–163). Because of the complex physiologic nature of the diseases involved, most of these diagnoses have multiple causes.

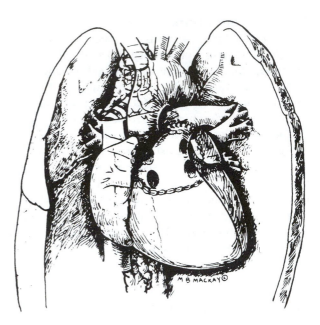

Figure 6–3. Anastamoses in the heart and lung procedure. *(Reproduced with permission from Myerowitz PD (1987).* Heart Transplantation. *New York: Futura Publishing Company), p 138.)*

Respiratory Management

Ineffective airway clearance may be caused by impairment of lymphatic drainage, phrenic nerve dysfunction, compromised respiratory mechanics, or immobilization. Problems with airway clearance make patients who have had heart-lung or lung transplants particularly vulnerable to respiratory infections (Gallagher & Lawrence, 1991; Cary, 1991). Management should be oriented toward prevention rather than treatment, because the mortality associated with these infections remains very high (Augustine, 1991; Hirt et al, 1993). Efforts are directed at keeping the airway clear of secretions to minimize the medium for infection. Weaning from the ventilator and extubation are initiated at the earliest possible time. Endotracheal suctioning with a flexible catheter is important. However, overly aggressive suctioning should be avoided to prevent trauma to the tracheal anastomosis.

Early mobilization and pulmonary toilet with effective pain management are essential to prevent atelectasis and optimize ventilation to the lungs (Ahrens & Powers, 1990). During the first 24 to 48 hours patients are positioned with the transplant side up to promote drainage and lung expansion. The physical therapy and respiratory therapy teams continue to follow patients throughout their course to promote activity, increase physical strength, and mobilize secretions. A moderate level of exercise can be expected (Levy et al, 1993). Assessment is continuous. It includes chest radiographs to monitor for pleural effusions, infiltrates, and pulmonary edema. Bronchoscopy is performed as needed to evaluate for infection and rejection and to assess anastamoses (Scott et al, 1991). Mucolytic therapy may be initiated depending on the amount and type of secretions (Boychuck & Malen, 1990). Chest physiotherapy is performed on an individual basis specific to the patient and conditions.

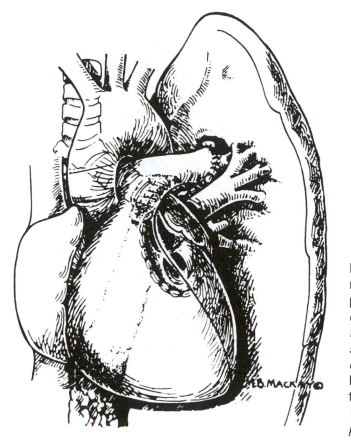

Figure 6–4. Anasta-moses in the single-lung procedure. *(Repro-duced with permission from Cooper JD, Patter-son GA. In: Wallwork J, ed (1989).* Heart and Heart-Lung Transplan-tation. *Philadelphia: W.B. Saunders Com-pany, p 500.)*

An incentive spirometer is used every day throughout the hospitalization and after discharge. The patient is required to monitor his or her progress with the spirometer and to report a decrease in ability because this may herald the onset of in-fection or rejection (Bjortuft et al, 1993). After discharge patients continue to be at risk for pulmonary complications. These complications are related not only to infec-tion and rejection but also to intraoperative ischemia. Interruption of bronchial cir-culation during the operation can lead to early as well as late airway complications, which increase morbidity and mortality (Frost et al, Cagle, 1993).

Fluid Volume Management

An excess in fluid volume may be related to interstitial fluid changes during cardio-pulmonary bypass, preexisting volume excess, decreased ability to excrete fluid, or disruption of pulmonary lymphatic drainage. Fluid volume excess may be com-pounded by a preexisting renal disease. The transplanted lung remains particularly susceptible to excess fluid volume, which can result in pulmonary edema. Fluid ad-ministration is kept to a minimum in the immediately postoperative period. Should

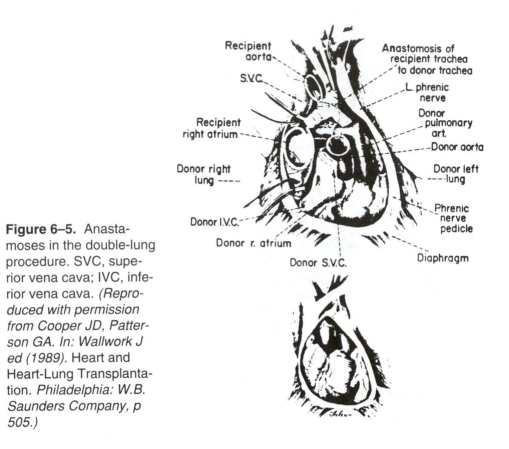

Figure 6–5. Anastamoses in the double-lung procedure. SVC, superior vena cava; IVC, inferior vena cava. *(Reproduced with permission from Cooper JD, Patterson GA. In: Wallwork J ed (1989).* Heart and Heart-Lung Transplantation. *Philadelphia: W.B. Saunders Company, p 505.)*

the patient demonstrate hemodynamic instability, vasoactive medications should be used before any fluid is given. Restriction of fluids to 1200 mL per day is recommended. Diuretics and low-dose dopamine as a renal artery vasodilator are often used (Parquin et al, 1993). Assessment includes routine arterial blood gas analysis; measurement of central venous, pulmonary artery, or left atrial pressures; daily measurement of weight; and measurement of intake and output. The serum bicarbonate level should be monitored frequently during diuretic therapy because patients may develop metabolic alkalosis. The goal is for the patient to be at or below preoperative weight.

Prevention of Infection

Infection constitutes a major cause of death among heart-lung and lung transplant patients (Ciulli et al, 1993; Frist et al, 1991). The patient is particularly vulnerable to infection in the immediately postoperative period. The mortality associated with early postoperative infection is 3% (Deusch et al, 1993). The most common bacterial infections are those due to *Klebsiella pneumoniae, P aeruginosa, Escherichia coli, S aureus,* and *Enterobacter cloacae* (Deusch et al, 1993). Several factors increase a

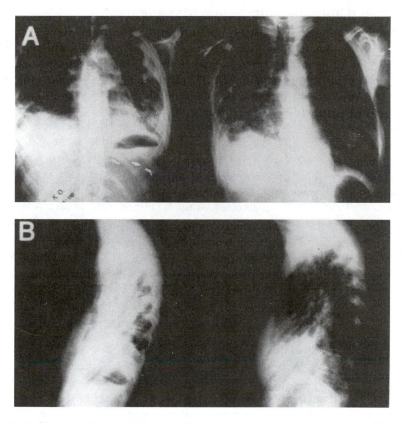

Figure 6–6. Chest radiographs of single and bilateral lung recipients. *(Repro-duced with permission from Egan TM, Kaiser LR, Cooper JD. (1989). Lung trans-plantation.* Curr Probl Surg. *26:709.)*

patient's susceptibility to infection. They include immunosuppressive therapy, the presence of invasive lines, the surgical incision, and endotracheal intubation. Iso-lation techniques vary among institutions; however, hand-washing and careful screening of visitors for infectious diseases have proved to be the most important measures in the prevention of infections (Muirhead, 1992). Vigilant observation of incisions and invasive line sites is important. Invasive lines should be discontinued as soon as possible and sites rotated when indicated. The patient may be unable to effectively and independently clear secretions. As soon as the patient is extubated, vigorous pulmonary toilet and mobilization should begin and be maintained through-out the hospital stay. It is important to monitor white blood cell (WBC) count and temperature trends because transplant patients do not demonstrate the normal phys-iologic responses to infection (Copeland, 1990; Swartz & Davis, 1992). Early identifi-cation of culprit organisms is essential to ensure appropriate antibiotic therapy (Deusch et al, 1993).

Rejection and Immunosuppression Management

Although immunosuppression causes serious infectious problems, it remains essential for the prevention of rejection. In heart-lung transplant patients, rejection of the heart is diagnosed with endomyocardial biopsies and rejection of the lungs is diagnosed with transbronchial or open lung biopsies (Ahrens & Powers, 1990). Rejection of the heart in the combined procedure does not occur as often as rejection of the lungs (Scott et al, 1990). Symptoms of lung rejection may include pulmonary infiltrates, poor arterial blood gas levels, dyspnea, low-grade fever, and elevated WBC count (Ahrens & Powers, 1990). In the first 6 weeks postoperatively, the patient usually experiences two to three rejection episodes. Transbronchial biopsies can provide valuable information to differentiate between infection, rejection, and lung injury. The symptoms of these conditions can mimic each other (Ahrens & Powers, 1990; Shumway et al, 1993). Bronchioalveolar lavage has been used in an attempt to diagnose the cause of respiratory complications. However, it, too, has not proved to be definitive in all cases. For patients who have negative cultures but show evidence of respiratory compromise, the usual course of treatment involves enhancement of immunosuppression. Should the patient's condition not improve despite treatment of rejection, an open lung biopsy may be warranted. Tables 6–5 and 6–6 present the various immunosuppression regimens relative to prevention and treatment of rejection.

Obliterative Bronchiolitis

Obliterative bronchiolitis is the most serious long-term complication of lung transplantation; it causes severe deterioration of lung function. The literature reports that obliterative bronchiolitis occurs in as many as 50% of patients who survive the first year after the transplant (Scott et al, 1991; Ahrens & Powers, 1990). To date, there has been little progress in isolating the cause of this complication. Some possibilities include chronic rejection, viral infection, cyclosporine toxicity, long-term denervation of the lung, the lack of lymphatics, or the loss of bronchial blood supply (Madden et al, 1992). Patients experience a cough and progressive dyspnea. Pulmonary infiltrates appear on a chest radiograph, and there is an obstructive pattern to pulmonary function tests. Scott and associates (1991) found a progressive fall in FEV_1. Obliterative bronchiolitis is diagnosed with fiberoptic bronchoscopy and transbronchial lung biopsy (Outlana et al, 1992). Bronchioles and pulmonary vessels show a pattern of extensive fibrosis. The blood vessels have fibrosis and atherosclerosis. This finding is consistent with a reduction in diffusing capacity and ventilation–perfusion (V/Q) imbalance (Outlana et al, 1992). Madden and colleagues (1992) found some improvement of symptoms in a small number of patients who received high-dose steroid therapy. Scott and co-workers (1990) believe closer monitoring with routine and diagnostic transbronchial lung biopsy may lead to the accurate diagnosis of acute rejection and therefore decrease the incidence of chronic rejection. Obliterative bronchiolitis continues to be an important cause of morbidity and mortality among these patients. It is mostly irreversible, and the only viable treatment option seems to be retransplantation. Current statistics for this procedure remain unfavorable. Mortalities for retransplantation are considerably higher for first-time procedures than for re-

TABLE 6–5. IMMUNOSUPPRESSION: MAINTENANCE PROTOCOL

Medication	Preoperative Dosage	Intraoperative Dosage	Postoperative Dosage	Comments
Cyclosporine	10 mg/kg orally once	—	10 mg/kg per day orally or 0.5–1 mg/kg per day IV	Level range = 200–400 mg/mL
Solumedrol	—	500 mg IV once	125 mg IV every 8 hours for 3 doses	—
Prednisone	—	—	0.4 mg/kg per day orally in divided doses	Begin on post-operative day 15 because of negative effects of steroids on healing
Azathioprine	—	—	2 mg/kg per day orally or IV	Hold for white blood cell count < 5000 cells/mm³
Rabbit antithymocyte globulin	—	—	1 dose a day IV for 5–7 days	Skin test before first dose; pre-medicate with steroids and diphenhy-dramine
TCR	—	—	Complete blood count with differential every day	T-cell check 3 times a week

TABLE 6–6. IMMUNOSUPPRESSION: REJECTION PROTOCOL

Medication	Dosage	Comments
Prednisone	100 mg/day in 3 divided doses then tapered by 5 mg/day until baseline reached	
Methylprednisolone	1 g/day for 3 days	Continue prednisone maintenance dose or taper during methylprednisolone pulse
Muromonab CD3	5 mg/day for 10–14 days	Premedicate with steroids and diphenydramine T-cell check 3 times a week Complete blood count with differ-ential every day
Rabbit antithymocytoglobulin	1 dose/day IV for 10–14 days	Same as muromonab-CD3

The type of medication used to treat rejection depends on the preference of the transplant center and the patient's level of rejection.

transplantation. Patients who survive to discharge, however, tend to have stable and satisfactory functional results (Novick et al, 1993).

A review of the research showed some similarities among patients who had obliterative bronchiolitis. Scott and co-authors (1991), in a review of 75 patients who underwent heart-lung transplants, found acute rejection more frequently, as diagnosed with bronchoscopy, in the chronic rejection patients with fibrosis than in those without fibrosis. Cytomegalovirus (CMV), herpes simplex virus (HSV), *Aspergillus, Pneumocystis carinii,* and bacterial pneumonias occurred with similar frequency in both groups. Bolman and associates (1991) reviewed 23% of survivors of heart-lung transplants and 19% of survivors of single-lung transplants who had obliterative bronchiolitis and found all but one of these patients to have an underlying diagnosis of pulmonary hypertension.

Cardiovascular Management

Decreased cardiac output may occur secondary to dysrhythmia, hyperthermia, preservation ischemia, or hypovolemia. Stabilization of the hemodynamic condition may take several hours postoperatively depending on the nature of the problems and related complications. Hemodynamic measurements helpful in making an assessment may include pulmonary artery pressures, pulmonary capillary wedge or left atrial pressures, and arterial and central venous pressures. Hemorrhage may intensify the instability in the blood pressure. Particularly important in the immediately postoperative period is control of bleeding, which may be related to platelet destruction due to cardiopulmonary bypass, inadequate heparin reversal, or disruption of intrathoracic adhesions or an anastomotic site. The nurse may have to administer blood, coagulation products, and various medications such as protamine or vitamin K.

Nutritional Management

Nutritional deficits may be related to increased metabolism or inability to digest and absorb nutrients. In addition to preoperative debilitation these patients have increased caloric requirements secondary to wound healing. Many patients have a decreased appetite the first few days after the operation, which further intensifies the problem. If the anorexia continues or vomiting occurs, hyperalimentation may be considered as a temporary measure to supply calories for wound healing and to maximize the strength of ventilatory muscles.

Patients with cystic fibrosis continue to experience digestive problems and require the enzyme pancrease. Patients who waited a long time for the transplant who had pre-existing nutritional deficits require frequent assessment of their nutritional needs. If gastrointestinal problems are not present, a gastric feeding tube may be placed for nutritional support to limit the number of intravascular devices used.

Psychosocial Concerns

Self-concept may be influenced by transplantation, the surgical wound, or the presence of invasive lines. During the pretransplant waiting period, patients may experience a multitude of emotions ranging from fear of death to hope for a new life. Patients with a chronic illness before transplantation may have had the opportunity to adapt to their disease. People who are acutely ill, however, may not have adjusted to the illness. For both types of patients, transplantation is a new and frightening experience (Maride, 1991). There are not many heart-lung or lung recipients with whom they can identify. As prepared as they may be and as eager as they are to receive the new organs, they experience many fears (Carr, 1990). "What will life be like?", "Will I be different?", and "How will I feel?" are some of the questions patients may ask. Their fear and excitement are part of the uncertainty that lies ahead.

After transplantation, patients may have feelings they cannot identify. If they are physically well, they usually are enthusiastic. Families may be unsure of how to treat the patient. They are happy about the transplant but are probably afraid of what lies ahead. This is a time for the nurses, social worker, and clinical nurse specialist or transplant coordinator to give continuous support to the patient and family. They should allow time for expression of feelings, asking questions, and expressing thoughts. The patient and family should have private time with each other without interruption.

Some patients may require the intervention of a psychiatrist or psychologist to help them through this period. Each patient should be assessed individually and the care plan adjusted to his or her needs. Patients respond differently depending on their stage of growth and development. The health care team should be prepared for a variety of questions, mood swings, and family dynamics.

Pain Management

Discomfort often occurs at the surgical incision. Recovery from anesthesia and pain management are the most important areas of concern in the immediately postoperative period. It may take 4 to 6 hours for the patient to arouse. Because weaning from the ventilator is an important consideration, the nurse should balance sedation and pain management with adequate strength for respiration. Low-dose sedatives and pain medications are often used, especially if the patient's condition is hemodynamically unstable. When the core temperature is close to normal, and the patient's condition is stable, sedatives can gradually be eliminated. With successful weaning, assessment of pain can lead to a plan for relief with medications or nonpharmacologic measures. Patient controlled analgesia may provide necessary pain relief once the patient is alert enough to manage this system.

FUTURE CONSIDERATIONS

With improved medical management, patients with cystic fibrosis, primary pulmonary hypertension, or Eisenmenger syndrome are living longer, more active lives. Heart-lung or lung transplants have been a consideration for a select group with end-stage pulmonary disease (Caine et al, 1991; Smyth et al, 1990). To date, approximately 1349 heart-lung procedures, 1144 single-lung, 521 double-lung, and 8 lobe transplants have been performed (Kaye, 1993).

Advances in heart-lung bloc preservation, tracheal anastamoses, immunosuppression medications, and postoperative care have improved the outcome for these patients (Ahrens & Powers, 1990). Bolman and associates (1991) showed an advantage of single-lung transplantation over heart-lung transplantation by comparing waiting times before transplantation. The average wait for a heart and lung was 394 days, and the wait for a single lung was 150 days. Because the number of centers performing heart transplantation is increasing, heart-lung transplantation will be even more rare than it is now because most of the suitable donor hearts are given to patients awaiting heart transplantation. Single-lung and double-lung transplants may become preferred over heart-lung transplants whenever possible because of this difficulty in procuring hearts *and* lungs. The question of whether it is ethical to replace a recipient's normal heart when there are patients with end-stage heart disease who may benefit has been addressed (Au et al, 1992). It is possible that heart-lung transplants may be performed strictly for patients with end-stage disease of the heart and lung.

In heart-lung, single-lung, and double-lung transplant patients there is a delicate balance between prevention of rejection and infection. Superimposed phrenic nerve damage, disruption of lymphatic drainage, and preexisting donor or recipient infections may tip this balance into a life-threatening situation. In isolation, any of these problems may be treatable. In combination they may be almost impossible to overcome. Continued investigation into the prevention of acute and chronic rejection while minimizing the risk of infection is an important direction for current and future research. Coordinated team activities will assist with timely assessment and early intervention for problems.

REFERENCES

Ahrens TS, Powers C (1990). Heart-lung transplantation. In: Smith SL, ed. *Tissue and Organ Transplantation: Implications for Professional Nursing Practice.* St. Louis: Mosby Year Book, 245–259.

Au J, Scott C, Hasan A, et al (1992). Bilateral sequential lung transplantation for septic lung disease: Surgical and physiologic advantages over heart-lung transplantation. *Transplant Proc.* 24:2652–2655.

Augustine S (1991). Organ and tissue transplantation. In: Gaedeke MK, et al, eds. *Organ and Tissue Transplantation: Nursing Care from Procurement Through Rehabilitation.* Philadelphia: Davis, 89–112.

Baum GL, Hershko EP (1989). Bronchiectasis. In: Baum GL, Wolinsky E, eds. *Textbook of Pulmonary Diseases.* Boston: Little Brown, 567–588.

Baumgartner WA (1990). Evaluation and management of the heart donor. In: Baumgartner WA, et al, eds. *Heart and Heart-Lung Transplantation.* Philadelphia: Saunders, 86–102.

Bjortuft O, Johansen B, Boe J, et al (1993). Daily home spirometry facilitates early detection of rejection in single lung transplant recipients with emphysema. *Eur Respir J.* 6:705–708.

Bolman RN, Shumway SJ, Estrin JA, Hertz MI (1991). Lung and heart-lung transplantation: Evolution and new implications, *Ann Surg.* 214:456–470.

Boychuck JE, Malen JF (1990). Lung transplantation. In: Smith SL, ed. *Tissue and Organ Transplantation: Implications for Professional Nursing Practice.* St. Louis: Mosby Year Book, 260–272.

Caine N, Sharples LD, Smyth R, et al (1991). Survival and quality of life of cystic fibrosis patients before and after heart-lung transplantation. *Transplant Proc.* 23:1203–1204.

Carr VH (1990). Managing the psychosocial responses of the transplant patient. In: Sigardson-Poor KM, Haggerty LM, eds. *Nursing Care of the Transplant Recipient.* Philadelphia: Saunders, 366–383.

Cary SS (1991). The pathology of heart and lung transplantation: An update. *J Clin Pathol.* 44:803–811.

Ciulli F, Tamm M, Dennis C, et al (1993). Donor-transmitted bacterial infection in heart-lung. *Transplant Proc.* 25:1155–1156.

Copeland JA (1990). Heart-lung and unilateral lung transplantation. In: Sigardson-Poor KM, Haggerty LM, eds. *Nursing Care of the Transplant Recipient.* Philadelphia: Saunders, 205–223.

Crystal RG, Bitterman PB, Rennard SI, et al (1984). Interstitial lung diseases of unknown cause. *N Engl J Med.* 310:235–244.

Deusch E, End A, Grimm M, et al (1993). Early bacterial infections in lung transplant recipients. *Chest.* 104:1412–1416.

Fishman AP (1992). Alpha-1-antitrypsin deficiency. In: Fishman AP. *Update: Pulmonary Diseases and Disorders.* New York: McGraw Hill, 19–35.

Friedman WF (1988). Congenital heart disease in infancy and childhood. In: Braunwald E, ed. *Heart Disease: A Textbook of Cardiovascular Medicine.* Philadelphia: Saunders, 941–1023.

Frist WH, Fox MD, Campbell PW, et al (1991). Cystic fibrosis treated with heart-lung transplantation: North American results. *Transplant Proc.* 23:1205–1206.

Frost AE, Keller CA, Cagle PT (1993). Severe ischemic injury to the proximal airway following lung transplantation: Immediate and long term effects on bronchial cartilage. *Chest.* 103:1899–1901.

Gallagher SL, Lawrence PA (1991). Heart-lung transplantation: The patient with cystic fibrosis. *Crit Care Nurs Q.* 13(4), 32.

Goldsmith MF (1990). Mother to child: First living donor lung transplant. *JAMA.* 264:2724.

Hardesty RL, Griffith BP (1987). Combined heart-lung transplantation. In: Myerowitz PD, ed. *Heart Transplantation.* New York: Futura, 126, 127.

Higgins N (1984). Epidemiology of COPD: State of the art. *Chest.* 85(Suppl):35–85.

Hirt SW, Hamm M, Schafers HJ, et al (1993). Patient rehabilitation following lung and heart-lung transplantation. *Transplant Proc.* 25:1296–1297.

Kaye MP (1993). The registry of the International Society for Heart and Lung Transplantation: Tenth official report—1993. *J Heart Lung Transplant.* 12:541–548.

Kirklin JW, Barratt-Boyes BG (1993). Primary cardiomyopathies and cardiac transplantation. In: Kirklin JW, ed. *Cardiac Surgery,* 2nd ed. New York: Churchill Livingstone, 1409–1432.

Kloner RA (1984). Pulmonary hypertension. In: Kloner RA, ed. *The Guide to Cardiology.* New York: Wiley, 475–482.

Levy RD, Ernst P, Levine SM, et al (1993). Exercise performance after lung transplantation. *J Heart Lung Transplant.* 12:27–33.

Madden B, Radley-Smith R, Hodson M, et al (1992). Medium-term results of heart and lung transplantation. *J Heart Lung Transplant.* 11:5241–5243.

Maride RA (1991). Psychiatric considerations in the cardiac transplant recipient. In: Hosenpud JD, et al eds. *Cardiac Transplantation: A Manual for Health Care Professionals.* New York: Springer-Verlag, 213–231.

McCarthy PM, Kirby TJ, White RD, et al (1992). Lung and heart-lung transplantation: The state of the art. *Cleveland Clinic J Med.* 59:307–316.

Muirhead J (1992). Heart and heart-lung transplantation. *Crit Care Nurs Clin North Am.* 4:97–109.

Novick RJ, Kaye MP, Patterson GA, et al (1993). Redo lung transplantation: A North American-European experience. *J Heart Lung Transplant.* 12:5–16.

Novitzky D, Cooper DKC (1990). Surgical technique of heterotopic heart transplantation. In: Cooper DKC, Novitzky D, eds. *The Transplantation and Replacement of Thoracic Organs: The Present Status of Biological and Mechanical Replacement of the Heart and Lungs.* Boston: Dordrecht Klower, 81–87.

Onofrio JM, Emory WB (1992). Selection of patients for lung transplantation. *Med Clin North Am.* 76:1207–1219.

Outlana BA, Higenbottom TW, Wallwork J (1992). Causes of exercise limitation after heart-lung transplantation. *Heart Lung Transplant.* 11:5244–5251.

Parquin F, Cerrina J, LeRoy F, et al (1993). Comparison of hemodynamic outcome of patients with pulmonary hypertension after double lung or heart–lung transplantation. *Transplant Proc.* 25:1156–1158.

Reitz BA (1990a). The history of heart and heart-lung transplantation. In: Baumgartner WA, et al eds. *Heart and Heart-Lung Transplantation.* Philadelphia: Saunders, 1–14.

Reitz BA (1990b). Heart and lung transplantation. In: Baumgartner WA, et al eds. *Heart and Heart-lung Transplantation.* Philadelphia: Saunders, 319–325.

Reitz BA, Wallwork J, Hunt SA, et al (1982). Heart-lung transplantation: A successful therapy for patients with pulmonary vascular disease. *N Engl J Med.* 306:557–563.

Renfroe DH (1992). Obstructive alterations in pulmonary function. In: Bullock BL, Rosendalh PB, eds. *Pathophysiology: Adaptations and Alterations in Function.* Philadelphia: Lippincott, 598–608.

Rubin LJ (1993). Primary pulmonary hypertension, *Chest.* 104:236–250.

Scott Hutter J, Stewart S, Higenbottom T, et al (1988). Heart-lung transplantation for cystic fibrosis. *Lancet.* 2:192–195.

Scott JP, Higenbottom TW, Clelland CA, et al (1990). The natural history of chronic rejection in heart-lung transplant recipients: A clinical, pathological and physiological review of 29 long-term survivors. *Transplant Proc.* 22:1474–1476.

Scott JP, Sharples L, Mullins P, et al (1991). Further studies on the natural history of obliterative bronchiolitis following heart-lung transplantation. *Transplant Proc.* 23:1201–1202.

Shennib H, Adoumie R, Noirclerc M (1992). Current status of lung transplantation for cystic fibrosis. *Arch Intern Med.* 152:1585–1588.

Shumway SJ, Hertz MI, Maynard R, et al (1993). Airway complications after lung and heart-lung transplantation. *Transplant Proc.* 25:1165–1166.

Smyth RL, Scott TW, Higenbottom B, et al (1990). The use of heart-lung transplantation in management of terminal respiratory complications of cystic fibrosis. *Transplant Proc.* 22:1472–1473.

Snider GL (1988). Chronic bronchitis and emphysema. In: Murray JF, Nadel JA, eds. *Textbook of Respiratory Medicine.* Philadelphia: Saunders, 1069–1106.

Swartz RO, Davis LA (1992). Cardiac transplantation. In: Vazquez M, et al eds. *Critical Care Nursing,* 2nd ed. Philadelphia: Saunders, 280–286.

Wallwork J ed. (1989). Indications for operation, patient selection and assessment. In: *Heart and Heart-Lung Transplantation.* Philadelphia: Saunders, 449–462.

Wilson SF, Thompson JM (1990). Infectious respiratory diseases. In: Wilson SF, Thompson JM, eds. *Respiratory Disorders.* St. Louis: Mosby Year Book, 186–194.

NURSING CARE PLAN 6–1. LUNG AND HEART AND LUNG TRANSPLANTATION

Nursing Diagnosis	Expected Outcomes	Nursing Interventions

Ineffective Airway Clearance
Related to
• Increased pulmonary secretions
• Anesthesia
• Pain
• Decreased mobility
 	
Impaired Gas Exchange
Related to
• Increased pulmonary secretions
	• Patient demonstrates effective coughing or other mechanism to remove airway secretions.
	• Patient maintains adequate gas exchange.
	• Patient reports decreased or absent dyspnea.
		• Frequently assess respiratory rate, effort, activity tolerance, and secretions.
		• Enhance airway clearance by
		  Placing the patient in the Fowler or side-lying position (lung transplant recipient should be transplant side up)
		  Instructing about and encouraging coughing and deep-breathing exercises.
		  Removing upper airway secretions and performing gentle suctioning if necessary.
		• Provide chest physiotherapy as ordered.
		• Give aerosol treatments as ordered.
		• Administer pain medication and therapy as needed. (patient-controlled analgesia per assessment).
		• Administer O_2 as needed.
		• Observe and report changes in amount, color, and quantity of sputum.
		(continued)

161

NURSING CARE PLAN 6–1. LUNG AND HEART AND LUNG TRANSPLANTATION (*continued*)

Nursing Diagnosis	Expected Outcomes	Nursing Interventions
High Risk for Infection	• Patient is free from bacterial and viral infections.	• Encourage pulmonary toilet activities as tolerated.
Related to		• Assess wound and invasive line sites according to protocol.
• Injection		• Assess temperature (elevations may be minor because of immunosuppression).
• Immunosuppression		• Mobilize patient as tolerated.
• Presence of invasive lines		• Provide wound and invasive line site care per protocol.
Defining Characteristics		• Disconnect invasive lines according to orders or protocol.
• Elevated temperature		
• Increased amount respiratory secretions		
• Purulent respiratory secretions		
• Redness, swelling, drainage from wound or invasive line sites		
Pain	• Patient expresses feelings of satisfactory pain management.	• Assess patient's pain level frequently by Observation of symptoms.
Related to		Discussion with patient about his or her pain.
• Surgical incision		• Discuss appropriate treatment with physician.
Defining Characteristics		• Implement pain management therapy according to orders.
• Complaints of pain		• Implement non-narcotic therapies such as relaxation techniques or music therapy, according to patient tolerance.
• Grimacing		
• Respiratory splinting		
• Inadequate coughing and deep breathing		

Altered Myocardial Tissue Perfusion

Related to

- Dysrhythmia
- Hyperthermia
- Preservation ischemia
- Hypovolemia

- Myocardial tissue perfusion is adequate or improved by the time the patient is transferred from the ICU.

- Monitor patient's cardiac output by

  Taking vital signs, including heart rate and rhythm, blood pressure

  Assessing pulses

  Assessing oxygenation status

  Calculating cardiac output and index, if pulmonary artery catheter is present

  Titrating vasoactive medications according to protocol

  Monitoring temporary pacing as necessary

  Monitoring intake and output

  Monitoring cardiac enzyme levels as necessary

  Monitoring patient complaints of chest

  pain or discomfort

7

Liver Transplantation

JoAnn Coleman
Barbara V. Wise
Melinda Mendoza
Cynthia A. Kaczmarek

The first liver transplant in a human became a reality in 1963. Twenty years later The Consensus Development Conference of the National Institutes of Health recognized liver transplantation as an accepted therapy for irreversible chronic liver disease. The number of patients receiving liver transplants has increased steadily since that time.

INDICATIONS

Patients who are referred for liver transplantation fall into three categories: (1) those with irreversible chronic liver disease; (2) those with primary malignant tumors of the liver and biliary tree; and (3) those with fulminant hepatic failure. Bilirubin concentrations greater then 10 mg/dL, a serum albumin concentration less than 2.5 mg/dL, and a prothrombin time (PT) greater than 5 seconds beyond the control value are clinical features predictive of the need for a liver transplant. Other criteria include incapacitating hepatic encephalopathy, recurrent variceal bleeding not controlled by sclerotherapy, intractable ascites refractory to medical therapy, and recurrent spontaneous bacterial peritonitis.

Cirrhosis due to a variety of causes is the leading indication for transplantation in adult patients. Primary biliary cirrhosis, primary sclerosing cholangitis, chronic active hepatitis, and autoimmune or cryptogenic cirrhosis are some of the causes of cirrhosis. Biliary atresia, Alagille syndrome, and inborn errors of metabolism such as α-1-antitrypsin deficiency are frequent indications for a liver transplant in children. A patient who is considered for a liver transplant usually has end-stage liver disease for which all other forms of therapy have failed.

LIVER DISEASES

Primary Biliary Cirrhosis

Primary biliary cirrhosis is an autoimmune disorder that causes slow, progressive destruction of bile ducts in the liver (Coleman et al, 1991). Most patients are middle-aged women who have no symptoms and who are able to lead active lives for a long period of time. Fatigue and pruritus are the usual presenting symptoms. At the time of diagnosis, pruritus may be accompanied by jaundice in 20% of the patients; 50 to 60% are without jaundice (Caplan, 1993). Other early symptoms include unexplained weight loss with right upper quadrant discomfort. The diagnosis is confirmed by a liver biopsy. However, an elevated alkaline phosphatase level and the presence of mitochondrial antibodies are clinically significant findings. Liver transplantation is considered to be an effective treatment of primary biliary cirrhosis; the success rate is 80 to 90% (Caplan, 1993).

Primary Sclerosing Cholangitis

Primary sclerosing cholangitis (PSC) is a chronic disease of unknown causation characterized by irregular narrowing of the bile ducts due to inflammation and scarring (Coleman et al, 1991). The disease is more common in men than women and is usually associated with inflammatory bowel disease, particularly chronic ulcerative colitis.

The clinical presentation of PSC include intermittent jaundice, pruritus, abdominal pain, fever, and chills. Patients with PSC have no symptoms, or exhibit clinical signs and symptoms that can lead to portal hypertension, ascites, variceal bleeding, and encephalopathy (Wiesner et al, 1993). Other conditions, such as common bile duct stones, hepatic duct stones, congenital strictures and cysts, cholangiocarcinoma, and malformations from previous biliary operations, can obscure the diagnosis of PSC. Definitive diagnosis is made by endoscopic retrograde cholangiopancreatography (ERCP) (Johlin, 1992).

The effectiveness of orthotopic liver transplantation for end-stage liver disease due to PSC has not been proved. However, it is recommended that a liver transplant be performed because PSC can progress to a malignant condition such as cholangiocarcinoma (Marsh et al, 1988).

Biliary Atresia

Biliary atresia is a congenital disease of unknown causation possibly related to a viral infection during intrauterine development or soon after birth (Sherlock & Dooley, 1993b). Biliary atresia results in inflammation and partial or complete absence of bile ducts. The infant becomes jaundiced by the first week of life and has an enlarged and hardened liver, pruritus, ascites, clay-colored stools, and tea-colored urine. Differential diagnosis of biliary atresia is made by liver biopsy and TcHida scan. However, it is confirmed during surgery by an intra-operative cholangiogram.

The most successful palliative treatment of biliary atresia is a hepatoportoen-terostomy or the Kasai procedure. This procedure uses the infant's own intestine to form a new conduit to drain the bile from the liver into the intestine (Coleman et al, 1991). However, 80% of patients eventually need a liver transplant because of recurrent cholangitis, progressive portal hypertension, and eventual liver failure.

Budd–Chiari Syndrome

The Budd–Chiari syndrome is hepatic venous outflow obstruction that results in congestion of the liver. It is manifested by abdominal pain, ascites, and an enlarged liver. The causes of Budd–Chiari syndrome can be attributed to myeloproliferative disorders, an increased thrombotic tendency associated with oral contraceptives and pregnancy, hematologic disorders such as polycythemia rubra vera and paroxysmal nocturnal hemoglobinemia, congenital hepatic venous webs, trauma, and tumors (Henderson, 1992).

Budd–Chiari syndrome can be acute or chronic. It can lead to portal hypertension with esophageal variceal bleeding and eventually liver failure if left untreated. The treatment of choice is a portosystemic shunt to decompress the congested liver. For patients with irreversible liver failure, however, a liver transplant with chronic anticoagulation is highly recommended (Halff et al, 1990).

Malignant Tumors

Primary hepatocelluar carcinoma (PHC) is a fatal malignant tumor that arises in the parenchymal cells of the liver. Worldwide, hepatitis B and C are risk factors for the development of PHC (Deutsch & Ahren, 1992). Other causes of the disease include environmental carcinogens such as aflatoxin, Thorotrast dye, contraceptives, steroids, and hormones such as estrogens. Cirrhosis from chronic liver injury appears to be the most important factor in the development of PHC (Deutsch & Ahren, 1992).

Patients usually present with fatigue, weight loss, right upper quadrant abdominal pain, and an abdominal mass. Measurement of serum α-fetoprotein levels, which is markedly elevated in patients with PHC, has been widely used as a screening test in populations at high risk for the disease.

Patients with PHC who cannot be treated do not survive more than 6 months (Coleman et al, 1991). The only curative treatment and hope for long-term survival is surgical resection with complete removal of the tumor. Transplantation for malignant liver tumors was performed in the early era of liver transplantation. However, recurrence rates of malignant hepatic tumors after transplantation have been disappointing. The recurrence rate of hepatocellular carcinoma is 40 to 75% (Hart et al, 1990). Lower recurrence rates have been noted in patients with fibrolamellar carcinoma and in patients in whom PHC was an incidental finding during transplantation for a nonneoplastic disease (Olthoff et al, 1990).

Treatment of malignant hepatobiliary tumors by liver transplantation continues to be controversial. Iwatsuki and associates (1991) reported a comparative analysis of patients with hepatocellular carcinoma treated with subtotal hepatic resection as opposed to liver transplantation. Recurrence rates were high in both groups. The study also concluded that better survival results will most likely be obtained with the use of nonsurgical anticancer therapy before and after surgical removal of the diseased liver. The study supported transplantation as superior to resection for patients with cirrhosis and for selected patients with tumor confined to the liver and not amenable to resection (Olthoff et al, 1990).

Carr and associates (1993) used pretransplant intrahepatic arterial chemotherapy for patients with extensive unresectable tumors. The therapy produced a statistically significant difference in survival rates and recurrence rates 1 year after transplantation.

It is believed that progress in preventing the recurrence of viral hepatitis and malignant hepatic tumors awaits the development of effective, specific antiviral and chemotherapeutic agents (Kahan, 1991). Careful patient selection is crucial to the success of either therapy.

Cholangiocarcinoma is a malignant tumor of the extrahepatic or intrahepatic biliary epithelium (Thung & Gerber, 1992). It is often found in patients with PSC. Other causes include fibrocystic disease, Thoratrast dye, anabolic steroids, and clonorchiasis (Sherlock & Dooley, 1993). The clinical features mimic those of hepatocellular carcinoma. However, α-fetoprotein level is not elevated (Sherlock & Dooley, 1993a).

Patients with cholangiocarcinoma appear to have a worse outcome than patients with PHC. Jenkins and associates (1989) reported a median survival time of 8 months and a 1-year survival rate of only 36% among patients who underwent transplants.

α-1-Antitrypsin Deficiency

α-1-antitrypsin deficiency is a metabolic disorder of the liver characterized by a decreased production of α-1-antitrypsin, a glycoprotein made by the liver. The deficiency is inherited in an autosomal recessive pattern and can lead to liver disorders such as neonatal hepatitis and cryptogenic cirrhosis and pulmonary disorders such as emphysema (Mezey, 1988).

Hepatitis

Hepatitis is an inflammation of the liver that can be acute or chronic. Hepatitis can be caused by a virus, a drug reaction, or alcohol abuse (Marx, 1993; Wright & Shelton, 1992). Five types of hepatitis have been identified by researchers.

Hepatitis A (infectious hepatitis) is transmitted primarily by the fecal-oral route. A high incidence of this virus is reported in underdeveloped areas that have poor sanitation and overcrowding. Hepatitis A rarely leads to chronic hepatitis or cirrhosis, but it may lead to fulminant hepatic failure in rare instances (Marx, 1993).

Hepatitis B virus (HBV) is transmitted in blood and body fluids and is commonly known as serum hepatitis. The virus is transmitted in a variety of ways, including needle-sharing, sexual relations, needlesticks, and blood transfusions. After a person is exposed to HBV, an infection occurs that usually involves some type of hepatocellular damage. In some cases, fulminant hepatic failure can occur.

Hepatitis C, also known as a non-A, non-B hepatitis, or posttransfusion hepatitis can lead to cirrhosis of the liver. It is transmitted in the same manner as hepatitis B and also can lead to fulminant hepatic failure.

Hepatitis D has been identified as being a delta virus that usually occurs as a co-infection with hepatitis B (Marx, 1993; Wright & Shelton, 1992). Hepatitis E has been identified in developing countries where there is a resistance to hepatitis A. It is transmitted enterically, usually through fecal contamination of water (Marx, 1993).

Alcoholic hepatitis, also called fatty hepatitis, Laennec cirrhosis, or nutritional cirrhosis is caused by chronic alcohol use. Injury occurs because the liver metabolizes alcohol instead of carbohydrates and glucose (Wright & Shelton, 1992). This results in fat deposition in the liver cells. The end result is hepatocellular destruction and cirrhosis. Alcoholics who are in need of a liver transplant are carefully screened to determine if there is a chance of recidivism. Each institution has a different policy specifying the length of abstinence required before transplantation. Data are not available to correlate length of abstinence and recidivism.

EVALUATION

The liver transplant evaluation is a complex process that has a multidisciplinary approach. This ensures that the evaluation is complete and nothing is missed. The evaluation has several purposes. First, the patient's liver disease is confirmed and a determination is made as to the severity of the disease. Second, health problems are identified and corrected so that the patient can be in the optimal state of health before the operation. Third, the patient is evaluated for any contraindications to transplantation, such as a cancerous lesion outside the liver parenchyma, alcoholism, or a positive test for the human immunodeficiency virus (HIV). During the transplant evaluation, a complete social and psychologic history is taken to determine if the patient has any problems that need to be addressed, such as depression or lack of family support.

Once it is determined that the patient is an appropriate candidate for liver transplantation, the patient is placed on the United Network for Organ Sharing (UNOS) waiting list. The patient is listed by blood type and status. Status is determined by the transplant surgeon in conjunction with the patient's hepatologist. There are four categories for listing a patient in need of liver transplant, as determined by UNOS.

Status 4 is the most critical. The patient is in the intensive care unit (ICU) and meets one of the following criteria. The patient is undergoing mechanical ventilation to protect the airway; is receiving dialysis because of renal dysfunction; has a PT greater than 25 seconds and rising; has Grade III to IV encephalopathy; is receiving vasopressors for maintenance of blood pressure; has uncontrollable variceal bleeding; or has primary graft non-function after a transplant. A status 3 patient is hospitalized and is receiving medical therapy to manage end-stage liver disease. Status 2 patients are at home waiting but under close medical supervision. Status 1 patients need a liver transplant but are currently able to perform activities of daily living.

Depending on his or her blood group and size, a patient can wait more than a year for a donor organ. At our institution, if a patient has blood type O, the average wait is 14 to 16 months. Patients who are in need of a liver transplant should be referred early in the disease to centers that perform this service in order to be activated on the national waiting list and gain waiting time.

There are absolute and relative contraindications to liver transplantation. Absolute contraindications include those associated with a high morbidity and mortality, such as advanced cardiac and respiratory disease. As liver transplantation continues to evolve, the absolute and relative contraindications have changed (Smith & Ciferni, 1990). Portal venous thrombosis is no longer an anatomic barrier to the procedure. A variety of maneuvers are used to remedy this situation, such as interposition of grafts of donor iliac arteries and veins.

A poor outcome is expected in patients who undergo transplants for viral hepatitis and malignant hepatic disease. Hart and associates (1990) reported recurrence of hepatitis B in 11 of 14 patients who survived longer than 2 months after a transplant. Recurrence of disease occurs 4 to 64 weeks after transplantation. Similar findings were observed by Read and colleagues (1991) in 45 liver transplant recipients who survived more than 60 days postoperatively. Thirty-seven of the 45 patients had reinfection of the graft with HBV. The recurrence rate of hepatitis B after liver transplantation varies according to the viral load and the clinical presentation of hepatitis B. Higher recurrence rates are reported among patients with chronic hepatitis (81%) than patients with chronic hepatitis and co-existent hepatitis D (16%). New HBV infections have been found in a small number of patients after transplants. A potential source is the donor (Lake et al, 1993). Samuel and associates (1991) suggested that HBV DNA positivity detected by molecular hybridization before the transplant is a useful indication of recurrent hepatitis B after transplantation. They reported that 13 of 14 patients who were positive for HBV DNA had reinfections, whereas 6 of 18 patients who were negative for HBV DNA had recurrences of HBV infections.

Hepatitis C does not occur as often as hepatitis B (Lake et al, 1993; Haagsma et al, 1991). Some possible explanations include a cause other than hepatitic C virus (HCV) because the lack of a specific diagnostic marker for HCV could have led to misdiagnosis of the original disease; the role of immunosuppression in the expression of the antibody response; or the possibility that the liver transplant is a cure of the viral infection (Read et al, 1991). Hepatitis C is responsible for most cases of hepatitis noted after a transplant. The most promising treatment of posttransplant hepatitis B or hepatitis C is hepatitis B immune globulin (HBIG).

SURGICAL PROCEDURES

Donor-Liver Recovery

A system of multiorgan procurement has been developed to recover as many organs as possible (heart, lungs, kidneys, pancreas, and liver) from each organ donor. During recovery of the liver, careful hemodynamic support of the donor is necessary to ensure optimal organ preservation and function (Staschak & Zamberlan, 1990). The goals of liver procurement are to (1) recognize an organ unacceptable for transplantation; (2) perform a technically perfect operation; (3) avoid warm ischemia; and (4) minimize cold ischemia of the donor liver (Smith & Ciferni, 1990). Both the donor and recipient operations require special training with an emphasis on recognition of anatomic variations, meticulous technique, and attention to detail.

In the donor hepatectomy, a midline incision from the sternal notch to the pubis allows wide exposure for careful visual inspection of and access to the abdominal and thoracic organs. When the donor liver is deemed suitable for transplantation, the recipient hospital is notified. The surgical team then begins simultaneous preparation of the liver transplant recipient for removal of the diseased liver (recipient hepatectomy).

Surgical removal of the donor liver involves isolating the liver from its supplementary structures by releasing the liver from the ligaments that secure it to the diaphragm and the anterior abdominal wall and dissecting the blood vessels and bile duct. The liver is flushed with cold preservation solution to prevent ischemia. When the liver is removed from the donor, it is placed on ice in a sterile plastic bag, put into a cooler, and transported to the receiving hospital (Zitelli, 1986). Although it may be preserved in this manner for up to 24 hours, the liver should be transplanted as soon as possible (Staschak & Zamberlan, 1990). Additional blood vessels are harvested from the donor because they may be needed for possible repair of the recipient's vessels. The recipient surgical team is kept informed of all phases of the donor hepatectomy, which enables them to plan the sequencing of the recipient operation (Staschak & Zamberlan, 1990).

Transplant Procedure

The orthotopic liver transplant takes 8 to 12 hours to complete and involves the removal of the recipient's diseased liver followed by implantation of the donor-liver allograft. The recipient is prepared by the insertion of multiple invasive monitoring devices and large-bore intravenous lines for rapid fluid and blood replacement. Proper padding of body parts and patient positioning on the operating table are critical to prevent peripheral nerve injuries and pressure-related tissue damage. The recipient is placed on a pressure diffusing mattress. Additional padding is placed under the sacrum, both heels, and the elbows. Because of the extended length of the procedure, preventive measures are taken to promote circulation and maintain adequate body temperature. Each of the recipient's legs and arms and the head are wrapped in plastic bags to maintain an adequate temperature.

Patients with chronic liver disease usually have a considerable degree of portal hypertension and coagulopathy, making hemorrhage a major risk during the recipient hepatectomy. Patients who have had previous upper abdominal operations often have adhesions vascularized with fragile collateral vessels. These fragile vessels contribute to the risk of hemorrhage. Patients with no previous operations or minimal portal hypertension may have little problem with this phase of the operation (Smith & Ciferni, 1990).

The recipient hepatectomy begins with opening of the abdomen with a bilateral subcostal incision and a midline extension, the so-called Mercedes incision. Before the diseased liver is removed, careful identification of the hepatic artery, portal vein, and common bile duct is performed. These structures are not divided until the donor liver has arrived in the operating room and has been carefully reinspected (Staschak & Zamberlan, 1990). The patient and family must be informed before consenting to the operation that the procedure may have to be aborted at this point if the condition of the donor or the donor liver deteriorates (Smith & Ciferni, 1990).

The recipient hepatectomy begins when the surgical team is assured that the donor liver is acceptable for transplantation. Vascular structures are clamped in the following order: hepatic artery, portal vein, suprahepatic vena cava, and infrahepatic vena cava. The diseased liver is removed en bloc. A venovenous bypass system may be used to allow normal hemodynamic values to be maintained while the recipient is without a liver. This is known as the anhepatic phase. Blood is drained through large-bore cannulas placed in the left common femoral vein and the portal vein and attached to a Y connector. A nonheparinized centrifugal pump provides venous return of systemic blood from the lower part of the body and abdominal viscera through a cannula placed in the left axillary or internal jugular vein. This bypass system helps prevent venous hypertension, circulatory instability, and excessive bleeding in adult liver recipients (Shaw et al, 1985; Griffith et al, 1985).

The donor liver is prepared for implantation at a back table by a second surgical team during the recipient hepatectomy. With the venovenous bypass system in place and the diseased liver removed, the donor liver can be inserted. The vascular anastomoses are performed in the following sequence: the suprahepatic inferior vena cava, the infrahepatic inferior vena cava, the portal vein, and the hepatic artery. After these anastomoses are completed, the portal venous blood flow is restored to the liver before the bypass system is discontinued. Hemostasis is obtained and the hepatic arterial anastomosis is completed. The anastomoses are inspected for any leaks before the biliary tree is reconstructed.

The biliary anastomosis is the final step. Anastomosis of the donor common bile duct to the recipient common bile duct, called a choledochocholedochostomy, is routinely performed using a T-tube to stent the anastomosis. Once the biliary anastomosis is completed, a cholangiogram is obtained to assess patency and to look for bile leaks. The T-tube is brought out the abdominal wall through a stab wound in the right upper quadrant and attached to a bile bag for external drainage. If the recipient's common bile duct cannot be used because of absent or diseased bile ducts (as in biliary atresia or sclerosing cholangitis), the donor common bile duct is anastomosed to a Roux-en-Y limb of jejunum, called a choledochojejunostomy (Fig 7-1). Three closed wound drains are strategically placed. One drain is placed on top of the right lobe of the liver, one drain on top of the left lobe of the liver, and one drain under the liver near the biliary anastomosis. These drains are brought out of the abdominal wall through stab wounds in the right abdomen. The abdominal incision is stapled closed, and the sites of the venovenous bypass shunts in the left femoral vein and left axilla or jugular vein are sutured. The recipient is taken directly to the ICU after the operation.

POSTOPERATIVE CARE

Postoperative care of a liver-transplant recipient can be categorized into three phases—the critical phase, the transitional phase, and the recovery phase. Nursing management requires assessment and problem-solving unique to each phase (see Nursing Care Plan 7–1, p 194).

Critical Phase
The critical phase begins when the patient leaves the operating room and enters the ICU. The ICU stay is usually 48 to 72 hours if there are no postoperative complica-

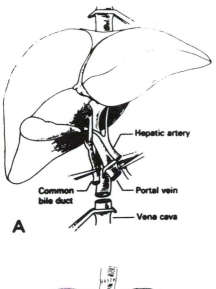

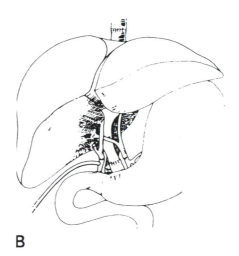

A

B

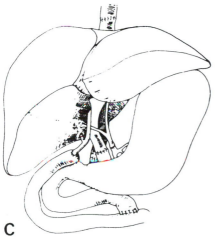

C

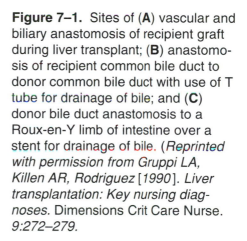

Figure 7–1. Sites of (**A**) vascular and biliary anastomosis of recipient graft during liver transplant; (**B**) anastomosis of recipient common bile duct to donor common bile duct with use of T tube for drainage of bile; and (**C**) donor bile duct anastomosis to a Roux-en-Y limb of intestine over a stent for drainage of bile. (*Reprinted with permission from Gruppi LA, Killen AR, Rodriguez [1990]. Liver transplantation: Key nursing diagnoses.* Dimensions Crit Care Nurse. 9:272–279.

tions. The nurse caring for the patient must carefully assess and monitor the patient to prevent complications. A liver transplant is a very complex operation. It puts the patient under a great deal of physiologic stress that is attributed not only to the complexity of the operation but also to the prolonged period of anesthesia, venovenous bypass, hypothermia, and hemorrhage that can occur during the intraoperative period (Smith & Ciferni, 1990). Preoperative conditions such as portal hypertension and coagulopathies can further complicate the postoperative course. During this time, the patient also undergoes massive fluid resuscitation, which can result in edema and fluid shifts. The patient also comes from the operating room with a variety of tubes and drains, including a central line, a pulmonary artery catheter, a T-tube, a Foley catheter, an arterial line, and several closed wound drains. The patient is intubated and mechanically ventilated. All this equipment helps the nurse to carefully monitor the patient for any sudden change in hemodynamic status.

Postoperative care of a liver-transplant recipient focuses on monitoring graft function, maintaining fluid and electrolyte balance, and supporting renal, respiratory, and cardiopulmonary function (Klein AS, unpublished, 1990). Emphasis should be placed on prevention of infection and rejection of the graft.

Liver Function

Graft function is monitored by bile production, which should begin in the operating room when the liver is revascularized. Bile is inspected through the T-tube, which is externalized during the immediately postoperative period. Measurements of bile drainage are obtained regularly. Color and consistency are inspected and documented. Normal bile is dark gold in color and somewhat sticky. Bile that is dark green with a muddy consistency can indicate a problem with liver function, such as ischemia or necrosis. The absence of bile is an indication of primary non-function (PNF) of the liver. Other manifestations of PNF are encephalopathy, elevated transaminase and bilirubin levels, uncorrectable coagulopathy, and hypoglycemia (Greig et al, 1989). Retransplantation is the only remedy.

Pediatric patients have very small bile ducts, which precludes the placement of a T-tube. Therefore, bile production is monitored with observation of bilirubin levels. If the levels are increased, indicating the obstruction of bile flow, stent placement or revision of the biliary tree may be required.

The most sensitive indicators of liver function are the measurement of PT and partial thromboplastin time (PTT) (Smith & Ciferni, 1990). In an adequately functioning liver the PT and PTT should decrease and return to normal values within the first few days after the operation. An increase in coagulation time indicates impaired synthetic function of the liver. It is important to ensure that no heparin is used in the preparation of maintenance fluid in arterial and central lines or pulmonary artery catheters, since coagulation times are already prolonged and the patient is already anticoagulated.

Liver enzymes and bilirubin can be expected to decrease to within normal ranges during the postoperative period. Measurement of liver enzymes such as transaminase enzymes alanine aminotransferase (ALT[SGOT]) and aspartate aminotransferase (AST[SGPT]), alkaline phosphatase, total and direct bilirubin, potassium, and glucose are used to monitor function. A sudden increase in the transaminases or bilirubin can be an indication of hepatic artery thrombosis (HAT). Should this occur, an emergency ultrasonographic duplex scan is needed to determine patency of the vessels (Smith & Ciferni, 1990). If HAT is diagnosed, a thrombectomy is the first line of treatment. If this is unsuccessful, the patient will need to be retransplanted.

If liver dysfunction continues for any reason and is not reversible with medical therapy, the only alternative is retransplantation.

Fluid and Electrolyte Abnormalities

It is not uncommon to see hypokalemia that requires replacement therapy during the postoperative period. This should be interpreted as a favorable sign. Hypokalemia is related to flushing with potassium-rich preservation solution, which causes an os-motic shift of potassium from the interstitial space into the cell.

Hyperkalemia, on the other hand, indicates cell death with release of intracellu-lar potassium into the bloodstream. When potassium levels are greater than 6.0 mmol/L, insulin may be administered to force potassium to re-enter the cell (Smith & Ciferni, 1990).

Hyperglycemia indicates that the new liver is functioning and able to convert glu-cose into glycogen and store it. A continuous insulin infusion may be required as a temporary measure to correct problems with hyperglycemia (Smith & Ciferni, 1990).

Metabolic complications in children include problems with hypoglycemia, hypocalcemia, hypokalemia, and hypomagnesemia. Hypoglycemia may be an early in-dication of PNF of the liver. Hypocalcemia is found in children who require massive transfusion of stored blood. Hypokalemia is related to the preservation solution, di-uretics, steroid therapy, and hypothermia.

Sommerauer and associates (1988) reported a high incidence of hypomagne-semia in children who received cyclosporine. Similarly, hypomagnesemia has been re-ported in clinical trials with FK506 (prograf). The children required both intravenous and oral replacement therapy. The hypomagnesemia may be related to preexisting chronic malnutrition, a frequent finding in children with chronic liver failure (Gruppi et al, 1990).

Fluid and electrolyte balance is carefully monitored. Patients may have a meta-bolic alkalosis that is often the result of blood replacement therapy. Citrates from blood products are often metabolized into bicarbonate. This can contribute to diffi-culty in weaning the patient from mechanical ventilation. In the presence of metabolic alkalosis, the patient usually hyperventilates and becomes hypercarbic (Smith & Ciferni, 1990). Metabolic alkalosis can be corrected with an intravenous infusion of hydrochloric acid.

Fluid volume management is a serious problem in the pediatric group because of the large surface area compared to weight (infants 0.1 m^2/kg). The large ratio leads to insensible water loss and an increased metabolic rate. Infants and children under-going operations experience fluid shifts from the intracellular and intravascular spaces into the peritoneum. Careful monitoring of output from wound drains, central ven-ous pressure (CVP), and abdominal girth is an essential part of nursing care. It is important to obtain as small a volume of blood as necessary for laboratory analy-sis; total blood volume for a child who weighs less than 10 kg is only 750 mL (Oleinik, 1990).

Neurologic Function

Neurologic complications can occur in patients with end-stage liver disease. In the im-mediately postoperative period, the neurologic status of the patient is an indicator of graft function. An hourly neurologic assessment is performed to determine if there are any changes in the patient's level of consciousness. Serum ammonia levels should be monitored. Elevated ammonia levels occur when the liver is unable to convert am-monia to urea, which can indicate the extent of hepatic injury and in turn affect the patient's level of consciousness. Neurologic assessment on the first postoperative day may be difficult because of the residual effects of anesthesia.

The neurologic assessment of children includes accurate Glascow Coma Scale Scores (revised for children younger than 5 years of age) and documentation of seizure activity. The development of seizures has been linked to hyponatremia, alkalosis, and use of immunosuppressive agents.

The brain of a developing child is highly vulnerable during the first few years of life, and this vulnerability may play a role in predicting long-term outcome after liver transplantation. The duration of the liver disease and deficiencies of fat-soluble vitamins A, D, E, and K may adversely affect intelligence. Stewart and associates (1988) compared children with early-onset and children with late-onset liver disease. They found that children with early-onset liver disease had lower scores on verbal and standardized intelligence tests. In addition, the children were of shorter stature and had a smaller head circumference. In another study, Stewart and associates (1991) compared the neuropsychologic outcomes of pediatric liver transplant recipients with those of children who had cystic fibrosis, a life-threatening chronic illness. The liver transplant group scored considerably lower in the area of academic functioning. Children who had undergone liver transplants had difficulty with higher-level abilities such as abstract thinking, logical analysis, and memory.

The reasons for the delay are not clearly understood. It may be the result of frequent absence from school or lack of supportive services in the school. Stewart and colleagues (1991) found that less than 30% of children with liver transplants had been referred for rehabilitation services. Prevention and treatment of developmental delays requires early recognition and referral to appropriate school services or an infant and toddler program.

Respiratory Function

The patient arrives in the ICU intubated. Mechanical ventilation is required in the immediately postoperative period to maintain adequate lung volume and normal gas exchange. As the patient begins to awaken from anesthesia, weaning from the ventilator is begun. The patient is usually extubated within 24 hours of admission to the ICU. Chest radiographs are taken—every 8 hours on day 1, then daily—to assess for infiltrates or pleural effusions. Right-sided pleural effusion is common because of subdiaphragmatic manipulation during the operation (Miller, 1988). Continuous pulse oximetry estimates the patient's ability to maintain adequate oxygenation of tissues without mechanical support. Good pulmonary toilet is emphasized, and the patient is encouraged and coached to cough and deep breathe and to use an incentive spirometer. Severe pulmonary complications are often observed in patients who were noted to have pulmonary compromise in the preoperative phase. Pleural effusions, lung disease, or excessive ascites may affect normal breathing and gas exchange. These patients often require longer periods of intubation and are more difficult to wean from the ventilator. Should a patient reach a point at which he or she needs continuous mechanical ventilatory support, a tracheostomy is considered.

Most children who have had a liver transplant have pulmonary compromise. Children are intubated and require assisted ventilation for an average of 3 days

(Sommerauer et al, 1988; McHugh, 1987). Younger children require higher-pressure support for ventilation. Pulmonary edema and atelectasis are frequent radiographic findings related to placement of a large organ in the subphrenic space and movement of ascitic fluid across the diaphragm.

Immunosuppression

Immunosuppressive therapy is begun in the preoperative phase. Immunosuppressive therapy usually consists of steroids, azathioprine, and cyclosporine. Immunosuppressive agents and their dosages vary among institutions. Steroids and azathioprine are administered intravenously in the postoperative period. These medications are converted to the oral route as the patient is able to tolerate oral liquids. Azathioprine is an antimetabolite that interferes with antibody production. One of the most common side effects of azathioprine therapy is bone marrow suppression; therefore white blood cell (WBC) counts should be closely monitored. If the WBC count is less than 2000 cells/mm³, azathioprine should be discontinued.

Cyclosporine is started in the preoperative period unless the patient has impaired renal function. Cyclosporine is administered intravenously and gradually converted to oral therapy when the patient is able to tolerate oral medications. Cyclosporine inhibits the specific T cells that respond to transplant antigens. The primary side effect of cyclosporine is nephrotoxicity. Nursing assessment includes careful monitoring of serum urea nitrogen and creatinine levels and daily measurement of weight, blood pressure, and urine output. The dose of cyclosporine may need to be adjusted to preserve renal function. Patients who are intolerant of cyclosporine because of impaired renal function, hirsutism, gingival hyperplasia, and hyperbilirubinemia may receive FK506. FK506 is a relatively new immunosuppressant agent that is still under study. FK506 has a mechanism of action similar to that of cyclosporine, but it is a more potent drug, requiring smaller doses to achieve the same level of immunosuppression as cyclosporine (Payne, 1992).

Infection

Infection continues to be a common problem after a transplant. Most patients are placed in protective isolation for the first 24 hours. Routine surveillance cultures for bacterial and viral organisms are obtained from wound-drain, urine, throat, and blood specimens. Patients receive prophylactic broad-spectrum antibiotics for 2 days to cover anaerobic and aerobic organisms. Strict sterile technique is used by the nurse when suctioning, handling wound drains, or providing wound care (Gruppi et al, 1990; Miller, 1988). Maintenance of skin integrity is important in the prevention of infection because any open area can be a source of infection. Hand-washing is an important and easy way to prevent the spread of infection. Water and foam mattresses may reduce pressure areas for patients who are immobile. Passive and active range-of-motion exercises should be initiated in the ICU.

The most frequent sites of bacterial infection are wound and operative sites. Gram-negative organisms are the most frequent bacteria found. Several factors contribute to the development of postoperative bacterial infections: a large abdominal incision, inadequate blood supply to the transplanted liver, invasive catheters and wound drains, and poorly functioning liver tissue. Release of gastrointestinal bacteria may cause systemic bacteremia (Vargo & Rudy, 1989). Most institutions have a protocol for the routine monitoring of body fluids in order to prevent and treat infections early.

A liver-transplant recipient is at risk for fungal infection. Disruption of the biliary tree or intestine causes the release of yeast from the gastrointestinal tract. Patients with autoimmune hepatitis who are given high doses of steroids in the preoperative period are at risk for acquiring a fungal infection. Two fungal organisms recognized in this population include *Candida albicans* and *Aspergillus*. Several factors associated with an increased risk for fungal infection include long-term administration of posttransplant antibiotics, bacterial infections, and the number of steroid boluses administered within 2 months of transplantation to treat rejection episodes (Vargo & Rudy, 1989).

Viral infection is a major threat to transplant patients. They are at risk for primary disease or a reactivation of a latent infection. Sources of viral infection include herpes zoster, Epstein-Barr virus (EBV), and cytomegalovirus (CMV). EBV infection may be manifested as a mild case of infectious mononucleosis or as severe lymphoprolifera-tive lesions (Vargo & Rudy, 1989). Recipients who are seronegative and receive a seropositive organ should receive intravenous immunoglobulin (IVIG) prophylacti-cally and undergo surveillance cultures to monitor for the development of CMV dis-ease. If the patient's CMV status changes, aggressive therapy with ganciclovir and reduced immunosuppression should be initiated (Broelsch et al, 1988; Superina et al, 1990; Tracey, 1992).

Cardiovascular Function

Cardiovascular complications include hypovolemia and hypertension. Right- and left-sided heart pressures and cardiac output are measured with a pulmonary artery catheter to facilitate the titration of fluids and vasoactive drugs. Liver-transplant pa-tients often have a high cardiac output and a low systemic resistance (Shaw et al, 1989). Chronic portal hypertension produces low right ventricular pressures. Large volumes of fluid and blood products infused during liver transplantation alter the cardiac output by increasing the work load of the right side of the heart.

Hypertension is commonly seen in the postoperative period. It is attributed to the stress of the operation as well as to hypervolemia, pain, and hypothermia (Smith & Ciferni, 1990). Hypertension is usually most severe in the first week after transplantation. The cause of this phenomenon is unclear; it is thought to be cyclosporine-related (Staschak & Zamberlan, 1990).

Hypotension that occurs in the immediately postoperative period is related to hy-povolemia. Factors that contribute to hypovolemia are massive fluid shifts related to an abdominal procedure, reaccumulation of ascites, and general malnutrition. Hypo-volemia is managed with volume expanders and blood products. Reexploration and repair of a bleeding site may be necessary if there is persistent hemorrhage (Smith & Ciferni, 1990).

The hypertension found in children who receive transplants is quite different from that in adults. The cause is probably multifactorial and may involve the release of angiotensin, a substance formed by the interaction of renin with angiotensin produced in the liver. Angiotensin is a powerful vasoconstrictor that is stimulated by a decrease in sodium and water. The combination of the renin-angiotensin mechanism and administration of steroids and cyclosporine results in an increase in blood pressure. The hypertension appears to be unrelated to pain, which is usually managed by continuous narcotic infusion or patient controlled analgesia. Hypertension has not been related to excessive fluid volume, which would be reflected in an elevated CVP (normal reading 3 to 14 mmHg). The hypertension can be controlled with antihypertensive drugs. Most children have transient episodes of hypertension that resolves within 3 months of transplantation because of changes in immunosuppressive therapy (Sommerauer et al, 1988).

Renal Function

It is not uncommon to see some type of renal dysfunction in the immediately postoperative period. Renal dysfunction is attributed to preexisting renal disease, intraoperative hypotension, hepatorenal syndrome, and antibiotic and cyclosporine toxicities. As doses are adjusted, renal function is restored. In cases of severe renal impairment, the patient may require dialysis, especially in the presence of fluid overload and hyperkalemia. Episodes of renal insufficiency are usually self-limiting and are managed with supportive measures. Resolution occurs within 3 to 4 weeks.

If a patient was known to have hepatorenal syndrome before transplantation, induction therapy with muromonab-GD3 or antithymocyte gammaglobulin (ATGAM), antirejection medications, may be initiated instead of cyclosporine to preserve renal function. Regardless of the drug used for induction therapy, levels must be monitored daily and dosages adjusted accordingly. Hepatorenal syndrome is characterized by severe hyponatremia that does not respond to fluid resuscitation. The clinical features of hepatorenal syndrome include renal vasoconstriction, reduced systemic vascular resistance, and elevated cardiac output (Amend, 1993). Hepatorenal syndrome results from persistent renal vasoconstriction.

Gastrointestinal Function

Assessment of gastrointestinal function is imperative for the early recognition of abdominal complications and promotion of adequate nutrition. The most common gastrointestinal complications are biliary leaks and strictures, which may occur at the anastomosis or the T-tube insertion site, and bleeding (Wood et al, 1985). A biliary leak is an early complication, whereas a stricture at the biliary anastomosis is a late finding. Biliary complications are usually related to ischemia or technical difficulties. Symptoms of a biliary leak include fever, chills, right upper quadrant pain, an elevated serum bilirubin level, and bilious drainage from wound drains. An aliquot of the wound drainage fluid is sent for detection of bilirubin. Additional diagnostic studies, such as cholangiography, are performed through the T-tube to assess for a biliary leak. In the absence of a T-tube, percutaneous transhepatic cholangiography and insertion of a percutaneous biliary catheter are performed to help control the leak.

Postoperative bleeding may be due to persistent coagulopathy, a biliary leak, stress ulcers, or prior problems with ascites and portal hypertension. Nasogastric tube drainage, stools, wound drainage, and hematocrit are monitored for evidence of bleeding.

Nutritional support is essential to promote adequate postoperative healing. In the immediately postoperative period patients are given nothing by mouth because of a surgically induced ileus. If the patient is intubated for a prolonged period of time, parenteral nutrition is initiated to provide calories and nutrition. When the patient is able to tolerate oral intake, the diet is advanced. When adequate intake of proteins and carbohydrates is maintained, healing occurs more effectively.

Children with end-stage liver disease are at risk for problems of malnutrition and growth failure. Supportive nutritional management leads to improved posttransplant outcomes. Children who are underweight and have nutritional deficits experience higher rates of death and postoperative complications (Shepherd et al, 1991). Parenteral nutrition is begun between the third and the fifth postoperative days. Supplemental tube feedings are administered and continued until adequate weight gain is documented. Careful management of nutritional deficits and early transplantation are recommended to minimize the deleterious effects of hepatic failure.

Rejection

Rejection of a transplanted liver is monitored by laboratory results and changes in patient status. Signs and symptoms include decreased bile flow and a change in bile color and consistency, fever, and elevation of liver enzymes levels. A liver biopsy is performed to gauge the amount of rejection or to distinguish rejection from another disorder, such as CMV infection or HAT, which also can cause a rise in enzyme levels.

Initial episodes of rejection are treated with steroid boluses. If this does not reverse rejection, OKT3 or ATGAM is added to the treatment regimen. OKT3 is a monoclonal antibody that blocks the ability of cells to recognize foreign antigens, inhibiting the generation and function of T cells. ATGAM is a polycloncal antibody that acts against T, B, and nonlymphoid cells. Treatment of rejection may greatly increase the patient's risk for acquiring an opportunistic infection. Prophylactic antibiotics and antiviral agents may be offered for 4 to 6 months after therapy to minimize this risk.

TRANSITIONAL PHASE

The transitional phase of recovery from a liver transplant begins when the patient is transferred to the surgical or transplant unit. The emphasis in this phase continues to be the prevention of infection and rejection. An important nursing role is to encourage patients to assume more of their own care.

The patient is taught to care for the T-tube and to self-administer medications. Side effects of medications and dosing schedules are reviewed. The family should be included in the teaching sessions to support the patient and to reinforce written and oral discharge instructions. Signs and symptoms of rejection and infection should be discussed. Patients are encouraged to be independent in their care several days before discharge.

Discharge instructions are provided for the families of infants and young children. Older school-age children and adolescents should be included in discharge planning.

Medication schedules and side effects are reviewed. Families are instructed to contact the transplant team if they see signs and symptoms of infection or rejection. They are also advised to avoid live virus vaccines for children who are immunosuppressed. Parents are instructed to contact the transplant team if their child is exposed to varicella-zoster virus (VZV; chickenpox). If the exposure occurred in the preceding 72 hours, varicella-zoster immune globulin (VZIG) should be administered to the child. If an immunosuppressed child presents with chickenpox, a 10-day course of intravenous acyclovir should be prescribed. Once the child's condition is stable, the acyclovir can be administered at home with the support of home-care nursing and an infusion company.

Specific information is provided to assist patients in reintegration into the community. Regular exercise, such as walking, is recommended. Heavy lifting and contact sports are discouraged until at least 6 to 8 weeks after the transplant. Patients are also advised to refrain from operating a motor vehicle until the incision is well-healed and the physician gives permission. A regular diet with no added salt is recommended. Patients may return to work or school 2 months after transplantation. Patients can resume sexual activity when they are comfortable. Women of child-bearing age are encouraged to wait 1 year before conceiving. After 1 year, female transplant recipients are usually taking low doses of immunosuppressants and the risks of rejection and infection are decreased.

The role of the nurse during the transitional period is to monitor and assess the patient for any postoperative complications. The nurse acts as a facilitator, allowing the patient to achieve an optimal level of functioning.

RECOVERY PHASE

The recovery phase begins when the patient leaves the hospital. Initially, patients are scheduled for weekly clinic visits. The patient undergoes routine blood-drawing to monitor for rejection. Doses of medication are adjusted according to the patient's clinical status and serum laboratory values. The patient must understand that reporting for regular examinations is a lifelong commitment and that rejection can occur at any time.

When the patient's condition is stable, clinic appointments are less frequent. Eventually the patient may be seen only once a year by the transplant physician. Routine medical care is provided by the referring physician. Although clinic visits are infrequent, blood work is monitored at least monthly.

PEDIATRIC LIVER TRANSPLANTATION

Reduced-Size Liver Transplants

Orthotopic liver transplantation has been an accepted treatment of end-stage liver disease in children since 1983. However, the survival rate among children with end-stage liver disease has been limited by the lack of availability of a size-matched donor. Because the waiting period for an appropriate donor is long, as many as 25% of potential recipients die while on the transplant waiting list. To alleviate this problem, transplantation with a reduced-size liver has been recommended (Kalayoglu et al, 1990; Bismuth & Houssin, 1984). Reduced-size liver transplantation (RSLT) was originally used to decrease problems due to intra-small or limited abdominal space in experimental heterotopic liver transplantation (Price et al, 1967). RSLT was then used for children who were critically ill and required immediate transplantation. Otte and associates (1988) reported the first large series of RSLT. The survival rate for the whole-liver group was 63%, compared with 76% for the RSLT group (Otte et al, 1990).

In 1984 Bismuth and Houssin performed a transplant on a 10-year-old boy who weighed 26 kg using a liver from a 75-kg donor. The child lived for 25 months. In 1986 Otte presented his experience with 10 children who underwent RSLT in Belgium. Eight of the 10 children lived (de Hemptinne et al, 1987). This encouraged transplant surgeons in the United States to consider RSLT as an option for young children with end-stage liver disease (Bismuth & Houssin, 1984).

Except for weight, the criteria for recipient selection are similar to the criteria used for whole-liver transplants. Priority is given to children with the most severe liver disease, a waiting time that exceeds 30 days, and those who are unresponsive to inpatient medical management. An attempt is made to match the donor and recipient for weight (Bismuth & Houssin, 1984; Otte et al, 1990).

Donor-recipient selection is complicated by the inability to accurately predict liver weight based solely on the donor's weight. There is a wide variation in the size and configuration of the left lateral segment of the liver (Woodle et al, 1990).

New surgical techniques and an understanding of the anatomy of the bile ducts, hepatic artery, and portal and hepatic veins have increased success with transplanting the left lobe or left lateral segment of the liver. Until specific guidelines are established, transplant surgeons will continue to work within their own experience.

Before the operation, the pediatric transplant team conducts a pretransplant evaluation that includes ABO compatibility; tissue typing; routine blood tests; vitamin levels of fat-soluble vitamins A, D, E, and K; screens for hepatitis A, B, and C; virologic screening for HSV, CMV, VZV, and EBV; screening for syphilis (rapid plasma reagin [RPR]); screening for toxoplasmosis; an electrocardiogram (ECG); chest radiography; and a duplex scan of the liver. Psychosocial screening is performed by a transplant social worker to identify potential financial or family problems that may preclude transplantation. Immunization records are obtained from the family. In addition to the regularly scheduled immunizations, children receive the hepatitis B series vaccine and pneumococcal vaccine (Woodle et al, 1990; Treacy, 1992).

Procurement of the donor liver is similar to the standard procedure used for recovery of a whole liver. Care is taken to preserve as much of the falciform ligament as possible. The liver is reduced by a formal lobectomy (right or left), or trisegmentectomy for left lateral segment implants, with ligation of the main vessels and ducts. Dissection of the bile-duct system occurs first; it includes a cholecystectomy, ligation of the cystic duct, and division of the right hepatic duct. Next, the arteries are dissected, including the aorta and celiac and hepatic arteries. Attention is then turned to the division of the portal vein and vena cava. If there is a large size discrepancy, the diameter of the vena cava can be tapered for right lobe or whole left-lobe implants, or the left hepatic vein can be used as a conduit to the vena cava for lateral segment implants (Fig. 7–2). The surgeon continues with a transection of the parenchyma and with ligation of the biliary and vascular structures, which are located along the transected surface. Finally, the remaining vascular structures are flushed with a preservation solution to check for possible leaks along the cut surface of the implant. If leaks are identified, they are repaired by individual ligation or sealed with fibrin tissue adhesive (Broelsch et al, 1988; de Hemptinne et al, 1988; Soubrane et al, 1990; Tracey, 1992; Woodle et al, 1990; Houssin et al, 1992; Badger et al, 1992; Tan et al, 1991).

The graft is implanted in the usual orthotopic position. The recipient hepatectomy on a pediatric patient may be complicated by previous surgical procedures, such

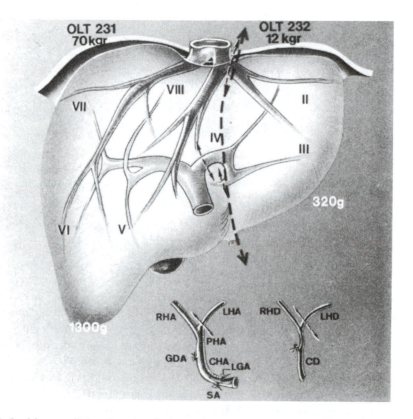

Figure 7–2. Liver splitting involved along the umbilical fissure. The right liver graft involved Couinaud segments IV to VIII (left medial and right medial and lateral segments). The left liver graft involved Couinaud segments II and II (left lateral segment). RHA, right hepatic artery; LHA, left hepatic artery; PHA, proper hepatic artery; GDA, gastroduodenal artery; CHA, common hepatic artery; LGA, left gastric artery; SA, splenic artery; RHD, right hepatic duct; LHD, left hepatic duct; CD, common bile duct; OLT, orthotopic liver transplant. (*Reprinted with permission from Otte et al* [*1990*]. Surgery. *St Louis: Mosby, p 606.*

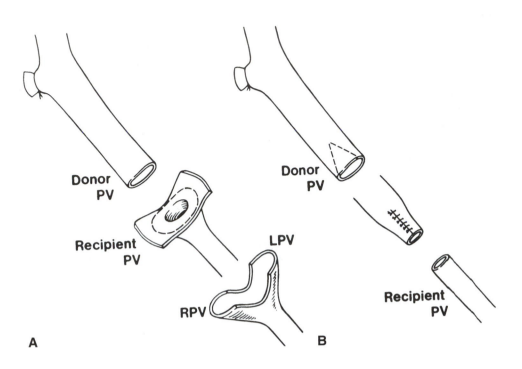

Figure 7–3. (A, B) Techniques of portal vein reconstruction in reduced-size liver transplant. PV, portal vein; RPV, right portal vein; LPV, left portal vein. (*Reprinted with permission from Kalayoglu M, et al [1990]. Experience with reduced size liver transplantation.* Surg Gynecol Obstet. *171:139–147.*)

as a portoenterostomy to manage biliary atresia. In this case, adhesions around the portal structures, the duodenum, the Roux-en-Y limb, and the colon are frequent findings. The vena cava of the recipient is preserved in its entirety for lateral-segment implants. Vascular anastomoses occur in the following order: suprahepatic inferior vena cava, infrahepatic inferior vena cava, portal vein, and hepatic artery. The portal vein and inferior vena cava are reconstructed with an end-to-end anastomosis and may require tapering if the donor and recipient size mismatch is apparent (Fig 7–3). An end-to-end anastomosis of the donor and recipient hepatic arteries is accomplished at this point, or a patch of the donor celiac trunk or aorta may be used to anastomose directly to the recipient aorta (Fig 7–4). To lessen the likelihood of vascular thromboses, low-molecular-weight dextran and subcutaneous heparin are given in the immediately postoperative period, when coagulation factors are normalizing. Children are prescribed aspirin therapy for 1 year after the transplant. The bile-duct reconstruction is usually accomplished with an end-to-side Roux-en-Y choledochojejeunostomy because the extrahepatic bile ducts from the transplanted segment are inadequate (Broelsch et al, 1988; Treacy, 1992; Woodle et al, 1990; Badger et al, 1992).

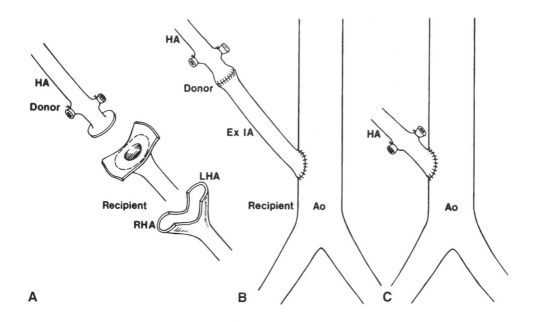

Figure 7–4. (A, B, and C) Techniques of arterial reconstruction in reduced-size liver transplant. HA, hepatic artery; RHA, right hepatic artery; LHA, left hepatic artery; Ex IA, external iliac artery ; Ao, aorta.

Complications

Complications of RSLT can be classified as either liver-related or non–liver-related. Liver-related complications include size mismatch, primary graft nonfunction, and biliary problems. Primary graft nonfunction occurs at approximately the same rate in whole-liver transplantation as in RSLT.

Size mismatch and determining the appropriate lobe to use as a reduced-size liver graft continue to present problems. If the size mismatch is not too great, the abdomen may be temporarily closed with synthetic graft material. If the liver is obviously too large, a second surgical team should be ready to transplant the donor liver into a larger recipient to avoid wasting a viable liver. Superina and associates (1990) reported a longer cold ischemia time in patients undergoing RSLT than in children receiving a whole-liver transplant. The recipient of a reduced-size liver is at increased risk for blood loss because of the extended procedure time (use of a second surgical team limits the operative time); the large transected surface of the donor liver; and preoperative problems with coagulopathy. The patient's condition preoperatively is probably the most important factor in determining the volume of blood that is lost. Careful ligation of vessels along the parenchyma can minimize postoperative problems with hemorrhage (Broelsch et al, 1988; Superina et al, 1990).

Biliary complications have historically been the leading cause of morbidity and mortality in pediatric liver transplantation. A biliary leak from the cut edge of the liver is a unique complication of RSLT. The most common biliary complications after transplants are leakage, an early complication, or stricture at the biliary-enteric anastomosis, a late finding. These complications are usually related to ischemia or technical difficulties. Biliary complications are diagnosed with either ultrasonography or percutaneous transhepatic cholangiography. The surgical management of obstruction involves revision of the choledochojejunostomy with insertion of a transhepatic biliary stent (Broelsch et al, 1988; Badger et al, 1992).

HAT is a common serious complication that leads to ischemia and biliary leakage. Factors that contribute to thrombosis include the intraoperative administration of fresh frozen plasma, an elevated hematocrit, rejection, a prolonged cold ischemia time, size of the recipient, and mismatch of donor and recipient vessels. Tan and associates (1991) reported an increased incidence of HAT when the donor weighed less than 15 kg. In a small series reported by Stevens (1992), the incidence of HAT in RSLT was compared with that of HAT in whole-liver grafts. It was determined that cadaveric left-lobe and left-lateral-segment grafts had a 15% incidence of HAT compared with 25% for whole-liver grafts in recipients younger than 2 years. The symptoms of HAT vary from no symptoms to elevated liver enzyme levels, acute liver failure, biliary leakage, or sepsis. Most of these children require surgical intervention involving a thrombectomy and anastomotic revision or retransplantation.

CMV infection continues to be the primary cause of non–liver-related complications. It is manifested as hepatitis, pneumonia, gastrointestinal bleeding, or retinitis. It has been suggested that CMV disease occurs more frequently in RSLT because of the use of adult donors in children (most children are CMV-seronegative whereas adult donors are usually CMV seropositive).

Split-Liver Transplants

Another technique used to overcome the shortage of available donor organs for the smallest recipients is the use of a split-liver transplant. This was proposed as an option to deal with two problems that occurred as result of RSLT for children. First, transplant surgeons were forced to choose between pediatric and adult recipients when it became possible to use adult donors for children. Second, given the shortage of donor organs, discarding a portion of viable liver parenchyma seemed wasteful. The split-liver graft differs from RSLT in that the division of the liver parenchyma and the vascular and biliary structures is carefully performed to obtain two viable grafts for two recipients. Recommendations for splitting the liver parenchyma are either through the umbilical fissure or through the main liver fissure (Fig 7–5). Langnas and associates (1992) recommended a hilar approach to split-liver grafts because it allows the surgeon to clearly identify the vascular anatomy without devascularizing the bile duct. The choice is based on the size and shape of the donor liver. Care should be taken to provide adequate liver tissue to maintain function for both recipients.

Initially surgeons who used split-liver grafts believed that the technique would solve the donor shortage problem by providing a two-for-one application. How-

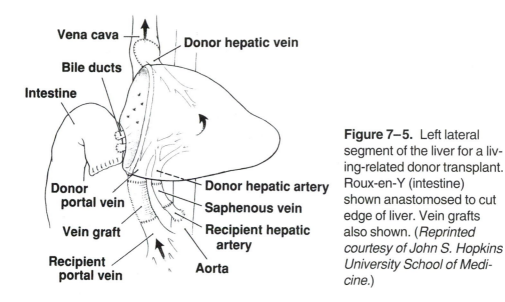

Vena cava

Donor hepatic vein

Bile ducts

Intestine

Donor portal vein

Donor hepatic artery

Saphenous vein

Vein graft

Recipient hepatic artery

Recipient portal vein

Aorta

Figure 7–5. Left lateral segment of the liver for a living-related donor transplant. Roux-en-Y (intestine) shown anastomosed to cut edge of liver. Vein grafts also shown. (*Reprinted courtesy of John S. Hopkins University School of Medicine.*)

ever, the complexity of the operation and the condition of the recipients led to a high incidence of morbidity and mortality; the complications included postoperative bleeding and biliary leaks. This technique is limited by the necessity of having an adequate number of surgical teams available and the need to follow UNOS guidelines to fairly distribute the organs (Emond et al, 1990; Otte et al, 1990; Merion & Campbell, 1991).

Living-Related Donor Transplants

The concept of living-related liver transplantation grew out of the need for appropriately sized donors for the smallest patients, those weighing less than 15 kg. The initial work done with RSLT and split-liver transplants established the feasibility and technique for using a portion of an adult liver in a pediatric recipient. However, the use of a healthy adult donor raised several ethical dilemmas. Ethical concerns include subjecting a healthy person to the complications of an operation, loss of income if the donor is the primary wage earner in the family, unknown outcome for the recipient and guilt felt by the donor if the recipient dies, and temporary abandonment of other children while the donor is hospitalized and recuperating. Reservations raised by ethicists about living organ donation include whether the donation can truly be made voluntarily. Family pressure may make it impossible to obtain voluntary consent to the operation (Caplan, 1993). Previous experience with a partial hepatectomy for benign tumors in patients without cirrhosis provided evidence that a partial resection was possible with minimal risk to the donor (Iwatsuki et al, 1990). It is well known that full regeneration of liver parenchyma occurs after a 50% resection (Kawasaki et al, 1992).

Surgical and psychologic risks should be presented to the donor before informed consent is obtained. A member of the health care team but not by a member of the transplant team should provide accurate information about obtaining a cadaveric donor. An advocate for the donor should be identified and should assist the donor throughout the evaluation process. The benefit to the donor is altruistic—being able to give a loved one the gift of life.

The donor evaluation involves blood tests, including routine hematologic and chemistry panels and electrolyte measurements, coagulation studies, hepatitis screening, tissue typing, virologic screening, and an HIV test. A physical examination is performed, and a three-dimensional computed tomographic scan of the liver is obtained to estimate the size of the left lateral lobe and its segments (segments smaller than 350 mL are most acceptable). Families are assessed for psychologic risk factors. Finally, angiography is performed to determine celiac and mesenteric vascular anatomy. When the evaluation is complete, the donor is referred to the blood bank for autologous transfusion.

Segments obtained from living donors are not comparable with those obtained from a cadaver. Segments from cadavers contain the entire hepatic artery and portal vein. The arterial reconstruction in transplants from living donors becomes a surgical challenge because of variations in normal anatomy and the small size of the vessels involved. Implantation of the donor liver is a modification of the technique used in split-liver transplantation. A saphenous vein graft from the donor or cadaver may be required as a replacement for an inadequate hepatic artery (see Figure 7–5). Limited resection of liver tissue and preservation of the hilar structures on the right side of the liver and gallbladder have prevented much of the trauma and scarring found in the initial procedures (Broelsch et al, 1992). Postoperative care follows the same protocols used for other liver-transplant patients.

Quality of Life

The long-term quality of life for children who have had liver transplants can be measured by a number of different variables. One variable is a decrease in the number of hospitalizations. Another factor is school performance. Findings indicate that only 50% of the children are in age-appropriate classrooms. Formal testing demonstrates an improvement in motor and social skills over pretransplant findings. Improved social skills allow a child more independence and responsibility at home and facilitate participation in sports. However, several authors report continued difficulties in establishing relationships with peers and feelings of loneliness. Changes in physical appearance as a result of medications also have a negative impact on a child's self-esteem (Bradford, 1991; Zamberlan, 1992; Zitelli et al, 1988).

Nurses can effectively reduce problems and improve the quality of life for pediatric liver-transplant recipients by using specific interventions. Nurses can provide emotional support and guidance for parents, siblings, and recipients. The family is counseled to "let go," especially as the child enters adolescence. The nurse offers suggestions for the use of cosmetics or clothing to enhance the child's appearance. Opportunities are provided for children and adolescents to discuss their fears, thoughts, feelings, and hopes for the future (Uzark, 1992). Children who have undergone transplantation are referred to an infant and toddler program or the appropriate school services.

Initially, children are followed closely by the transplant team with biweekly blood drawing and measurements of drug levels. When liver function returns to normal and drug levels are stable, children return once a month for clinic visits. Children need to be encouraged to return to school, assume appropriate household responsibilities, and pursue their regular activities.

Caring for a child who has had a liver transplant and the family involves helping them accept that they have exchanged a fatal disease for a chronic condition. Because the number of long-term survivors is increasing, more information is available regarding the quality of life after liver transplantation. One study compared quality of life before and after liver transplantation. There was a substantial improvement in physical health, including ambulation, mobility, and body care, and in psychosocial health, including social interaction, communication, alertness, and emotional behavior (Tarter, et al, 1991). Similar studies by Haagsma and associates (1991) and Bonsel and colleagues (1992) concluded that liver transplantation contributes positively to the quality of life of surviving patients.

Although liver transplantation has many positive effects, factors associated with this treatment may have a negative impact on quality of life. One example is the adverse effects of immunosuppression. Liver-transplant patients who suffered from ongoing rejection, renal failure, hypertension, cyclosporine, and steroid toxicity, which can cause numbness, tingling sensation, tremors, headaches, hair growth, mood swings, depression, and insomnia, had their medication switched from cyclosporine to FK506. The study by Wagner and associates (1991) concluded that there was improvement in general health and quality of life after the conversion. The continued search for better immunosuppressants should help resolve these adverse effects.

Another negative factor is the low employment rate among this patient population. Potential employers may be hesitant to hire liver-transplant recipients because of concerns about absenteeism and high health insurance claims. More documentation is needed to show that the rapid development and refinement of liver transplantation, the use of specific immunosuppressants with fewer adverse effects, and the use of prophylactic drugs for bacterial, viral, and fungal infections should decrease the frequency and duration of hospitalization. Such findings should have an important bearing on prospective employers' decisions to provide gainful work to transplant recipients.

Conclusion

Alternative surgical procedures such as RSLT and living-related-donor transplants have come about as the demand for solid organ transplants has increased. Advances in immunosuppressive medications to decrease the incidence of rejection and produce fewer side effects are on the horizon. The management of malignant hepatobiliary tumors by combined therapies including liver transplantation, chemotherapy, and radiation therapy is being attempted. As changes occur in adult and pediatric liver transplantation, so too will nursing care continue to evolve.

REFERENCES

Amend WJC (1993). Pathogenesis of hepatorenal syndrome. *Transplant Proc.* 25:1730–1733.

Badger IL, Czerniak A, Beath S, et al (1992). Hepatic transplantation in children using reduced size allograft. *Br J Surg.* 79:47–49.

Bismuth H, Houssin D (1984). Reduced-sized orthotopic liver graft in hepatic transplantation in children. *Surgery.* 95:367–370.

Bonsel GJ, Essink–Bot ML, Klompmaker IJ, Slooff MJH (1992). Assessment of the quality of life before and following liver transplantation. *Transplantation.* 53:796–800.

Bradford R (1991). Children's psychological health status—the impact of liver transplantation: A review. *J R Soc Med.* 84:550–553.

Broelsch CE, Emond JC, Thistlethwaite JR et al (1988). Liver transplantation with reduced-size donor organs. *Transplantation.* 45:519–523.

Broelsch CE, Whitington PF, Emond JC, et al (1992). Liver transplantation in children from living related donors. *Ann Surg.* 214:428–437.

Caplan A (1993). Must I be my brother's keeper? Ethical issues in the use of living donors as sources of liver and other solid organs. *Transplant Proc.* 25:1997–2000.

Carr BI, Selby R, Madariaga J, et al (1993). Prolonged survival after liver transplantation and cancer chemotherapy for advanced-stage hepatocellular carcinoma. *Transplant Proc.* 25:1128–1129.

Coleman JA, Mendoza MC, Bindon-Perler P (1991). Liver diseases that lead to transplantation *Crit Care Nurs,.* 13:41–50.

de Hemptinne B, Salizzoni M, Tan KC, Otte JB (1988). The technique of liver size reduction in orthotopic liver transplantation. *Transplant Proc.* 20(Suppl 1):508–511.

de Hemptinne B, de Ville de Goyet J, Kestens PJ, et al (1987). Volume reduction of liver graft before orthotopic liver transplant: Report of 11 cases. *Transplant Proc.* 19:3317–3322.

Deutsch J, Ahren D (1992). Hepatocellular carcinoma. In: Rector WG, ed. *Complications of Chronic Liver Disease.* St. Louis: Mosby Year Book, 161–181.

Emond JC, Whitington PF, Thistlethwaite JR, et al (1990). Transplantation of two patients with one liver: Analysis of a preliminary experience with "split liver" grafting. *Ann Surg.* 212:14–22.

Greig PD, Woolf GM, Abecassis M, et al (1989). Treatment of primary liver graft non-function with prostaglandin E results in increased graft and patient survival. *Transplant Proc.* 21:2385–2388.

Griffith BP, Shaw BW, Hardesty RL et al (1985). Veno-venous bypass without systemic anticoagulation for human liver transplantation. *Surg Gynecol Obstet.* 160:270–272.

Gruppi LA, Killen AR, Rodriquez W (1990). Liver transplantation: Key nursing diagnoses. *Dimens Crit Care Nurs.* 9:272–278.

Haagsma EB, Klompmaker IJ, Verwer R, Slooff MJH (1991). Long term results after liver transplantation in adults. *Scand J Gastroenterol.* 26(Suppl 188):38–43.

Halff G, Todo S, Tzakis AG, et al (1990). Liver transplantation for the Budd-Chiari syndrome. *Ann Surg.* 211:43–49.

Hart J, Busuttil RW, Lewin KJ (1990). Disease recurrence following liver transplantation. *Am J Surg Pathol.* 14(Suppl 1):79–91.

Henderson MJ (1992). Vascular disorders. In: Gitnick G, ed. *Diseases of the Liver and Biliary Tract.* St. Louis: Mosby Year Book, 421–445.

Hicks FD, Larson JL, Ferrans CE (1992). Quality of life after liver transplant. *Res Nurs Health.* 15:111–119.

Houssin D, Soubrane O, Boillot O, et al (1992). Orthotopic liver transplantation with a reduced-size graft: An ideal compromise in pediatrics? *Surgery.* 111:532–42.

Iwatsuki S, Starzl TE, Sheahan DG, et al (1991). Hepatic resection versus transplantation for hepatocellular carcinoma. *Ann Surg.* 214:221–229.

Iwatsuki S, Todo S, Starzl TE (1990). Excisional therapy for benign hepatic lesions. *Surgery.* 171:240–246.

Johlin FC (1992). Diseases of the biliary tract. In: Gitnick G, ed. *Diseases of the Liver and Biliary Tract.* St. Louis: Mosby Year Book, 539–593.

Jenkins RL, Pinson CW, Stone MD (1989). Experience with transplantation in the treatment of liver cancer. *Cancer Chemother Pharmacol.* 23:S104–S109.

Kahan BD (1991). The evaluation of liver transplantation. *Transplant Immuno.* 7:2.

Kalayoglu M, D'Alessandro AM, Sollinger HW, et al (1990). Experience with reduced-size liver transplantation. *Surg Gynecol Obstet.* 171:139–147.

Kawasaki S, Makuuchi M, Ishizone S, et al (1992). Liver regeneration in recipients and donors after transplantation. *Lancet.* 339:580–581.

Lake JR, Wright T, Ferrell L, et al (1993). Hepatitis C and B in liver transplantation. *Transplant Proc.* 25:2006–2009.

Langnas AN, Marujo WC, Inagaki M, et al (1992). The results of reduced-size liver transplantation, including split livers, in patients with end-stage liver disease. *Transplantation.* 53: 387–391.

Marsh JW, Iwatsuki S, Makowka L, et al (1988). Orthotopic liver transplantation for primary sclerosing cholangitis. *Ann Surg.* 207:21–25.

Marx JF (1993). Viral hepatitis: Unscrambling the alphabet. *Nursing 93.* 1:34–42.

McHugh MJ (1987). Intensive care aspects of organ transplantation in children. *Pediatr Clin North Am.* 34:187–201.

Merion RM, Campbell DA (1991). Split liver transplantation: One plus one doesn't equal two. *Hepatology.* 14:572–574.

Mezey E (1988). Chronic liver disease: Alcoholic liver disease, chronic hepatitis, cirrhosis. In: Harvey AM et al, eds. *The Principles & Practice of Medicine,* 22nd ed. Norwalk: Appleton & Lange, 861–863.

Miller HD (1988). Liver transplantation: Postoperative ICU care. *Crit Care Nurse.* 8:19–31.

Oleinik SS (1990). Care of the critically ill child after liver transplantation. *Focus Crit Care.* 17:300–307.

Olthoff KM, Millis JM, Rosove MH, et al (1990). Is liver transplantation justified for the treatment of hepatic malignancies? *Arch Surg.* 125:1261–1266.

Otte JB, de Ville de Goyet J, Alberti D et al (1990). The concept and technique of the split liver in clinical transplantation. *Surgery.* 107:605–612.

Otte JB, Yandza T, de Ville de Goyet J, et al (1988). Pediatric liver transplantation: Report on 52 patients with a 2-year survival of 86%. *J Pediatr Surg.* 23:250–253.

Payne JL (1992). Immune modification and complications of immunosuppression. *Crit Care Nurs Clin North Am.* 4:43–57.

Price JB, Voorhees AB, Britton RC (1967). Partial hepatic autotransplantation with complete revascularization in the dog. *Arch Surg.* 95:59–64.

Read AE, Donegan E, Lake J, et al (1991). Hepatitis C in liver transplant recipients. *Transplant Proc.* 23:1504–1505.

Samuel D, Bismuth A, Serres C, et al (1991). HBV infection after liver transplantation in HBsAg positive patients: Experience with long-term immunoprophylaxis. *Transplant Proc.* 233:1492–1494.

Shaw BW, Byers WS, Stratta RJ, et al (1989). Postoperative care after liver transplantation. *Semin Liver Dis.* 9:202-230.

Shaw BW, Martin DJ, Marquez JM, Kang, YG, et al (1985). Advantages of venous bypass during orthotopic transplantation of the liver. *Semin Liver Dis.* 5:344-348.

Shepherd RW, Chin SE, Cleghorn GJ, et al (1991). Malnutrition in children with chronic liver disease accepted for liver transplantation: Clinical profile and effect on outcome. *J Pediatr Child Health.* 27:295-299.

Sherlock S, Dooley J (1993a). Hepatic tumors. In: Sherlock S, Dooley J, eds. *Diseases of the Liver and Biliary System.* London: Blackwell, 503-531.

Sherlock S, Dooley J (1993b). The liver in infancy and childhood. In: Sherloch S, Dooley J, eds. *Diseases of the Liver and Biliary System.* London: Blackwell, 434-451.

Smith SL, Ciferni M, (1990). Liver transplantation. In: Smith SL, ed. *Tissue and Organ Transplantation: Implications for Professional Nursing Practice* St. Louis: Mosby Year Book, 273-300.

Sommerauer J, Gayle M, Frewen T, et al (1988). Intensive care course following liver transplantation in children. *J Pediatr Surg.* 23:705-708.

Soubrane O, Dousset B, Ozier Y, et al (1990). The choice of the reduction technique for orthotopic liver transplantation in children using a reduced-size graft. *Transplant Proc.* 22:1487-1488.

Staschak S, Zamberlan K (1990). Liver transplantation: Nursing diagnoses and management. In: Sigardson-Poor KM, Hagerty LM, eds. *Nursing Care of the Transplant Recipient.* Philadelphia: Saunders, 140-179.

Stevens LH, Emond JC, Piper JB, et al (1992). Hepatic artery thrombosis in infants. *Transplantation.* 53:396-399.

Stewart SM, Hiltebeitel C, Nici J, et al (1991). Neuropsychological outcome of pediatric liver transplantation. *Pediatrics.* 87:367-376.

Stewart SM, Uauy R, Kennard BD, et al (1988). Mental development and growth in children with chronic liver disease of early and late onset. *Pediatrics.* 82:167-172.

Superina RA, Strasberg SM, Grieg PD, Langer B (1990). Early experience with reduced-size liver transplants. *J Pediatr Surg.* 25:1157-1161.

Tan KC, Malcolm GP, Reece AS, Calne RY (1991). Surgical anatomy of donor right trisegmentectomy before orthotopic liver transplantation in children. *Br J Surg.* 78:805-808.

Tarter RE, Switala J, Arria A, et al (1991). Quality of life before and after orthotopic hepatic transplantation. *Arch Intern Med.* 151:1521-1526.

Thung SN, Gerber MA (1992). Benign and malignant neoplasms of the liver. In: Gitnick G, ed. *Diseases of the Liver and Biliary Tract.* St. Louis: Mosby Year Book, 389-404.

Treacy S (1992). Reduced size liver transplantation for infants and children. *Crit Care Nurs Clin North Am.* 4:235-42.

Uzark K (1992). Caring for families of pediatric transplant recipients: Psychosocial implications. *Crit Care Nurs Clin North Am.* 4:255-261.

Vargo RL, Rudy EB (1989). Infection as a complication of liver transplant. *Crit Care Nurse.* 9:52-62.

Wagner FS, Depee J, Johnson N, et al (1991). Changes in quality of life following conversion from cyclosporin to FK506 in orthotopic liver transplant patients. *Transplant Proc.* 23: 3032-3034.

Wiesner R, Parayko ML, Larusso NF, Ludwig J (1993). Primary sclerosing cholangitis. In: Schiff L, Schiff ER, eds. *Diseases of the Liver.* Philadelphia: Lippincott, 441-426.

Wood RP, Shaw BW, Starzl TE (1985). Extrahepatic complications of liver transplantation, *Semin Liver Dis.* 5:377-384.

Woodle ES, Budzinski J, Pitman M, et al (1990). Reduced-size liver transplantation. *AORN J.* 52:252–260.

Wright JE, Shelton BK (1992). *Desk Reference for Critical Care Nursing.* Boston: Jones and Bartlett.

Zamberlan K (1992). Transplantation: Children's quality of life. *Matern-Child Nurs J.* 20:170–219.

Zitelli BJ (1986). Pediatric hepatology: A three year experience with cyclosporine and steroids. In: Winters PM, Yang YG, eds. *Hepatic Transplantation.* New York: Praeger, 61–73.

Zitelli BJ, Miller JW, Gartner JC, et al (1988). Changes in life-style after liver transplantation. *Pediatrics.* 82:173–180.

NURSING CARE PLAN 7–1. LIVER TRANSPLANTATION

Nursing Diagnosis	Expected Outcomes	Nursing Interventions

Altered Nutrition: Less than Body Requirements
 	
Related to
• preexisting malnutrition
• Poor appetite
 	
Defining Characteristics
• Minimal food intake
• Weight loss
	• At the time of discharge the patient is able to state one way of increasing nutritional intake.	• Implement measures to prevent malnutrition
		  Monitor weights every day
		  Count calories
		  Allow family to bring home-cooked foods as long as they are within dietary restrictions
		  Obtain nutrition consult to identify areas of knowledge deficit regarding the quality of intake by discharge
		  Provide high-calorie or protein supplement drinks as ordered
		  Provide total parenteral nutrition (TPN) as ordered
		• For pediatric patients
		  Monitor weight daily
		  Record calorie count for 3 days
		  Administer multivitamins
		  Provide nasogastric or gastrostomy tube feeding if patient unable to take adequate calories (infant 100 cal/kg a day)
		  Monitor albumin and total protein
		  Provide TPN if needed
		  At discharge give regular diet for age, no added salt.

High Risk for Infection

Related to

- Hospitalization and compromised immune response

Defining Characteristics

- Fever
- Redness, warmth, purulent drainage, swelling of suture lines or catheter sites
- Persistent cough, sore throat, rales, rhonchipleuritic chest pain
- Headache, change in mental status
- Nausea and vomiting, diarrhea, abdominal pain
- Dysuria, urgency

- A patient who is free from infection on admission remains free from infection throughout hospitalization.

- Inspect all catheter and line insertion sites, suture lines, wounds and oral cavity daily.
- Perform suture line, wound drain, and T-tube site care with hydrogen peroxide once a day.
- Monitor for signs and symptoms of respiratory infection.
- Monitor for signs and symptoms of central nervous system (CNS) infection.
- Monitor for signs and symptoms of gastrointestinal (GI) infection.
- Monitor for signs and symptoms of urinary tract infection.
- Monitor vital signs according to protocol.
- Perform surveillance cultures according to protocol.
- Enforce appropriate infection control measures and isolation techniques.
  Perform good hand-washing
  Limit visitors
  Allow no cut flowers at beside
- Instruct patient that while he or she is taking high doses of immunosuppressants to
  Avoid people who have obvious sources of infection (ie, flu, measles, mumps)
  Avoid crowded areas such as movie theaters, public transportation, airports

(continued)

NURSING CARE PLAN 7–1. LIVER TRANSPLANTATION (*continued*)

Nursing Diagnosis	Expected Outcomes	Nursing Interventions
		• Administer acyclovir 200 mg orally twice a day for 3 months as prophylaxis against herpes simplex virus (HSV) infection. Administer trimethoprim-sulfamethoxozole (TMP-SUX) tablet orally on Monday, Wednesday, and Friday for 3 months as prophylaxis against urinary tract, wound, and lung infections.

		• For pediatric patients
		  Report exposure to varicella virus
		  Administer acyclovir IV for 10 days.

		• For both adult and pediatric patients
		  Administer no live virus vaccines
		  Administer intravenous immune globulin (IVIG) according to protocol for patients who are cytomegalovirus (CMV) seronegative and receiving a CMV seropositive organ
		  Provide protective isolation if white blood cell (WBC) count < 2000/mm^3

Ineffective Individual Coping

Related to

- Prolonged hospitalization
- Rejection
- Alteration in body image due to operation, side effects of immunosuppressants

Defining Characteristics

- Noncompliant behaviors
- Social isolation
- Inability to sleep
- Loss of appetite

- The patient states onset of feelings and symptoms and correlates them with events and life changes.
- The patient verbally identifies who or what is responsible for the problem.
- The patient lists at least one option for managing stress.

- Encourage patient to verbalize feelings, questions, and concerns about liver function.
- Discuss treatments during a rejection episode.
- Inform patient of progress of treatment.
- Explain to patient that untoward side effects of immunosuppressants are temporary and dose-related.
- Offer emotional support and initiate appropriate referrals, to social worker, a psychologist or psychiatrist.
- Allow patient to talk to other transplant patients who could provide support.
- Encourage patient to participate in own care, eg, activities of daily living (ADLS), administration of medication
- Encourage patient to use previously successful coping mechanisms.
- For pediatric patients
  Foster independence in adolescent
  Discuss medication compliance
  Encourage use of cosmetics, depilatories, and appropriate weight control measures

(continued)

NURSING CARE PLAN 7–1. LIVER TRANSPLANTATION (*continued*)

Nursing Diagnosis	Expected Outcomes	Nursing Interventions
• Knowledge Deficit: Health care practices	• The patient, family, or both verbalize knowledge related to the disease process, treatments, and health care practices.	• Discuss discharge teaching with patient, family, or both.
Defining Characteristics		• Conduct discharge teaching early but when patient exhibits minimal anxiety.
• Noncompliant behavior	• Patient, family, or both demonstrate skills related to therapies and health care practices by discharge.	• Conduct teaching in an environment conducive to learning.
• Nervousness		• Follow procedure for self-medication.
	• They know how to administer medication and perform T-tube care.	• Instruct patient and family on the care of T tube (provide preprinted instructions). Initiate appropriate referral, eg, a visiting nurse.
	• Patient and family verbalize appropriate reporting mechanism should problems develop after discharge.	• Instruct patient on signs and symptoms of infection and rejection.
		• Discuss clinic follow-up visits and frequency of blood work after discharge.
		• Provide patient with medical alert application form.
		• Provide patient with telephone numbers of whom to call after discharge for problems or concerns.
		• For both adult and pediatric patients Instruct patient and family about the need for prophylactic antibiotics before dental work
		Encourage patient to receive appropriate follow-up care with gynecologist

198

Refer patient to occupational or physical therapist during long-term hospitalization

- For pediatric patients

  Provide prescriptions to family at least 24 hours before discharge

  Review administration of medication

  Provide family with syringes for oral administration.

  Discuss return to school, no contact sports

  Referral to infant stimulation program, initially to receive therapy in home while immunosuppression at maximum levels

  Acquire appropriately sized cuff for infants and children to monitor blood pressure

8

Renal Transplantation

Mary Jo Holechek
Myrlin O. Agunod
Denise Burrell-Diggs
Jacqueline K. Darmody

The number of people living with end-stage renal disease (ESRD) has increased dramatically since the early 1970s. In 1989, it was estimated that 202,000 people had a diagnosis of ESRD (United States Renal Data System [USRDS], 1991). By the year 2000, the number of people with ESRD is expected to increase to 240,000 (Levinsky & Rettig, 1991). In 1972 the Social Security Act was amended to cover the medical costs associated with ESRD for eligible patients under the auspices of the Medicare program. Currently, 93% of all patients with ESRD are eligible for coverage under this program, the remaining 7% must cover the costs of ESRD privately (USRDS, 1991).

The diagnosis of ESRD can be overwhelming for both the patient and family. Severe kidney failure leads to important changes in lifestyle. The decreased energy level, need for dialysis, and health problems associated with renal failure can alter the ability to work and perform basic daily activities, conduct interpersonal relationships, and maintain financial stability. Since the 1960s there have been a variety of options available to keep people with renal failure alive and functioning. These options include hemodialysis, peritoneal dialysis, and transplantation. Of the three, transplantation offers the best chance for resumption of a near normal lifestyle.

This chapter discusses the major causes of ESRD and the options available to patients with ESRD, focusing on renal transplantation. The risks, benefits, survival rates, and quality of life associated with each treatment are considered. The pretransplant evaluation process, operative procedure, postoperative care, complications, and discharge planning for renal transplant recipients are presented.

CAUSES OF END-STAGE RENAL DISEASE

The three most common causes of ESRD are diabetes mellitus, hypertension, and glomerular nephritis. According to the USRDS (1991), diabetes and hypertension represent 60% of all causes of ESRD and accounted for the greatest number of new patients starting on dialysis between 1986 and 1989. Other common causes include pyelonephritis, congenital disorders, hereditary diseases, systemic diseases, nephrotoxins, urologic disorders, cancer, trauma, stenosis or occlusion of renal veins or arteries, and hemolytic disorders (Flye, 1989; Jacobsson and Cohan, 1991; USRDS, 1991) (Table 8–1). Regardless of the cause of renal failure, once a diagnosis of ESRD has been made, the patients along with their families must select the treatment option that best meets their physical, psychologic, and social needs.

TREATMENT SELECTION

In selecting a treatment option, patients must give consideration to the following: cost, benefits and risks, survival rate, quality of life, and availability of the treatment. To facilitate the decision-making process, patients and their families must be provided with adequate information to make an informed decision.

According to the USRDS (1991), in 1989 approximately 60% of the 163,069 known Medicare-eligible patients with ESRD were undergoing hemodialysis. Fifty eight percent were on in-center hemodialysis and 2% on home hemodialysis. Nearly 10% were undergoing continuous ambulatory peritoneal dialysis (CAPD) or continuous cycling peritoneal dialysis (CCPD). Twenty-five percent of the patients (40,812 patients) underwent transplants.

Cost

The estimated annual cost for each Medicare-supported patient with ESRD in 1989 was about $37,800, $30,900 of the bill being covered by Medicare and the remainder being the responsibility of the patient and private insurers (USRDS, 1991). According to the United Network for Organ Sharing (UNOS) (1991a), the median cost of a renal transplant procedure in 1988 was $39,625. Levinsky and Rettig (1991) reported that the annual cost during the first year after a transplant was $56,000 but that the annual cost fell to approximately $6000 a year thereafter. These figures show that the cost of 5 years of dialysis is $189,000, whereas the cost of the of the first 5 years of treatment for a patient who has undergone a renal transplant is $80,000 and is $30,000 every 5 years thereafter. Cost may or may not influence the decision for or against transplantation depending on the patient's income, private insurance, and availability of state and federal funds.

Benefits, Risks, and Survival Rates

Each of the treatments has inherent benefits and risks that can have an impact on selection. In-center hemodialysis provides two to three treatments a week of 2 to 4

TABLE 8–1 CAUSES OF END-STAGE RENAL DISEASE

Systemic Diseases
Hypertension
Diabetes mellitus
Amyloidosis
Henoch–Schönlein purpura
Systemic lupus erythematosis

Nephrotoxins
Lead
Intravenous drugs
Analgesics

Urologic Disorders
Calculi
Reflux
Neurogenic bladder

Stenosed or Occluded Renal Veins or Arteries

Congenital Disorders
Hypoplasia
Aplasia

Hereditary Disorders
Alport Syndrome
Polycystic kidney disease
Pyelonephritis

Cancer
Renal cell carcinoma
Multiple myeloma
Wilms tumor

Trauma

Hemolytic Disorders
Hemolytic uremic syndrome
Thrombotic thrombocytopenic purpura

hours in a controlled environment and requires varying degrees of patient participation. Home hemodialysis provides the same treatment at the patient's convenience but puts the burden of responsibility for the treatment on the patient and a partner. The risks or burdens associated with hemodialysis include the need for 9 to 12 hours of treatment per week; dependence on health care professionals; leaving home for treatment; hypotension or cramping; vascular access; only moderate control of uremic symptoms; and scheduling problems, which may preclude employment.

CAPD or CCPD affords more freedom and independence because patients can provide their own treatments at home, but it is not problem-free. Both CAPD and

CCPD require several hours each day. The primary problems associated with peritoneal dialysis include performing daily exchanges and the risk of peritonitis. Peritoneal dialysis also provides only moderate control of uremic symptoms.

Transplantation, if successful, allows the greatest opportunity for a normal lifestyle. There are many clear benefits to transplantation, including eliminating the need for expensive, time-consuming, and involved dialysis treatments; decreased dietary restrictions; and more complete resolution of uremic symptoms. Sutton and Murphy (1989) emphasized, however, that transplantation is not a perfect solution because some dietary restrictions continue, medications with unwanted side effects are required, and some problems such as bone disease and hypertension may persist.

Unfortunately, as with the other treatments, transplantation is not risk-free and there is no guarantee that a newly transplanted kidney will function. The risks of transplantation include rejection, infection, cardiovascular problems, increased incidence of malignancies, hypertension, steroid-induced complications (avascular necrosis, diabetes mellitus, weight gain, cataracts, gastrointestinal bleeding, and ulcers), liver dysfunction secondary to azathioprine, renal artery or vein thrombosis or stenosis, urine and bladder leaks, ureteral necrosis, lymphocele formation, and death (Burdick, 1990; Harasyko, 1989; Jacobsson & Cohan, 1991; Rao & Anderson, 1988; Sequeira & Cutler, 1992; Shapiro & Simmons, 1992; Tilney, 1982). The list of complications is long, and although the incidence of many of the complications is low, the potential recipient must be aware of them. Hauser and associates (1991) reported that patient awareness of possible problems allows them to develop strategies to manage the problems before they occur.

Fear of rejection and death can cause significant stress both before and after transplantation (Blagg, 1983; Sutton & Murphy, 1989). To deal with this fear, it would be important to discuss all treatment modalities and their complications as well as how transplantation has improved over the years.

From 1988 to 1989, the USRDS (1991) reported a remarkable improvement in graft survival. Since 1984, improved graft survival has been the trend, coincident with the introduction of cyclosporine (USRDS, 1991). Other factors believed to improve graft and patient survival rates include increased surgeon experience, improved surgical and tissue-typing techniques, more selective transplant candidate criteria, new immunosuppressive drugs (Fischel et al, 1991; House & Thompson, 1988), and new pharmacologic agents for treating infections common to patients who are immunosuppressed (Schweitzer et al, 1991).

Potential recipients should understand that patient and graft survival rates are an estimate influenced by a number of variables. Studies by Burton and Wall (1987) and Vollmer and associates (1983) showed no significant differences in patient survival rates across treatment modalities. However, data since the inception of cyclosporine reflect longer patient survival rates for transplant recipients than for dialysis patients. Matas (1991), using Medicare data, reported that diabetics undergoing dialysis have a 79 to 83% patient survival rate after 1 year of treatment, which decreases with age, 25 to 30% survival rate after 5 years of treatment. For patients without diabetes, 1-year survival rates of 92 to 95% were reported, the rates also decreasing with age.

After 5 years of treatment, the survival rate among patients without diabetes was 68 to 79%. Flye (1989) reported an overall mortality of 10% for all patients during the first year of dialysis.

UNOS (1990) reported that the patient survival rate was 92.5% and the graft survival rate 77.3% one year after transplantation for all recipients of cadaveric renal grafts in 1990. For all recipients of transplants from living-related donors, the patient survival was 96.8% and the graft survival rate was 89.6% 1 year after transplantation. The graft survival rate among blacks 1 year after transplantation was only 75% (Cecka & Terasaki, 1990). Zhou and associates (1990) compared 1-year graft survival rates among Asians, whites, and blacks on the UCLA registry who received cadaveric transplants between 1985 and 1989 and found survival rates of 83% among the Asians, 78% among the whites, and 71% among the blacks.

Many factors are thought to account for the differences in survival rates among different patients. Ranjan and associates (1991) reported that having a cadaveric donor, being black, having insulin-dependent diabetes mellitus, and lack of compliance adversely affected long-term graft survival rates. The USRDS (1991) cited other facts that can impact graft survival, including pretransplant blood transfusions, duration of warm and cold ischemia time, pulsatile perfusion time, panel reactive antibodies (PRA), human leukocyte antigens (HLA), patient demographics, and immunosuppressive therapy.

HLA typing has been implicated as a reason for the disparity in survival rates among different ethnic groups (Kasiske et al, 1991; Zhou et al, 1990). Black recipients have many more HLA mismatches than other patients because most donors are white. UNOS (1991b) reported that only 9.5% of the donors between 1989 and 1990 were black, whereas, 20.3% of the patients on the waiting list were black. UNOS (1992a) further reports that 20% of blacks have antigens that preclude donation from nonblack donors. Other factors found to impact survival rates adversely were inability to produce urine within 1 hour of transplantation and early rejection (Cecka & Terasaki, 1990).

Considering these data, transplant recipients, especially recipients of kidneys from living-related donors, have the best survival rates among patients with ESRD. However, only the healthiest dialysis patients are selected for transplantation, leaving more acutely ill patients to continue with dialysis (USRDS, 1991).

The statistics that influence the treatment selection may seem complicated to patients. Patients should be provided with the transplant center statistics specific to their age group, race, physical condition, and cause of ESRD. Wing (1984) reported that often a treatment is selected because of its impact on lifestyle rather than morbidity and mortality statistics.

The incidence of malignancies in transplant recipients is approximately 6% (Penn, 1990). Transplant recipients do not experience a greater frequency of neoplasms common to the general public such as lung, prostate, colon, rectal, and breast cancer, but they do experience a higher incidence of skin and lip cancers, non-Hodgkin lymphoma, and Kaposi sarcoma (Penn, 1989; Sequeira & Cutler, 1992; Stuart, 1978). Skin cancers among transplant recipients are mostly squamous cell carcinomas, whereas the general population usually develops basal cell carcinoma (Liddington et al, 1989;

Sequeira & Cutler, 1992). This increased incidence is associated with intense immunosuppression (Penn, 1990). Potential recipients must weigh the risk of the increased incidence of cancer against the benefits of freedom from dialysis.

Potential candidates must also reflect on the other side effects of immunosuppression. Steroids can lead to cataracts, aseptic avascular necrosis, diabetes mellitus, weight gain, and gastrointestinal complications (Harasyko, 1989; Rao & Anderson, 1988; Shapiro & Simmons, 1992). Cyclosporine is nephrotoxic and can cause hypertension (Haraskyo, 1989; Shapiro & Simmons, 1992). Azathioprine has been associated with liver dysfunction (Haraskyo, 1989; Shapiro & Simmons, 1992).

Surgical and technical problems include renal artery and vein stenosis or thrombosis, ureteral or bladder leaks, ureteral necrosis, and lymphocele formation (Burdick, 1990; Haggerty & Sigardson-Poor, 1990; Jacobsson & Cohan, 1991; Perryman & Stillerman, 1990; Shapiro & Simmons; 1992). Despite the number of possible complications, most can be corrected. Presentation of the risks of transplantation is not meant to frighten or dissuade potential recipients. Discussion of complications should help the patients have realistic expectations of transplantation.

Quality of Life

The data regarding which treatment provides the best quality of life are inconsistent (Hauser et al, 1991; O'Brien et al, 1986). The issue is complicated by the fact that transplant recipients are often selected by virtue of their good health, compliance, and youth, leaving older, less healthy, noncompliant patients to continue with dialysis. The definition of quality of life can further cloud the issue depending on whether it is defined by physical activities such as the ability to work or be active or according to psychosocial criteria (Hauser et al, 1991). Controlling for these variables is important when comparing quality of life across the various treatment groups.

Parfrey and associates (1987) found no significant difference on subjective measures between dialysis and transplant patients, but the transplant patients had a significantly better objective quality of life. Blagg (1983) found no significant difference in quality of life between transplant patients who received cadaveric kidneys and hemodialysis patients. Recipients of kidneys from living-related donors reported the best quality of life of the three groups. Johnson and associates (1982) and Kalman and colleagues (1983) found no significant differences between transplant and dialysis groups. The poorest quality of life was reported by transplant patients whose grafts had failed and who had resumed dialysis (Bremer et al, 1989).

Because the quality of life studies are inconclusive, they neither support nor rule out the option of transplantation. What should be considered is that all decisions regarding transplantation are individual and must be based on the candidates' perceptions of an acceptable quality of life.

Availability of Treatment

A final consideration when selecting a treatment is availability. Hemodialysis and peritoneal dialysis are available throughout the United States to all who are in need. Renal transplantation, on the other hand, is a limited resource restricted by the number of living-related and cadaveric donors.

As of May 1992 (UNOS, 1992b), 20,741 patients with ESRD were on the waiting list for a renal transplant. The average waiting time increased from 430 days during 1988 and 1989 to 465 days in 1990 and 1991 (UNOS, 1992d). Older patients of any race (UNOS, 1992d) and blacks (Kallich et al, 1990) wait longer for transplantation than do whites and younger patients. The estimated waiting time for blacks is twice that of whites. The number of deaths of all patients on the waiting list increased from 757 in 1988 to 935 in 1990 (UNOS, 1992c).

Donor kidneys are allocated by a complex rating system that takes into account waiting time, HLA matching, PRA, medical urgency, and geographic proximity of donor to recipient (Starzl et al, 1987). Potential recipients must understand that this system and overall organ availability dictate organ distribution. In 1991, of more than 21,000 patients on the waiting list, only 9949 patients received renal transplants (Department of Health and Human Services [DHHS], 1991). Candidates must clearly understand the disparity between these numbers and how it can affect waiting time.

Once the potential transplant recipients and their families decide that transplantation is the appropriate option, the pretransplant evaluation process can begin. The pretransplant evaluation includes assessment of physiologic, psychologic, and sociologic factors.

RECIPIENT AND DONOR EVALUATION

Assessment Criteria

An extensive patient assessment and careful selection are essential to a successful transplant outcome. Patient records such as recent health history and report of a physical examination, dialysis records, renal biopsy reports, and psychologic evaluation are used as a basis for an initial assessment. The need for medical consultation and any surgical intervention is addressed.

There are a few absolute contraindications to transplantation; these include active malignancy, substance abuse, and infections. Some patients may not be considered for transplantation until existing problems such as cholelithiasis, heart disease, and oral infections have been corrected. It is believed to be of less risk to a patient to correct these problems before transplantation because immunosuppression can impede wound healing and increase the severity of infections.

Most transplant candidates are undergoing dialysis at the time of transplantation. In some special situations, pediatric patients or patients with ESRD who have a slow decline in renal function may undergo transplantation before dialysis therapy is indicated. Katz and associates (1991) analyzed 85 preemptive renal transplant cases and found that although there are definite benefits to transplantation before dialysis, such as preventing the debilitating effects of dialysis and decreasing the rehabilitation period postoperatively, lack of compliance with medications, medical visits, and dietary restrictions can be problems.

The guidelines used as an initial screening for potential transplant recipients at Johns Hopkins Hospital are listed below. Patients who meet these criteria proceed to the full assessment.

The Johns Hopkins Hospital Guidelines for Patient Selection

1. Age evaluated case by case
2. No underlying untreated systemic disease
3. No active infection
4. Well-controlled diabetes and hypertension
5. No evidence of malignancy
6. No history of mental illness
7. No history of recent substance abuse
8. Compliance with medical recommendations

(From the Johns Hopkins Hospital Surgical Sciences Solid Organ Transplant Programs, June 1992.)

Physiologic Assessment

Each transplant candidate's physical profile is examined closely. Very young and old patients can undergo renal transplants. Extremes of chronologic age are not necessarily a limiting factor. General physical condition is of more concern than age. Morbid obesity precludes transplantation until weight is lost. A contract is used to achieve this goal.

Several diseases can recur in a transplanted kidney. Determining if a patient has a recurrent disease is essential. Patients must understand that certain diseases, such as glomerulonephritis, can recur quickly, whereas changes associated with diabetes mellitus can take a long time to recur (Flye, 1989). Patients with diseases that may recur must understand that their success with transplantation may be limited. After consideration of these general criteria, a more specific systemic assessment should take place.

Cardiovascular Assessment. Patients with cardiovascular conditions are at great risk for complications after a transplant. Fischel and associates (1991) found that most of their patients with good kidney function who died suffered from a cardiac condition that may have been due to transplantation or immunosuppressive therapy. Because of the increased mortality among transplant patients who suffer from cardiovascular disease, a careful pretransplant cardiovascular screening is essential. Severe cardiac vessel or valve disease that cannot be surgically corrected is a contraindication to transplantation. Advanced cardiomyopathies also preclude transplantation. Active cardiac infections such as pericarditis and endocarditis rule out the option of transplantation until they are resolved.

Patients with ESRD with a history of hypertension are usually treated with medication, dietary and fluid restrictions, and dialysis. If hypertension is malignant or cannot be controlled by standard therapy, bilateral native nephrectomies may be recommended to prevent hypertensive damage to the graft.

Respiratory Assessment. Postoperative immunosuppression leaves a patient susceptible to infection. Therefore, any existing respiratory infections must be totally resolved before the patient can be placed on the waiting list. Tuberculosis has a high incidence of reactivation after transplantation (Sever et al, 1991). It must be established that any patients with a history of tuberculosis have received adequate treatment.

Infection Assessment. Infection is a contraindication to transplantation because the immunosuppression required postoperatively can lead to a fulminant infection. Fischel and associates (1991) found that there has been a decrease in transplant failure related to acute rejection or deaths due to infection because of better immunosuppression management, particularly with cyclosporine. Also, with the introduction of less toxic yet powerful antibiotics, deaths due to opportunistic organisms such as *Pneumocystis, Nocardia, Listeria* and *Toxoplasma* have decreased (Schweitzer et al, 1991). At this time, presence of the human immunodeficiency virus (HIV) is a contraindication to transplantation because of the serious concerns of immunosuppressing an already immunocompromised patient.

Genitourinary Assessment. A urologic evaluation is performed to assess for the presence of any lower urinary tract abnormalities. These can include outflow obstruction and ureteral or urethral reflux. These abnormalities are usually identified by performing a voiding cystourethrogram (VCUG). Sometimes, a cystometric evaluation is indicated to determine if there is bladder dysfunction. Any obstructions or chronic reflux can result in infection, which will be exacerbated by immunosuppression.

Surgical correction is the usual approach to lower urinary tract abnormalities. For congenital abnormalities such as posterior urethral valves or neurogenic bladder dysfunction, an ileal conduit may be constructed in preparation for a transplant. Frequent catheterization after transplantation is the usual management of other types of bladder dysfunction (Flye, 1989). Bilateral nephrectomies are indicated for patients with recurrent urinary tract infections, polycystic kidney disease with bleeding and infection, and urinary reflux with infection. This is to prevent introduction of an existing chronic infection into the transplanted kidney.

Gastrointestinal Assessment. Careful screening and early treatment of ulcerative gastrointestinal disease is essential to prevent gastrointestinal bleeding and perforation after transplantation. Steroids can cause gastrointestinal bleeding and perforation; therefore, identification of the potential risk for these problems is important. Common causes of death in the first year after transplantation are peptic ulcer disease, ischemic bowel disease, or perforated viscus (Bia & Flye, 1989b).

Immunosuppressive agents, particularly azathioprine and cyclosporine, are hepatotoxic. It is therefore important to assess the patient's history of liver disease before the transplant. Some patients may require close monitoring and alterations in the standard immunosuppressive therapy to prevent hepatic complications. Bia and Flye (1989b) found that there is a high incidence of acute hepatitis within the first year after a transplant. They noted that patients who have hepatitis B virus (HBV) before or after a transplant have more than a 50% risk for cirrhosis.

Endocrine Assessment. The endocrine assessment includes evaluation of the thyroid and parathyroid glands and the pancreas. Hyperparathyroidism develops in patients with ESRD as a result of impaired calcium absorption and phosphate excretion.

This condition results in bone demineralization as the parathyroid glands produce parathyroid hormone (PTH) in response to hypocalcemia. As PTH demineralizes the bones, the serum calcium level increases at the expense of bone integrity. Hyperparathyroidism can be managed medically with drugs and dietary alterations, but if therapy is not successful, a subtotal parathyroidectomy may be required to stop bone demineralization. Reasonable control of calcium and phosphate levels must be achieved preoperatively to prevent calcium deposition in the lungs, which is associated with postoperative steroid therapy, and to limit bone disease, which is worsened by steroid use.

For diabetic patients, the endocrine evaluation focuses on the patient's general condition and the extent of the disease. Diabetics often have severe atherosclerotic heart disease, neurogenic bladders, neuropathy, and retinopathy. A thorough evaluation is required; it involves cardiologic, urologic, neurologic, ophthalmologic, and vascular studies.

Fischel and associates (1991) found that diabetics treated with cyclosporine experienced long-term success. Several factors contributed to these results, including early recognition and treatment of cardiovascular disease in diabetics in the pretransplant phase and better immunosuppression management, which decreased the incidence of infection without increasing the incidence of rejection.

Malignancy Assessment. Malignant neoplasms are difficult to manage in an immunosuppressed patient. Any incurable or active malignancies are absolute contraindications to transplantation. A patient must be free of malignant neoplasms for a minimum of 2 years before being considered for a transplant.

Immunologic Assessment. HLA typing for A,B,C and DR loci and ABO group testing are performed on both the recipient and the donor. The PRA level is determined in the recipient. Immediately before transplantation, a final crossmatch is completed by mixing the donor lymphocytes with the recipient's serum to test for cell agglutination. If lysis occurs, preformed circulating antibodies to the donor are present in the recipient. This is referred to as a positive crossmatch, and should the graft be transplanted, it would be rejected immediately.

A potential recipient with a high PRA level or degree of antibody sensitization usually has a long wait for a negative crossmatch with a cadaveric donor (Flye, 1989). Regular monthly screening is important to detect changes in antibody titers, because the presence of antibodies varies in the serum over time.

Psychologic Assessment

The impact of being chronically ill is great for patients with ESRD. These patients are forced to adjust to radical changes in lifestyle, such as incorporating dialysis into their daily routine, taking numerous medications, and adhering to a rigid diet to survive. These changes can cause patients with ESRD feel as if they have lost control. Restrictions can also lead to the development of lack of compliance with therapy as patients attempt to show that they can control their own lives. It is essential that a patient's psychologic status and mental capabilities be screened carefully before transplantation to ensure that they can adhere to the posttransplant treatment regimen. For patients with psychologic or mental impairment that precludes independent living, family support is essential for a successful transplant. Problems or changes that may be viewed as stressful should be discussed with both recipient and family. Discussing how they will cope with these issues can help prepare them in the event that problems develop (Hauser et al, 1991).

Compliance Assessment. Missing treatments or appointments or not following the dietary or medication regimen may indicate an inability or unwillingness to adhere to posttransplant guidelines. At the Johns Hopkins Hospital, patients with documented lack of compliance must sign and adhere to a contract for a minimum of 3 to 6 months before transplantation. In our experience failure to identify and deal with lack of compliance preoperatively can have serious consequences in the posttransplant period.

Substance Abuse Assessment. There is much concern for candidates who abuse drugs or alcohol. In general, these patients are not considered candidates unless they can demonstrate abstinence and ongoing rehabilitation treatment. Many programs require patients with a history of substance abuse to be drug-free and to undergo random urine and blood tests. We have found that requiring a patient to sign and follow a contract for 3 to 6 months is often helpful.

Social Assessment

Family Assessment. Adjustments in dealing with ESRD affect both the patient and family. With proper resources and support, they may be able to deal with dialysis and transplantation, but for some it can be difficult. The ability of the patient and family to deal with problems must be determined before the transplant. Families should be prepared for transplant complications, including rejection and changes in mood and mental status, which can occur during immunosuppressive therapy. To form realistic expectations, they must be made aware that sometimes the patient's recovery is slow. The family must be supportive and willing to help the patient, but they must realize the patient must be encouraged to be independent. Above all both patient and family must understand that although a successful transplant promises the greatest chance to return to a normal lifestyle, it requires work and frequent follow-up visits and is not without problems.

Lack of a support system is not a definite contraindication to renal transplantation, but it is a risk factor. It is recognized that the chronicity of ESRD and the impact of the physical limitations and complications after a transplant can affect one's psychologic stability. However, our experience at the Johns Hopkins Hospital shows that if a family or friend provides appropriate support to a patient, there is less fear and anxiety during hospitalization and increased motivation for self-care and cooperation with the staff. This can lead to faster recovery and facilitate the patient's discharge home. The nursing and medical staff must provide ongoing education to and open communication with the family to alleviate the fears and anxieties the family shares with the patient. This interaction among patients, family, and nursing and medical staff reduces concerns and allows easier discharge planning and better follow-up care after the transplant.

Financial Assessment. The financial concerns and resources of a patient should be discussed and identified during the evaluation period. Medicare covers the cost of the transplant operation, any transplant-related admissions, and follow-up care. Medicare also covers immunosuppressive medications for 1 year. Medicare eligibility for kidney transplantation lasts 36 months after a successful transplant (Health Care Financing Administration, 1991). After this, payment is the responsibility of the patient, private insurers, or state agencies. Forty-seven states provide Medicaid coverage for outpatient immunosuppression, as do 90 to 98% of private insurers (DHHS, 1991). Lack of full insurance coverage does not preclude transplantation, but necessitates careful planning to determine alternative methods of payment or insurance sources.

Some patients are employed while undergoing dialysis. Usually an important concern is their ability to return to employment after transplantation. In our experience, patients who can return to work usually experience fewer financial worries and higher self esteem. Some patients may choose not return to work because doing so would decrease their medical disability income or would exceed income restrictions to qualify for government assistance programs. The transplant team's awareness regarding these financial issues facilitates referral to government assistance agencies. Vocational rehabilitation should be offered to patients qualified to return to work.

DETERMINATION OF DONOR SOURCE

Cadaveric Donor

After the pretransplant evaluation is completed and a patient is accepted for transplantation, he or she is placed on the UNOS list. Participation in a support group can be helpful. It increases the patient's awareness that other patients are also waiting and sharing the same experience.

Living Donor

When a compatible living donor is identified, an evaluation process similar to the recipient's is initiated. The donor must have a compatible blood and tissue type, be at least 18 years of age, and be able to consent to donation. The medical evaluation includes nephrologic and urologic consultations to assess the integrity and function of the genitourinary tract. Other consults, such as cardiologic or endocrinologic, may be required as indicated. Routine tests include blood chemistry, hematologic screening, serologic screening, screening for HIV, HBV, hepatitis C virus (HCV), and cytomegalovirus (CMV); chest radiography; glomerular filtration rate (GFR); renal sonography and arteriography; an electrocardiogram (ECG); and urine tests for protein, creatinine, and culture and sensitivity. As for the recipient, severe cardiac, gastrointestinal, or respiratory disease, active infection or malignant disease, and genitourinary abnormalities preclude donation. In addition, a potential donor with diabetes, HIV infection, hepatitis B or C, or impaired renal function will be rejected. These criteria protect both the donor and the recipient.

The psychologic evaluation of a donor is important. It determines the donor's emotional and mental stability. It also identifies the donor's motives and willingness to donate. If a potential donor is reluctant, a meeting with the psychologist or psychiatrist should be scheduled. At this meeting, it should be emphasized that donation is voluntary and that one must be physically, mentally, and emotionally fit to donate. If for any reason the donor is not mentally or emotionally fit or has any reservations, that person is not considered suitable to make the donation. If a suitable living-related donor is not identified, the situation is discussed with the recipient, and he or she is placed on the UNOS list to wait for a cadaveric donor.

Once a cadaveric transplant donor or a living-related donor is found, the patient moves to the next stage in the process, preoperative preparation. This stage is followed rapidly by the transplant procedure and the recovery phase.

RENAL TRANSPLANT OPERATION

Preoperative Care

Living Related Donors and Recipients. At least 1 month before the operation, a hepatitis B panel is obtained for the donor and the recipient. The week before the transplant, a final crossmatch is done and the donor undergoes a preoperative renal arteriogram to detect any vascular defects that may preclude transplantation. The donor and recipient are usually admitted to the hospital the day before the operation. The night before the operation, azathioprine is administered to initiate the recipient's immunosuppression.

The recipient should undergo hemodialysis the day before the operation. If the patient is undergoing peritoneal dialysis, it should continue until about 2 hours before the operation and be followed by complete drainage and capping of the Tenckhoff catheter. The morning of the operation, if the recipient has any hemodialysis access, a sign should be taped to the access arm stating "no procedures" to prevent trauma to the access during the operative procedure. Prophylactic antibiotics are given to protect against postoperative infection.

Because this is an anxiety-producing yet hopeful time for both the donor and the recipient, psychologic support is a critical part of preoperative nursing care. Living-related transplantation allows for extensive psychologic preparation of the involved parties, but the fear of rejection and surgical complications can still be a major concern at this time (Gharbieh, 1988; Weems & Patterson, 1989).

Cadaveric Recipients. Preparation of a recipient of a cadaveric transplant is similar to that of a recipient of a transplant from a living-related donor, except that activities are carried out within a shorter period of time and the final crossmatch is not done until the patient reaches the transplant facility. If the patient has hyperkalemia or fluid overload, dialysis may be required preoperatively. It usually takes 4 to 6 hours for the final crossmatch to be completed. If the final crossmatch is negative, azathioprine is administered, and final preparations are made to move the patient to the operating room.

Once in the operating room, the patient is anesthetized. General anesthesia is preferred (Shapiro & Simmons, 1992), but if the patient has eaten in the immediately preoperative period, epidural anesthesia may be indicated to reduce the risk of aspiration.

Transplantation Procedure

Regardless of the source of the donor kidney, the procedure for the transplant is the same. The anesthetized recipient has a urinary catheter in place. Before the operation, the bladder is flushed with several hundred milliliters of an antibiotic solution. Flushing the bladder in this manner helps reduce bacterial contamination when the bladder in incised. After the flushes are complete, 100 to 200 mL of the antibiotic solution is left in the bladder, and the catheter is clamped. This distends the bladder, making it easier to locate during the surgical procedure (Flye, 1989).

The transplanted kidney is usually placed extraperitoneally in the iliac fossa of the recipient (Tilney, 1982) through an incision that originates above the iliac crest and terminates above the symphysis pubis. The muscle layers and fascia are incised and the peritoneum is retracted medially, making a small opening in which to place the kidney. Because it is close to the blood vessels and the bladder, this anterior superficial placement facilitates vascular and ureteral anastomoses. It also makes the transplanted kidney readily accessible for assessment or biopsy (Perryman & Stillerman, 1990).

In choosing on which side to place the donor kidney many factors are considered. It is preferred to place the donor kidney on the contralateral side in the recipient. This placement facilitates vessel anastomoses (Flye, 1989; Tilney, 1982) and puts the renal pelvis in an anterior position. This anterior placement of the pelvis makes reoperations easier. Because most additional operations affect the urinary collecting system, anterior is believed to be the most effective placement. If contralateral placement is contraindicated, the kidney can be placed on the ipsilateral side. At some centers, if ipsilateral placement is used, the kidney may be placed upside down with the ureter gently bent downward to keep the pelvis and ureter anterior (Tilney, 1982); other centers prefer the normal upright positioning of the transplanted kidney.

If a transplanted kidney is placed on the left side of the body, it must be kept in mind that diverticulitis could obscure the diagnosis of rejection and vice versa (Tilney, 1982). Many centers try to avoid the use of the left iliac fossa in patients older than 40 years for this reason because, if needed, sigmoid resection would be extremely difficult.

A left iliac fossa placement also results in a slower return of bowel function because the lumen of the sigmoid colon is small and the stool is formed, whereas the right intestinal lumen is large and the stool more liquid. Because of the slower recovery from ileus with a kidney transplant on the left side, a nasogastric tube may be required postoperatively. If a diabetic patient is likely to receive a pancreatic transplant at a later date, the kidney is placed on the left because the pancreas must go on the right to prevent kinking of the portal vein.

A final major consideration in selecting a transplant site is whether or not other operative procedures have been performed. The surgeon avoids the site of previous transplants and abdominal operations when possible because of possible scarring and stenosis of blood vessels required for transplantation and the presence of adhesions.

Once the site is selected and the wound is opened, the donated kidney is ready for placement. The surrounding lymphatic vessels must be carefully ligated. Failure to do so results in the formation of a lymphocele, which can compress the newly transplanted kidney or ureter, impairing function (Flye, 1989). The iliac and hypogastric vessels are then dissected free. The arterial anastomosis is completed first by one of two approaches. The donor renal artery can be anastomosed end to end to the recipient's internal iliac (hypogastric) artery (Fig 8–1A) or end to side to the recipient's external iliac artery (Fig 8–1B) (Shapiro & Simmons, 1992; Shapter & Yonkman, 1979). In female recipients, the end-to-end anastomosis to the internal iliac artery is preferred because it provides a better anastomosis. In male recipients, the end-to-side anastomosis to the external iliac artery is preferred because it avoids ligation of the internal iliac artery, which can lead to impotence.

Occasionally there are multiple arteries. In this situation, the multiple arteries may be anastomosed separately to a patch of donor aorta and the patch sutured to the side of the recipient's vessel (Fig 8–2A). An alternative is that the multiple donor vessels may be anastomosed to the main donor renal artery, and this vessel can then be anastomosed to the recipient's artery (Fig 8-2B). Anastomosing and patching of multiple arteries is usually done immediately after organ harvesting.

For the venous anastomosis, the donor renal vein is sutured end to side to the recipient's external iliac vein. Multiple veins are not common, but if present one vein can be ligated or a bifurcated vein graft can be done (Shapiro & Simmons, 1992).

After the vascular anastomoses are complete, the vascular clamps are removed and perfusion of the kidney and urine production are assessed (Jacobsson & Cohan, 1991). Diuretics are usually administered to enhance urine flow which should start within minutes of revascularization (Perryman & Stillerman, 1990). Revascularization is usually completed within 30 minutes.

If the newly transplanted kidney is perfusing and producing adequate urine, the ureteral anastomosis is performed usually by one of the three following techniques. The first is a ureteroneocystostomy, which is usually made using the Politano-Ledbetter technique (Fig 8–3). An incision is made in the bladder to facilitate the internal bladder anastomosis of the donor ureter. A submucosal tunnel is made near the trigone. The tunneled ureter runs through the bladder wall for about 1 cm and then enters the bladder. The end of the ureter is folded back over the bladder wall and sutured (Shapiro & Simmons, 1992). This procedure prevents urine reflux because when the bladder contracts on urination, the ureter is compressed by the bladder wall. A fairly long ureter is required for this procedure.

A second technique, which is ideal when the donor ureter is short, involves making an extravesical ureteroneocystostomy (Fig 8–4). A 2.5-to-3 cm incision is made in the dome of the bladder. The ureter is sutured to the mucosa and then the muscle layer is approximated, the first layer forming a submucosal tunnel (Shapiro & Simmons, 1992). There is an increased incidence of reflux with this technique (Flye, 1989).

The third technique, ureteroureterostomy, is used when a recipient has known bladder contamination or has had repeated bladder procedures (Perryman & Stillerman, 1990) or if the blood supply to the donor ureter has been interrupted (Shapiro & Simmons, 1992) (Fig 8–5). The donor ureter is anastomosed to the recipient's native

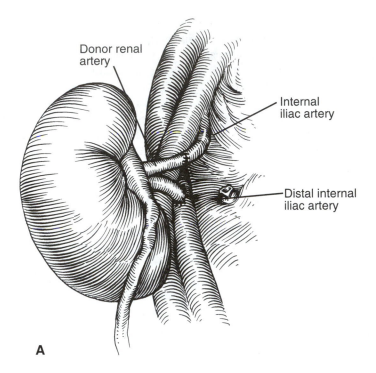

Donor renal artery

Internal iliac artery

Distal internal iliac artery

A

Figure 8–1. (A) End-to-end anastomosis of donor renal artery to recipient internal iliac (hypogastric) artery. The distal internal iliac artery is ligated. **(B)** End-to-side anastomosis of donor renal artery to recipient external iliac artery. *(From Sabiston DC, Gordon RG [1994]. Atlas of General Surgery. Philadelphia: Saunders.)*

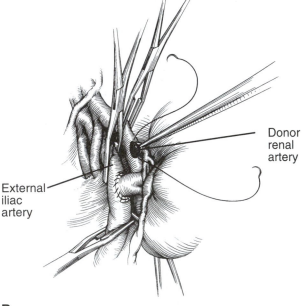

Donor renal artery

External iliac artery

B

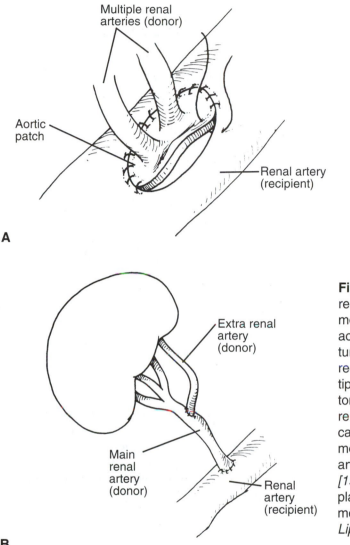

Multiple renal
arteries (donor)

Aortic
patch

Renal artery
(recipient)

A

Extra renal
artery
(donor)

Main
renal
artery
(donor)

Renal
artery
(recipient)

B

Figure 8–2. (A) Multiple renal arteries anastomosed to cuff of donor aorta. The patch is sutured to the side of the recipient artery. **(B)** Multiple donor arteries anastomosed to the main renal artery. The vessel can then be anastomosed to the recipient's artery. *(From Cerilli GJ [1988].* Organ Transplantation and Replacement. *Philadelphia: Lippincott.)*

ureter. This eliminates the need to open a scarred or contaminated bladder and allows blood to be supplied to the ureter.

If a patient has an ileal loop, the full thickness of the ureter is anastomosed to the intestine. Interrupted absorbable sutures are used (Flye, 1989; Shapiro & Simmons, 1992).

Throughout the operative procedure, it is desirable to keep the central venous pressure (CVP) just above normal to ensure adequate perfusion and hydration sufficient for urine production (Flye, 1989; Jacobsson & Cohan, 1991). It is also important

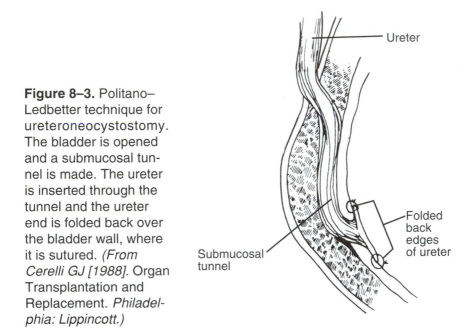

Figure 8–3. Politano–Ledbetter technique for ureteroneocystostomy. The bladder is opened and a submucosal tunnel is made. The ureter is inserted through the tunnel and the ureter end is folded back over the bladder wall, where it is sutured. *(From Cerelli GJ [1988].* Organ Transplantation and Replacement. *Philadelphia: Lippincott.)*

to maintain the patency of any internal vascular access. A blood pressure of 140 mm Hg systolic is recommended at the time of release of the cross-clamp (Shapiro & Simmons, 1992).

After all of the anastomoses are complete, the wound is irrigated with an antibiotic solution, and a small drain is placed in the lower quadrant on the side of the transplant. The wound is closed in layers and dressed. The patient is then transferred to the postanesthesia or critical care unit for recovery. The entire procedure can require 2 1/2 to 4 1/2 hours. Perryman and Stillerman (1990) report that the intraoperative mortality at most centers is less than 0.1%.

POSTOPERATIVE CARE OF THE RENAL TRANSPLANT RECIPIENT

Nursing care of the renal transplant recipient is challenging and rewarding. Acute assessment skills and effective teaching techniques are necessary to help the patient progress from the immediately postoperative period through discharge and toward outpatient management.

A number of potential complications can occur after renal transplantation. These include fluid and electrolyte imbalances, acute tubular necrosis (ATN), rejection, infection, and arterial, venous or ureteral complications (Burdick, 1990; Flye, 1989; Jacobsson & Cohan, 1991; Shapiro & Simmons, 1992) (see Nursing Care Plan 8–1, p XXX).

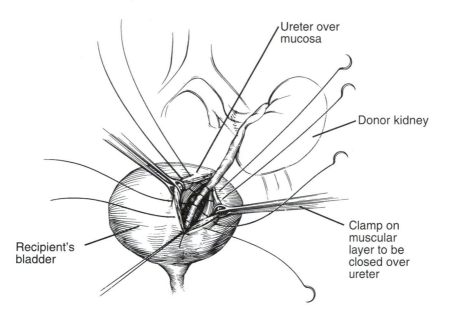

Ureter over mucosa

Donor kidney

Clamp on muscular layer to be closed over ureter

Recipient's bladder

Figure 8–4. Extravesical ureteroneocystostomy. Incision made in bladder dome and the donor ureter sutured to bladder mucosa. Muscle layer closed over ureter forming submucosal tunnel. *(From Sabiston DC, Gordon RG [1994].* Atlas of General Surgery. *Philadelphia: Saunders.)*

Several weeks to months after a kidney transplant, additional complications may occur. These include technical complications such as ureteral stenosis, renal artery stenosis, and development of a lymphocele (Bia & Flye, 1989b; Burdick, 1990; Flye, 1989; Haggerty & Sigardson-Poor, 1990). Additional long-term complications include hypertension, bone problems, gastrointestinal complications, cataract formation, cyclosporine nephrotoxicity, malignancy, and infection (Bia & Flye, 1989a,b; Harasyko, 1989). Liver disease, hyperlipidemia, erythrocytosis, chronic rejection, and de novo and recurrent glomerulonephritis also can develop (Bia & Flye, 1989b).

Alteration in Fluid Volume

During the immediately postoperative period, maintenance of adequate perfusion of the newly placed kidney is paramount to optimize function. If the kidney functions, there may be an immediate diuresis of more than 100 mL/hour because of a large osmotic load secondary to the ability of the new kidney to filter urea. Rapid diuresis can also result from intraoperative overhydration or renal tubular dysfunction due to prolonged ischemic time which prevents the kidney from concentrating urine normally (Flye, 1989; Haggerty & Sigardson-Poor, 1990). Adequate fluid replacement is necessary to prevent hypotension, which could lead to oliguria and impaired renal function.

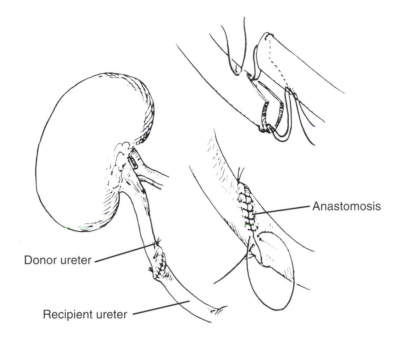

Figure 8–5. Ureteroureterostomy. Donor ureter anastomosed to recipient native ureter. *(From Morris PJ [1984].* Kidney Transplantation: Principles and Practice. *Orlando: Grune & Stratton.)*

If the transplant does not function immediately, overhydration can lead to pulmonary edema and necessitate administration of diuretics or the initiation of acute hemodialysis or hemofiltration (Flye, 1989).

Intravenous fluid replacement varies among transplant centers. The amount of intravenous fluid replacement usually is matched to urine output. The fluid of choice is normal saline solution or 0.45 normal saline solution with or without dextrose depending on the serum glucose levels (Burdick, 1990; Flye, 1989; Shapiro & Simmons, 1992).

Nursing assessment for fluid balance includes vital signs, intake and output, daily weight, CVP, heart and lung sounds, and the presence or absence of edema (Gharbieh, 1988).

Alteration in Elimination

Oliguria in a kidney transplant recipient is a complication that requires immediate attention. A decrease or total lack of urine output during the initial postoperative period can be the result of a number of conditions. These include clots in the urinary catheter, hypovolemia, ATN, rejection, or technical complications, such as renal artery or vein thrombosis, hemorrhage, and urine leaks (Burdick, 1990; Gharbieh, 1988).

Clotting in the urinary catheter is a common cause of decreased urine output and is easily remedied by irrigation with sterile normal saline solution. Sometimes changing the catheter is required to alleviate the problem (Gharbieh, 1988). Hypovolemia can occur as the result of rapid diuresis. If hypovolemia is not treated with an infusion of intravenous fluids, oliguria may occur.

If the urine output remains low after ruling out catheter clots and hypovolemia as the cause, ATN should be considered. ATN is the major cause of early nonfunction in cadaveric kidney transplants, involving 30 to 50% of all recipients (Tilney, 1988). Factors associated with the increased likelihood of ATN include length of cold preservation time, prolonged warm ischemic time, reperfusion injury, or premortem donor incidents such as hypotension and cardiac or pulmonary arrest (Jacobsson & Cohan, 1991).

When ATN is suspected as the cause of decreased urine volume, the evaluation includes renal ultrasonography to rule out obstruction or perinephric fluid collection. A radionuclide scan is done to rule out obstruction of blood flow, urine leak, or rejection (Gharbieh, 1988).

Burdick (1990) wrote that in cases of severe ATN, renal scans may be repeated on a weekly basis to monitor for decreasing blood flow, which is an indicator of developing rejection. During this period of ATN, the patient will need hemodialysis or peritoneal dialysis until there is a decline in the creatinine level and urine output increases. Cyclosporine is associated with an increased incidence and duration of ATN (Jacobsson & Cohan, 1991). Therefore, the use of cyclosporine at the Johns Hopkins Hospital is delayed until postoperative day 5 and only given if urine output is adequate. If ATN is considered likely, muromonab-CD3 (Orthoclone OKT3; a monoclonal anti-T-cell antibody) or lymphocyte immune globulin, an antithymocyte gamma globulin (ATGAM), is used for induction therapy.

Rejection

Despite advances in immunology, tissue-typing, crossmatching techniques, and immunosuppressants, rejection remains a major cause of transplant graft loss. Rejection can be categorized into four types based on the time of onset. These include hyperacute, accelerated, acute, and chronic rejection (Jacobsson & Cohan, 1991; Shapiro & Simmons, 1992).

Hyperacute rejection occurs immediately after revascularization of the transplanted kidney and is caused by the recipient's preformed antibodies' reacting to antigens on the donated kidney. The transplanted kidney becomes irreversibly damaged and must be removed. Pretransplant crossmatching screens for these preformed antibodies in a potential recipient (Jacobsson & Cohan, 1991; Shapiro & Simmons, 1992).

Accelerated rejection often occurs after an initial period of urine output, between 2 and 5 days after transplantation. Urine output abruptly declines, making rejection difficult to distinguish from ATN. A renal scan may be useful to make this diagnosis. In the case of accelerated rejection, the renal scan shows poor flow; in ATN it shows adequate flow. Sometimes a renal biopsy is performed to confirm the diagnosis. Treatment usually consists of high-dose steroids, followed by muromonab-CD3 if the steroids are not effective (Jacobsson & Cohan, 1991; Shapiro & Simmons, 1992).

Acute rejection commonly occurs within the first 2 weeks after transplantation, but it can occur after months or even years. A diagnosis of acute rejection is based on clinical signs, such as a rising creatinine level, oliguria, fever, weight gain, and graft tenderness. A renal flow scan and renal biopsy are useful in making the diagnosis of acute rejection (Jacobsson & Cohan, 1991; Shapiro & Simmons, 1992). At the Johns Hopkins Hospital, treatment consists of an intravenous bolus of steroids. If this is not effective in reversing the acute rejection, then muromonab-CD3 is given for a course of 10 to 14 days. Muromonab-CD3 has been proved to be 94 to 95% effective in reversing acute rejection in a number of studies (Norman et al, 1987; Thistlewaite et al, 1988). During the course of treatment with muromonab CD3, the dosages of prednisone, azathioprine, and cyclosporine are reduced to prevent overimmunosuppression.

A number of adverse reactions the patient may experience during muromonab-CD3 therapy may require nursing intervention. Pulmonary edema is the most serious adverse reaction; it occurs most often in patients who are fluid overloaded before administration. It is recommended that a patient have a clear chest radiograph within 24 hours of administration of muromonab-CD3 and that the patient's weight not be more than 3% over the dry weight. If the weight is more than this, hemodialysis is initiated to remove excess fluid (Moir, 1989; Wyszynski et al, 1989). Vital signs are taken frequently during the initial administration. Vital signs are monitored every 4 hours during the subsequent days of treatment. Additional adverse reactions include fever, generalized aches and pains, nausea, vomiting, diarrhea, and anorexia (Moir, 1989; Wyszynski et al, 1989). Patients should be premedicated with oral acetaminophen and diphenhydramine before the first dose of muromonab-CD3. Methylprednisolone is administered intravenously 4 to 6 hours before the first dose of muromonab-CD3. These medications help minimize the fever and chills often experienced by patients who receive muromonab-CD3.

Nausea, vomiting, and diarrhea can lead to dehydration. Intake and output, daily weight, and laboratory values should be carefully monitored to avoid problems with electrolyte imbalances. Patients may be given prochlorperazine (Compazine) to help with nausea and vomiting. An antidiarrheal agent such as diphenoxylate hydrochloride with atropine sulfate (Lomotil) may be administered for diarrhea. Intravenous fluids may be used in severe cases if dehydration becomes a problem.

Chronic rejection usually occurs late in the posttransplant period, although it can occur as early as several weeks after transplantation (Jacobsson & Cohan, 1991). Chronic rejection is a poorly understood phenomenon even though it is one of the principal causes of graft loss. One study conducted by Schweitzer and associates (1991) showed that chronic rejection accounted for 45% of all the grafts lost at the University of Minnesota during the last 20 years.

The clinical signs of chronic rejection are similar to those of ESRD. Often proteinuria is the first indicator, followed by a rising serum creatinine level and decreased creatinine clearance. Hypertension and fluid retention with weight gain may be seen. As renal function deteriorates, anemia, acidosis, and hyperphosphatemia may occur. A renal biopsy confirms the diagnosis of chronic rejection. Chronic rejection is irreversible and may progress over a period of years, or renal function may decline rapidly (Jacobsson & Cohan, 1991; Shapiro & Simmons, 1992). Plans for retransplantation and interim dialysis are made once the GFR is less than 40% of normal.

As is evident, rejection and ATN continue to be important problems inhibiting successful transplantation beginning from the moment of revascularization to years after transplantation. In addition to ATN and rejection, a number of early postoperative complications result from the operation itself. These include complications involving the artery, vein, or ureter. Vascular complications include hemorrhage, thrombosis, infarction, and aneurysm formation. A late vascular complication is renal artery stenosis. The most common technical problem during the immediately postoperative period involves the ureter. Leaks from the ureteroneocystostomy site can occur during the early postoperative period. This may produce a urine leak from the wound and, later, a urinoma (Burdick, 1990; Shapiro & Simmons, 1992).

Symptoms of early postoperative vascular complications include a sudden decrease in or cessation of urine output, a drop in hematocrit, pain at the graft site or in the back radiating to the flank, graft swelling, proteinuria, hematuria, and ipsilateral leg swelling. Symptoms of ureteral necrosis, stenosis, or obstruction include decreased urine output, fever, graft tenderness, wound drainage, and ipsilateral leg swelling (Jacobsson & Cohan, 1991). Diagnosis of these technical problems requires various radiologic studies. Ultrasonography is used to detect perinephric fluid collections. Arteriography and venography are used to diagnose vascular problems.

Treatment consists of surgical intervention to correct the arterial, venous, or ureteral problem. In the case of hemorrhage and renal artery thrombosis, nephrectomy may be required because of kidney damage due to prolonged ischemic time (Jacobsson & Cohan, 1991).

Alteration in Electrolyte Balance

Electrolyte balance is an important consideration during the immediately postoperative period. When initial function with rapid diuresis occurs, there is risk for hypokalemia. Hyponatremia may occur because the kidney has decreased concentrating ability. Treatment consists of administration of potassium supplements or intravenous normal saline solution.

Hyperkalemia can occur during the early postoperative period when function of the transplanted kidney is delayed. The risk for hyperkalemia is compounded by the administration of blood, the trauma of the operation, and the nephrotoxic effects of cyclosporine (Jacobsson & Cohan, 1991). Prompt treatment of hyperkalemia with the administration of glucose and insulin, bicarbonate, and calcium can help avert cardiac arrhythmias. Some transplant centers may use sodium polystyrene sulfonate (Kayexalate) administered orally or as an enema, but it should not be given to patients with an ileus. Hemodialysis is often initiated, even during the first few postoperative hours, to treat hyperkalemia (Burdick, 1990; Flye, 1989; Haggerty & Sigardson-Poor, 1990). If hemodialysis is required, attempts are made to minimize heparinization to avoid increasing the risk of postoperative bleeding. To monitor the effects of heparin on bleeding, the wound drain should be left in place until after the first dialysis, if dialysis is required within 24 to 36 hours after the transplant (Burdick, 1990).

Even when renal function exists, kidney-transplant recipients are prone to electrolyte imbalances mostly due to the effects of cyclosporine on the renal tubules. Hypomagnesemia, hypophosphatemia, hyperkalemia, acidosis, and sodium retention may occur. Treatment consists of supplementation with oral magnesium, phosphorus, or an alkalizer and neutralizing buffer (sodium citrate and citric acid/Bicitra) as indicated. Hyperkalemia is controlled with a low-potassium diet and polystyrene sulfonate (Jacobsson & Cohan, 1991).

Management of Immunosuppression

The goal in the use of immunosuppression is to protect the patient from rejection while minimizing the side effects of the immunosuppressants. Advances in immunosuppression, such as cyclosporine, have improved patient graft survival and have made renal transplantation an excellent choice for patients with ESRD. Immunosuppressive drug therapies vary among transplant centers, but frequently used protocols use triple-drug therapy consisting of azathioprine, prednisone, and cyclosporine (Flye, 1989).

Monitoring of immunosuppressantive drug therapy consists of observing for and minimizing the side effects of the various drugs. Often these do not become apparent for months to years after transplantation, but several important side effects can occur during the immediately postoperative phase.

Administration of cyclosporine must be carefully monitored because of its nephrotoxic effects. The first dose of cyclosporine is delayed until the fifth postoperative day because of its association with ATN. Serum levels are monitored by radioimmunoassay (RIA), and the dosage is adjusted to achieve a therapeutic trough level of 100 to 250 ng/mL (Johns Hopkins Surgical Sciences, 1992a). Symptoms of cyclosporine toxicity include a rise in creatinine level and possibly a decrease in urine output.

Azathioprine has been associated with myelosuppression. Therefore, the patient's white blood cell (WBC) count must be monitored daily. A count below 400 cells/mm^3 may warrant discontinuation of the drug until the WBC count returns to normal (Shapiro & Simmons, 1992).

Prednisone has multiple side effects related to dose and duration. These include cataract formation, aseptic avascular necrosis of the femoral head, vertebral compression fractures, gastrointestinal problems, muscle wasting, and Cushing syndrome (Shapiro & Simmons, 1992). One side effect that can become apparent during the initial postoperative phase is steroid-induced diabetes. It may occur in as many as 10% of patients (Bia & Flye, 1989b).

Risk for Infection

Infection is a major complication of immunosuppression. It contributes substantially to the morbidity and mortality of renal transplantation (Cohen et al, 1988). Transplant recipients are at increased risk for infection because of immunosuppressive drug therapy. A continuous effort is made to balance the amounts of immunosuppressants given to achieve adequate prevention of rejection while trying to avoid compromising the patient's ability to fight infection.

Five factors commonly predispose renal transplant recipients to infection (Doran & Rubin, 1990). These include granulocytopenia, cellular immune dysfunction, humoral immune dysfunction, obstruction of natural body passages, and breech of body barriers. Transplant recipients are prone to different infections at different times during the posttransplant period. Early postoperative infections are commonly bacterial infections of the surgical wound, urinary tract, lung, and intravenous catheters. Early removal of invasive lines, sterile technique with dressing changes and catheter irrigations, strict hand-washing by health care professionals, and vigorous pulmonary toilet all help prevent these infections (Haggerty & Sigardson-Poor, 1990). Surveillance cultures of urine are done routinely during the immediately postoperative period to test for bacteria, CMV, herpes simplex virus (HSV), and varicella-zoster virus (VZV) infections.

After the immediately postoperative period, usually 1 to 6 months after the transplant, fungal and viral infections are common. Oral or esophageal candidiasis is a common occurrence (Shapiro & Simmons, 1992). Patients are treated prophylactically with nystatin suspension or clotrimazole troche. A viral infection common during this period is HSV infection, which is usually seen as oral, genital, or skin lesions. Oral acyclovir may be given for the first 6 months after the transplant to prevent this infection. Epstein–Barr virus (EBV) and CMV infections also may occur during the first 6 months after a transplant. EBV infection is manifested by symptoms of fever, malaise, and rising antibody titer. EBV infection can progress to a full-blown lymphoproliferative disorder. The only treatment is discontinuation of immunosuppression (Shapiro & Simmons, 1992).

CMV infection is the most common viral infection. Doran and Rubin (1990) wrote that 60 to 90% of all renal-transplant recipients demonstrate laboratory or clinical evidence of CMV infection in the first posttransplant year. CMV infection can occur in numerous organs, including the kidney, liver, colon, lungs, and retina. CMV infections are treated with systemic ganciclovir (Shapiro & Simmons, 1992). Some centers give ganciclovir prophylactically. In an attempt to prevent CMV infections at the Johns Hopkins Hospital, renal-transplant recipients are given oral acyclovir for the first 3 months after transplantation. Oral acyclovir has been shown to reduce the incidence of CMV disease in renal-transplant recipients (Balfour et al, 1991). In addition, patients who are CMV-seronegative and receive a CMV-seropositive organ are given a course of CMV immune globulin.

DISCHARGE TEACHING

An important function of the transplant nurse is to prepare the patient for discharge and for a lifetime of self-monitoring and care. The topics included in the discharge teaching are medications, diet, activity, signs and symptoms of infection, signs and symptoms of rejection, conditions requiring notification of a physician, personal care, and follow-up appointments.

Patients are taught about the indications, doses, and side effects of medications. Supervised self-administration of medications is begun during hospitalization. Written materials are provided to reinforce teaching and assist the patient in keeping track of medications on a daily basis. In addition to the immunosuppressant, most patients are discharged with a prescription for a multivitamin containing zinc, a stool softener, a magnesium supplement, and a drug to inhibit gastric secretion.

Transplant recipients are encouraged to follow a no-added-salt diet to minimize the sodium-retaining effect of prednisone. Some patients may need to restrict potassium intake because of the hyperkalemic effect of cyclosporine. Fluid restriction depends on the degree of renal function at the time of discharge. Because of the effect

TABLE 8–2 SIGNS AND SYMPTOMS OF INFECTION AND REJECTION

Infection	Rejection
Temperature over 101°F	Temperature over 101°F
Wound drainage	Flu-like symptoms: chills, joint and muscle aches, restlessness
Redness of incision	
Pain in incisional area	Tenderness over kidney
Cloudy, foul-smelling urine	Weight gain of 4–5 lb a day
Pain with urination	Swelling of hands, feet, legs, and eyelids
White coating on tongue	Decreased urine output
	High blood pressure
	Rise in blood urea nitrogen and creatinine levels

of prednisone on the appetite, transplant recipients often struggle with weight gain during the posttransplant period. A dietician counsels each patient before discharge and provides them with an individualized diet.

Activity restrictions include avoiding heavy lifting for 3 months and avoiding driving for 4 weeks after the operation. Patients are advised to avoid activities that could cause trauma to the kidney, such as contact sports. Regular exercise is encouraged to help control weight. Patients are advised to minimize stress to hips and knees because of the risk for aseptic avascular necrosis from long-term steroid use.

Routine health-maintenance activities are encouraged. These include dental examinations twice a year; procurement of a medic-alert bracelet; and for women, an annual gynecologic examination with a Papanicolaou smear, monthly self examinations of the breasts, and avoidance of pregnancy during the first posttransplant year.

Probably the most important information for the transplant recipient is the signs and symptoms of infection and rejection. These are listed in Table 8–2. Early detection of these complications yields the most positive outcomes.

CARE AFTER DISCHARGE

Renal transplantation is looked upon by many as a cure of ESRD. In truth, it is a treatment requiring a life-time of medical follow-up care. After discharge, a renal-transplant recipient must begin a regular routine of medications, clinic follow-up visits, and blood tests. Before leaving the hospital, each patient receives instructions about these routines. It is this type of management that offers the patient and the transplant team the best chance for long-term successful graft function and early detection of possible complications.

Immunosuppressive medications are gradually decreased after the transplant until the patient is taking maintenance doses. The schedules to taper these medications vary among different transplant centers and depend on the patient's renal function.

The clinic visits allow the transplant team to assess the patient's understanding of medication doses, schedules, and signs and symptoms of any complications.

Clinic visits also provide an opportunity to review any previous patient teaching. The patient and family's understanding of activity restrictions, medications, laboratory tests, diet, and the follow-up regimen can be assessed. Additional teaching can be provided at this time as needed.

Most renal transplant recipients experience one or more complications after discharge. During the first year after transplantation, complications generally include infections, rejection, obesity due to steroids, cardiovascular problems, or problems related to the side effects of medication. Many late complications are related to the long-term use of immunosuppressive medications.

Infection

Infections generally occur more often in patients taking immunosuppressive medications than in the general population. Urinary tract infections are the most common type of bacterial infection seen in transplant recipients (Harasyko, 1989). Patients are often asymptomatic, which is why regular urine cultures are important for detection. Many transplant centers treat patients with prophylactic antibiotics, which helps to decrease the frequency of these infections (Jacobsson & Cohan, 1991). Patients with urinary tract infections are usually given outpatient treatment with oral antibiotics. Fungal and viral infections can be a problem after discharge and are discussed in the Postoperative Care section of this chapter and in Chapter 2.

Rejection

Rejection is one of the most important concerns for renal-transplant recipients. During clinic visits and by assessment of laboratory values the physician and transplant coordinators monitor for early signs of rejection. Early treatment of acute rejection is critical. Rejection can be confirmed with sonography and a renal biopsy. The biopsy is an important diagnostic tool to differentiate rejection from cyclosporine nephrotoxicity or recurrent from de novo disease.

Cardiovascular Problems

The most common cardiovascular problem seen in renal-transplant recipients is hypertension. The cause is often multifactorial. Hypertension can be related to cyclosporine, obesity, fluid retention, renal artery stenosis, and rejection (Bia & Flye, 1989b; Haggerty & Sigardson-Poor, 1989; Harasyko, 1989). Hypertension may respond to adjustments in cyclosporine dosage, weight loss, sodium restriction, or diuretic therapy. Antihypertensive medications are commonly used to control hypertension in long-term recipients of renal-transplants.

Renal artery stenosis can cause severe hypertension and renal dysfunction. An audible bruit is often heard over the transplanted kidney, but the diagnosis should be confirmed with arteriography. Intervention includes balloon dilation of the artery, though sometimes surgical intervention is necessary (Harasyko, 1989; Haggerty & Sigardson-Poor, 1989).

Renal Vein Thrombosis

Renal vein thrombosis is a rare complication after transplantation. Symptoms include graft swelling, proteinuria, oliguria, anuria, and edema of the lower extremities. Treatment includes thrombectomy and anticoagulant therapy. However, renal function is often lost, and a transplant nephrectomy is required (Haggerty & Sigardson-Poor, 1990; Jacobsson & Cohan, 1991).

Liver Function Abnormalities

Abnormal liver function has been reported in 10 to 35% of renal-transplant recipients. It often leads to the development of acute hepatitis or chronic liver disease (Bia & Flye, 1989b). Acute hepatitis is usually caused by a virus or it can be the result of azathioprine therapy. It usually resolves in a few weeks or with a reduction in drug doses. Acute hepatitis can develop into chronic liver disease. Although chronic liver disease has some viral associations, its development is not fully understood. Chronic liver disease has caused the death of as many as 20% of renal-transplant recipients 5 or more years after transplantation (Bia & Flye, 1989b).

Steroid-Associated Problems

The long-term use of steroids can cause a variety of problems in renal-transplant recipients. In addition to the complications discussed elsewhere, other complications that develop over time include avascular necrosis and cataracts. Avascular necrosis can occur in 10 to 20% of renal-transplant recipients receiving long-term steroid therapy (Bia & Flye, 1989b). The most common complaint is severe pain, which usually affects the hips and occasionally the knee joints. Although early diagnosis and intervention can help to decrease symptoms, many patients ultimately require total hip replacements. Cataracts occur in one-fourth to one-third of renal-transplant recipients. There is no other treatment of cataracts other than lens removal.

Excessive weight gain is a major problem for renal transplant recipients. Consultation with a nutritionist is important to help recipients with meal planning and weight loss. Excessive weight gain seems to be less of a problem when lower doses of steroids are used. Loss of body image can be a problem for a patient who gains large amounts of weight and has cushingoid features as a result of steroid therapy.

Malignancies

Most malignancies diagnosed after a transplant respond to therapy. The types of malignant tumors usually found in transplant recipients include lymphomas, Kaposi and other sarcomas, carcinomas of the kidney, vulva, and perineum, and hepatobiliary tumors (Penn, 1990). Studies also indicate that there is an increased incidence of lymphoma and Kaposi sarcoma and a decreased incidence of skin cancers, uterine cervical cancers, and cancers of the vulva and perineum among patients treated with cyclosporine than those treated with azathioprine or cyclosphosphamide and prednisone. Patients treated with monoclonal antibodies have a higher incidence of lymphomas than other patients (Penn, 1990).

Malignancies in transplant recipients are treated by conventional methods. Treatment for renal-transplant recipients, unlike liver or heart recipients, may also include withdrawal of immunosuppression because there is the option to return to dialysis.

This may be a permanent return to dialysis or a temporary measure until it is safe to consider retransplantation (Penn, 1990).

Recurrence of Primary Renal Disease

Several types of renal disease can recur in a transplanted kidney. Most of these are types of glomerulonephritis. The type with the highest degree of recurrence is type II mesangiocapillary glomerulonephritis. It recurs about 88% of the time. The second most frequently recurring disease, seen in about 50% of patients, is IgA nephropathy (Bia & Flye, 1989b). Other types known to recur include focal glomerulosclerosis, crescentic glomerulonephritis, Henoch–Schönlein purpura, systemic lupus erythematosus, and antiglomerular basement membrane disease (Bia & Flye, 1989b). Having a renal disease that has recurred does not necessarily exclude a patient from receiving a second organ, because in most cases failure of the transplanted kidney occurs slowly. Retransplantation however, should be carefully considered for recurrent diseases such as focal sclerosis and type II mesangiocapillary glomerulonephritis, since these diseases lead to rapid loss of graft function (Bia & Flye, 1989b). Glomerulonephritis also can occur as a de novo disease in a transplanted kidney.

Despite the numerous complications associated with transplantation, most can be easily treated. Most patients feel the freedom from dialysis is worth the risks. Currently only the most healthy patients undergo transplants. Perhaps in the future with new treatments for complications, better immunosuppressive medications, and more donor sources, renal transplantation can be an option for all patients with ESRD.

FUTURE ISSUES IN KIDNEY TRANSPLANTATION

Medications

Because current immunosuppressive medications, though effective against rejection, have many side effects, ongoing efforts are underway to find better immunosuppressive drugs. One drug now in clinical trials for liver and kidney transplant recipients is FK506. Initial reports indicate that FK506 has mechanisms of action similar to those of cyclosporine and can be given at lower dosages. So far, FK506 seems to be less nephrotoxic than and does not cause the hypertension, hyperuricemia, hypercholesterolemia, or gingival hyperplasia seen with cyclosporine (Thomson, 1990).

Another drug being studied in animal trials is rapamycin. Rapamycin has been found to be more potent than cyclosporine and FK506 (Lake, 1990). Rapamycin also exhibits antifungal and antitumor properties (Calne et al, 1989). A third drug, 15-deoxyspergualin, is being tested for effectiveness in treating steroid-resistant rejection (Amemiya et al, 1990). Other new immunosuppressive agents in various phases of study include cyclosporine G and brequinar sodium (Kahan, 1992; Matas, 1991).

Donors

Because of the lack of availability of living-related donors and the shortage of cadaveric donors, some transplant programs are examining alternative means of obtaining donors. Methods of using kidneys from donors whose hearts are not beating are being evaluated. Kidneys from a patient who has died would be perfused with a rapid high-flush pressure in situ using Belzer solution through a tube inserted into the patient's femoral artery soon after death has been declared. Continuous hypothermic peritoneal perfusion would then be instituted after insertion of two peritoneal dialysis catheters to maintain the core temperature of the organs for 5 hours after death (UNOS, 1992f). The option of kidney donation would be offered to the patient's next of kin, and if consent were not obtained, the nonmutilated body would be released to the family. This would provide the opportunity for organ donation to patients otherwise who would have been missed.

Another option being considered in some transplant centers is the use of living unrelated donors. According to Rutger J. Ploeg, M.D., Ph.D. of the University of Wisconsin-Madison Medical School, "The use of living unrelated kidney donors could increase the organ supply, shorten waiting time and reduce overall health care cost by eliminating the need for dialysis" (UNOS, 1992e, p 6). Although all living kidney donors undergo thorough physical and psychologic evaluations to minimize any risks to their health, the use of living-unrelated kidney donors can be the subject of many ethical discussions, as was the use of living-related donors in the past. The immunosuppressive properties of cyclosporine and the use of donor-specific blood transfusions are making this an option for patients with ESRD at the University of Wisconsin (UNOS, 1992e). These results and the longer waiting time for cadaveric kidneys will cause more transplant centers to consider this option for their patients.

New donor sources, improved preservation techniques, and improved immunosuppressive medications are making the option of renal transplantation available to more patients with ESRD.

REFERENCES

Amemiya H, Suzuki S, Ota K, et al (1990). A novel rescue drug, 15-dexoyspergualin: First clinical trials for recurrent graft rejection in renal recipients. *Transplantation*. 49:337–343.

Balfour HH Jr, Fletcher CV, Dunn D (1991). Prevention of cytomegalovirus disease with oral acyclovir. *Transplant Proc*. 23(Suppl 1):17–19.

Bia MJ, Flye MW (1989a). Infectious complications in renal transplant patients. In: Flye MW, ed. *Principles of Organ Transplantation*. Philadelphia: Saunders, 294–306.

Bia MJ, Flye MW (1989b). Long term follow-up of the renal transplant patient. In: Flye MW, ed. *Principles of Organ Transplantation*. Philadelphia: Saunders, 307–333.

Blagg, C (1983). Dialysis or transplantation? *JAMA*. 250:1072–1073.

Bremer BA, McCauley CR, Wrona RM, Johnson JP (1989). Quality of life in end-stage renal disease: A reexamination, *Am J Kidney Dis*. 13:200–209.

Burdick J (1990). Complications of renal transplantation. In: Marshall FF, ed. *Urological Complications*, 2nd ed. St. Louis: Mosby Year Book, 183–200.

Burton PR, Wall J (1987). Selection adjusted comparison of life expectancy of patients on continuous ambulatory peritoneal dialysis, hemodialysis, and renal transplantation. *Lancet*. 1:115–118.

Calne RY, Lim S, Samaan A, et al (1989). Rapamycin for immunosuppression in organ allografting. *Lancet* 2:227.

Cecka JM, Terasaki PI (1990). The UNOS scientific renal transplantation registry—1990. In: Terasaki PJ, ed. *Clinical Transplants 1990* Los Angeles: UCLA Tissue Typing Laboratory, 1-10.

Cohen J, Hopkin J, Kurtz J (1988). Infectious complications after renal transplantation. In: Morris PJ, ed. *Kidney Transplantation: Practice and Principles*. Philadelphia: Saunders, 533-573.

Department of Health and Human Services (DHHS) (1991). *Questions and Answers About Organ Transplantation*. Rockville, Md: Division of Organ Transplantation.

Doran M, Rubin RH (1990). Infection in the renal transplant patient: New approaches to treatment in a compromised host. *Nephrol Nurs. Update.* 2:1-8.

Fischel R, Payne W, Gillingham K, et al (1991). Long-term outlook for renal transplant recipients with one year function. *Transplantation.* 51:118-122.

Flye MW (1989). Renal transplantation. In: Flye MW, ed. *Principles of Organ Transplantation.* Philadelphia: Saunders, 264-293.

Gharbieh PA (1988). Renal transplant: Surgical and psychologic hazards. *Critical Care Nurse.* 8:58-71.

Haggerty LM, Sigardson-Poor K (1990). Kidney transplantation. In: Sigardson-Poor KM, Haggerty LM, eds. *Nursing Care of the Transplant Recipient.* Philadelphia: Saunders, 114-139.

Harasyko C (1989). Kidney transplantation. *Nurs Clin North Am.* 28:851-863.

Hauser ML, Williams J, Strong M, et al (1991). Predicted and actual quality of life changes following renal transplantation. *ANNA J* 18:295-303.

Health Care Financing Administration (1991). *Medicare Coverage of Kidney Dialysis and Kidney Transplant Services* (DHHS Publication No. HCFA 10128). Baltimore, Md: US Government Printing Office.

House RM, Thompson TL (1988). Psychiatric aspects of organ transplantation. *JAMA.* 260:535-539.

Jacobsson PK, Cohan JL (1991). Kidney transplantation. In: Williams BA, et al eds. *Organ Transplantation: A Manual for Nurses* New York: Springer, 81-128.

Johns Hopkins Hospital Surgical Sciences (1992). *Johns Hopkins Hospital Transplant Immunosuppression Protocol.* Baltimore: Johns Hopkins Hospital.

Johnson JP, McCauley CR, Copley JB (1982). The quality of life of hemodialysis and transplant patients. *Kidney Int.* 22:286-291.

Kahan BD (1992). *Immunosuppressive Therapy.* Presented at the Second Annual Postgraduate Course: Transplant Immunobiology, Immunosuppression Complications, Tolerance, Preservation, New York, November 1992.

Kallich JD, Wyant T, Krushat M (1990). The effect of DR antigens, race, sex and peak PRA on estimated median waiting time for a first cadaver kidney. In: Terasaki PI, ed. *Clinical Transplants 1990.* Los Angeles: UCLA Tissue Typing Laboratory, 311-318.

Kalman TP, Wilson PG, Kalman CM (1983). Psychiatric morbidity in long term renal transplant recipients and patients undergoing hemodialysis. *JAMA.* 250:55-58.

Kasiske B, Neylan J, Riggio R, et al (1991). The effect of race on access and outcome in transplantation. *N Engl J Med* 324:302-307.

Katz S, Kerman R, Golden D, et al (1991). Preemptive transplantation: An analysis of benefits and hazards in 85 cases. *Transplantation.* 51:351-355.

Lake KD (1990). Immunosuppressive therapy: What's new? Presented at the Meeting of Advances in Transplantation, Washington, DC, October 1990.

Levinsky NG, Rettig RA (1991). Special report: The Medicare end stage renal disease program: A report from the Institute of Medicine. *N Engl J Med.* 324:1143-1148.

Liddington M, Richardson A, Higgins R, et al (1989). Skin cancer in renal transplant recipients. *Br J Surg* 76:1002-1005.

Matas AJ (1991). Where do we go from here? Long-term kidney transplant outcome. *Contemp Dial Nephrol* 12:18-21.

Moir EJ (1989). Nursing care of patients receiving Orthoclone OKT3. *ANNA J* 16:327-366.

Norman DJ, Shield CF, Barry JM, et al (1987). Therapeutic use of OKT3 monoclonal antibody for acute renal allograft rejection. *Nephron.* 46(Suppl 1):41-47.

O'Brien ME, Donley R, Flaherty MJ, Johnstone B (1986). Therapeutic options in end stage renal disease: A preliminary report. *ANNA J.* 13:313-318.

Parfrey PS, Bullock VS, Henry S, et al (1987). Symptoms in end stage renal disease: Dialysis vs. transplantation. *Transplant Proc.* 19:3407-3409.

Penn I. (1989). Risk of cancer in the transplant patient. In Flye MW, ed. *Principles of Organ Transplantation.* Philadelphia: Saunders, 634-643.

Penn I (1990). Occurrence of cancers in immunosuppressed organ transplant recipients. In: Terasaki PJ, ed. *Clinical Transplants 1990.* Los Angeles: UCLA Tissue Typing Laboratory, 53-62.

Perryman JP, Stillerman PU (1990). Kidney transplantation. In: Smith SL, ed. *Tissue and Organ Transplantation: Implications for Professional Nursing Practice.* St. Louis: Mosby Year Book, 176-209.

Ranjan D, Burke G, Esquenazi V, et al (1991). Factors affecting the ten-year outcome of human renal allografts: The effect of viral infections. *Transplantation.* 51:113-117.

Rao KV, Anderson R (1988). Long term results and complications in renal transplant recipients: Observations in the second decade. *Transplantation.* 45:45-52.

Schweitzer EJ, Matas AJ, Gillingham KJ, et al (1991). Causes of renal allograft loss: Progress in the 1980s, challenges for the 1990s. *Ann Surg.* 214:679-688.

Sequeira LA, Cutler RE (1992). Occurrence of cancer in transplant recipients. *Dial Transplantat.* 21:143-151.

Sever M, Steinmuller D, Hayes J, et al (1991). Pericarditis following renal transplantation. *Transplantation.* 51:1229-1232.

Shapiro R, Simmons RL (1992). Renal transplantation. In: Starzl T, et al, eds. *Atlas of Organ Transplantation.* New York: Gower, 4.1-4.21.

Shapter RK, Yonkman FF (1979). *Kidneys, Ureters, and Urinary Bladders*, 3rd ed. Summit, NJ: CIBA Pharmaceutical Company.

Starzl TE, Hakala TR, Tzakis A, et al (1987). A multifactorial system for equitable selection of cadaver kidney recipients. *JAMA.* 257:3073-3075.

Stuart F (1978). Selection, preparation and management of kidney transplant recipients. *Med Clin North Am.* 62:1381-1397.

Sutton TD, Murphy SP (1989). Stressors and patterns of coping in renal transplant patients. *Nurs Res.* 38:47-49.

Thomson AW (1990). FK-506: Profile of an important new immunosuppressant. *Transplant Rev.* 4:1-13.

Tilney N (1982). Surgical considerations of renal transplantation. In: Tilney N, Lazarus M, eds. *Surgical Care of the Patient with Renal Failure.* Philadelphia: Saunders, 184-211.

Tilney NL (1988). The early course of a patient with a kidney transplant. In: Morris PJ, ed. *Kidney Transplantation: Principles and Practice.* Philadelphia: Saunders, 263-283.

Thistlewaite JR, Stuart JK, Mayes JT, et al (1988). Use of a brief steroid trial before initiating OKT3 therapy for renal allograft rejection. *Am J Kidney Dis.* 11:94-98.

UNOS (1990). *Annual Report of the U.S. Scientific Advisory Board for Organ Transplantation and the Organ Procurement and Transplantation Network 1990.* Richmond: UNOS.

UNOS (1991a). National cooperative transplantation study completed. *UNOS Update.* 7:1, 4-5.

UNOS (1991b). Racial distribution of donors and transplant candidates. *UNOS Update.* 7:11.

UNOS (1992a). Enlightenment to black concerns influences kidney recipient to start committee. *UNOS Update.* 8:12.

UNOS (1992b). Waiting list characteristics. *UNOS Update.* 8:36-37.

UNOS (1992c). Deaths on waiting list. *UNOS Update.* 8:31-37.

UNOS (1992d). Median waiting time. *UNOS Update.* 8:37-40.

UNOS (1992e). Living unrelated kidney donation advocated. *UNOS Update.* 8:6-8.

UNOS (1992f). The non-heartbeating cadaveric donor: A solution to the organ shortage crisis. *UNOS Update.* 8:32-34.

United States Renal Data System (USRDS) (1991). *USRDS Annual Data Report.* Bethesda: National Institutes of Health.

Vollmer WM, Wahl PW, Blagg CR (1983). Survival with dialysis and transplant. *N Engl J Med.* 308:1553-1558.

Weems J, Patterson ET (1989). Coping with uncertainty and ambivalence while awaiting a cadaveric renal transplant. *ANNA J.* 16:27-31.

Wing AJ (1984). Choosing a dialysis therapy: A narrative summary of a panel discussion. *Am J Kidney Dis.* 4:256-259.

Wysynski EA, Jenkins DL, Hart TD (1989). Nursing considerations in patients receiving OKT3 for acute renal allograft rejection. *Contemp Dial Nephrol.* 10:16-28.

Zhou YC, Cecka JM, Terasaki PI (1990). Effect of race on kidney transplants: In Terasaki PI, ed. *Clinic Transplants 1990.* Los Angeles: UCLA Tissue Typing Laboratory, 447-459.

NURSING CARE PLAN 8–1

Nursing Diagnosis	Expected Outcomes	Nursing Interventions
Altered Urinary Elimination	• The patient produces a urine volume sufficient to maintain fluid and electrolyte balance before discharge.	• Maintain urinary catheter; irrigate as needed.
Related to	Urine output is approximately two-thirds intake.	• Assess and document clots in urine.
• Acute tubular necrosis (ATN)	Chemistry and electrolyte values are within normal limits for a new transplant recipient.	• Measure and document intake and output.
• Rejection		• Assess bladder for distention.
• Vascular hemorrhage, stenosis, thrombosis, or aneurysm		• Assess and document vital signs.
• Ureteral obstruction or leak		• Assess patient for pain around site of transplant.
		• Assess blood chemistry and electrolyte values.
Defining Characteristics		
• Decreased urine output		
• Pain, graft tenderness		
• Hematuria		
• Bladder distention		
• Hypotension		
• Clots in urinary catheter		
• Elevated blood urea nitrogen (BUN) and creatinine levels		
• Electrolyte abnormalities		
High risk for fluid volume deficit	• The patient achieves stabilization of fluid volume before discharge	• Assess skin turgor and mucous membranes for signs of dehydration.
Related to	Urine output is approximately two-thirds of intake	• Measure and document intake and output.
• Osmotic diuresis with functioning kidney	Urine specific gravity is between 1.010–1.025.	• Measure and record weight daily.
• Administration of diuretics		• Monitor vital signs and CVP.
		• Administer fluids as ordered by physician.
Defining Characteristics		
• Decreased central venous pressure (CVP), weight, and blood pressure		

234

- Decreased urine output
- Increased hemoglobin and hematocrit

Fluid Volume Excess

Related to

- ATN
- Rejection

Defining Characteristics

- Fluid intake greater than urine output
- Increased CVP, weight, respirations, blood pressure, heart rate
- Decreased urine output
- S3 heart sound
- Adventitious breath sounds
- Distended neck veins
- Edema (pulmonary and peripheral)
- Pink, frothy sputum

High Risk for Electrolyte Imbalance

Related to

- Decreased kidney function
- Blood transfusion
- Aggressive diuresis
- Effects of cyclosporine

Defining Characteristics

- Cardiac arrhythmias
- Nausea and vomiting
- Muscle aches, tingling

- The patient achieves a decrease or stabilization of fluid volume.
  Pulse, blood pressure, and respiratory rate approach normal for age and condition.
  Peripheral edema is reduced or absent.
  Output is approximately two-thirds of intake.
  Urine specific gravity is 1.010–1.025.
  Patient is within 2 kg of established dry weight.

The patient achieves stabilization of electrolytes before discharge.
  Sodium, potassium, and magnesium levels are within normal limits with dietary restrictions or medications

- Assess and document status of breath sounds, heart sounds, mucous membranes, skin turgor, peripheral edema, and neck veins.
- Measure and record daily weight.
- Measure and document intake and output.
- Assess urine specific gravity every shift
- Monitor vital signs and CVP.
- Elevate head of bed if patient is in respiratory distress.
- Administer diuretics as ordered and evaluate response.
- Restrict fluids and sodium intake as ordered.

- Monitor patient for cardiac arrhythmias, nausea, vomiting, muscle aches, and tingling.
- Instruct patient about dietary restrictions.
- Instruct patient about medication supplementation, if needed.

(continued)

NURSING CARE PLAN 8–1 (*continued*)

Nursing Diagnosis	Expected Outcomes	Nursing Interventions
Pain *Related to* • Surgical incision • Fluid overload *Defining Characteristics* • Patient complaint • Grimacing • Increased heart rate and blood pressure • Edema • Shortness of breath	The patient achieves effective management of pain before discharge and is free of excessive fluid overload. Pain tolerance is sufficient for activities of daily living. Patient identifies at least one pain-relieving technique, such as medication, devices, physical measures, and psychologic interventions. Patient is free of excessive peripheral edema and shortness of breath	• Assess and document pain and fluid status. • Administer pain medication and document patient's response. • Promote pain relief measures such as splinting of wound, positioning.
Knowledge deficit *Related to* • Renal transplantation and related health care practices • Effects of immunosuppressants and other medications • Diet • Activity limitations • Signs and symptoms of infection and rejection	• The patient has increased knowledge related to renal transplantation, treatments, and health care practices. Patient verbalizes a basic knowledge of renal transplantation and related health care before discharge. Patient demonstrates ability to take prescribed medications properly by discharge. Patient states activity limitations, signs and symptoms of infection, and signs and symptoms of rejection.	• Instruct patient to monitor daily weight, temperature, and blood pressure. • Observe patient preparation and self-administration of medications. • Instruct patient on the indications and side effects of medications. • Instruct patients on symptoms of rejection. • Instruct patient about diet, activity restrictions, sexuality, and health maintenance practices. • Document patient teaching and evidence of learning.

Potential for infection

Related to

- immunosuppression
- invasive catheters, IV lines, and drains
- surgical wound
- uremia
- diabetes

Defining Characteristics

- increased temperature and pulse
- purulent drainage of wound
- redness of IV sites or wound
- white coating on tongue
- cloudy, foul smelling urine
- green or yellow sputum
- patient complaint of pain on urination
- elevated WBC
- appearance of herpetic lesions

- The patient who is free from infection on admission will remain so throughout hospitalization.
  - urine is clear and there are no complaints of dysuria
  - clear respiratory secretions
  - normal temperature
  - IV sites and surgical incisions are without redness, drainage or odor
  - WBC is WNL
  - oral cavity is clear
- The patient will have no untreated infections prior to discharge.

- Inspect and document appearance of all catheters, drains, IV insertion sites, suture lines, wounds, and oral cavity daily.
- Assess and document appearance of urine and sputum.
- Perform suture line and drain site care with hydrogen peroxide using sterile technique.
- Monitor vital signs, especially temperature.
- Send urine for culture and sensitivity every Monday and Thursday; for virologic tests every Monday to rule out CMV, HSV, and varicella-zoster virus
- Enforce appropriate infection control measures
  - Hand-washing according to CDC guidelines
  - Mask and glove isolation for 24 hours postoperatively
  - No cut flowers at bedside
  - Patient surroundings clean
- Remove all indwelling catheters as soon as possible

9

Bone Marrow Transplantation

Jane C. Shivnan
Karen V. Ohly
Janet L. Hanson

Bone marrow transplantation (BMT) is a challenging modality with wide application for the treatment of malignant and nonmalignant disorders. Several decades of research in BMT have advanced it as the preferred method of intervention for selected diseases (Thomas, 1992). Medical efforts are continuously aimed at improving the long-term survival of recipients of BMT. As integral members of the transplant team, BMT nurses are faced with immense challenges. Their contribution to patient care has expanded with time. They not only care for patients undergoing highly complex state-of-the-art treatment programs but also assist patients with multiple issues of survivorship and reintegration into society.

HISTORICAL PERSPECTIVES

Early Efforts

The earliest reports of the administration of human bone marrow to patients occurred at the turn of the 19th century. At that time, attempts were made to treat selected patients with bone marrow failure disorders by either injecting them with or feeding them viable marrow cells (Wingard, 1991; Santos, 1983). Although these attempts were largely unsuccessful because of a lack of knowledge of immunology and tissue typing, this early inquiry paved the way for more rigorous scientific study in the 20th century.

In the 1940s and 1950s, it was noted that excessive exposure to radiation was associated with failure of the bone marrow. Laboratory research with canine models used both autologous and allogeneic bone marrow reinfusions to rescue animals after large doses of radiation (Thomas, 1992; Thomas et al, 1959). The Vinca nuclear reactor incident in Yugoslavia in the late 1950s highlighted an early attempt at human BMT when physicians treated several exposed workers by transfusions of allogeneic bone marrow cells (Wingard, 1991).

Many of the efforts in human BMT in the late 1950s and early 1960s were performed in patients with end-stage diseases, including aplastic anemia, leukemia, and immune deficiency disorders. However, because the initial results were dismal, efforts at allogeneic transplants in humans were temporarily abandoned. It was not until the discovery of the human leukocyte antigen (HLA) system in the 1960s and its application to histocompatibility typing that medical research was able to resume in human transplantation (Thomas, 1992). At that time, it became possible to select HLA-matched sibling donors.

Modern Bone Marrow Transplantation

Recent medical research and developments in ancillary fields facilitated supportive care through antibiotics and blood transfusions, conditioning regimens, and control of graft-versus-host disease (GVHD). These advances also contributed to the resurgence of interest in human BMT in the late 1960s. The application of BMT in the treatment of aplastic anemia, leukemia, and immunodeficiency syndromes widened, and improved results and better survival rates were reported by the mid 1970s (Wingard, 1991).

Since the early 1970s both clinical interest and the volume of bone marrow transplants performed have grown exponentially. By 1986, it was reported that more than 250 BMT centers were handling thousands of cases annually (Bortin & Rimm, 1989). The use of allogeneic transplantation has increased at a rate of more than 600 patients and 25 transplant teams annually (Bortin, et al, 1992). Advances in the development of patient selection criteria have further improved long-term disease-free survival rates. In addition, several new areas of clinical investigation have evolved in the past decade, including the use of unrelated or partially matched donors and the use of intensive chemotherapy for refractory solid tumors.

TYPES OF MARROW TRANSPLANTATION

The type of BMT used for treatment is contingent on several factors. These factors include the underlying illness, availability of a histocompatible donor, and current clinical indications.

Autologous

Autologous transplantation is the use of the patient's own bone marrow for treatment. The bone marrow is removed from the patient during an operative harvesting procedure and is cryopreserved for later use after the administration of a prescribed high-dose preparatory regimen. Bone marrow purging is sometimes used as a strategy to remove tumor cells from the bone marrow when tumor contamination is present or considered likely.

Syngeneic

Syngeneic transplantation is the use of an identical twin's bone marrow for treatment. Theoretically, if an identical twin is used as the donor, the patient does not incur the risk for GVHD after treatment. It has been reported, however, that GVHD may provide an antileukemic benefit, known as the graft-versus-leukemia effect (Vogelsang, 1990). In support of this phenomenon, higher relapse rates of leukemia have been reported in this population (Klingemann & Phillips, 1991).

Allogeneic

Allogeneic transplantation is the use of marrow from an HLA-matched donor, most often a sibling, for the transplant. With a decreasing national birthrate, however, only 35% of patients in the United States can anticipate having an HLA-identical sibling (Beatty, 1992). GVHD is also a major limitation of allogeneic transplantation.

Unrelated Matched and Partially Matched Transplants. With the hope of making BMT more accessible to patients who lack an HLA-matched sibling, many centers have begun exploring the use of partially matched or unrelated donors. Advances in histocompatibility testing have enabled researchers to define disparity between patient and donor. In general, as the disparity between the donor and recipient increases, the rate, incidence and severity of GVHD increase, the risk for graft failure increases, and the survival rate decreases (Beatty, 1992). Nevertheless, for some patients, undergoing a possibly curative unrelated donor transplant may be the best therapeutic alternative, in spite of high morbidity risks.

Donor registries established in the United States and abroad assist in the search for HLA-matched unrelated donors. The National Marrow Donor Program in the United States has a registry of more than 200,000 donors. More than 35 transplant centers in the United States and around the world participate in both transplants and ongoing research through this program (Weinberg, 1991). The International Bone Marrow Transplant Registry reported in its 1988–1990 survey that 14,745 patients received allogeneic transplants; 1153 (8.0%) were from unrelated donors (Bortin et al, 1992). The use of unrelated donor volunteers continues to rise.

CURRENT CLINICAL APPLICATIONS OF BONE MARROW TRANSPLANTATION

BMT is used to treat a wide variety of malignant and nonmalignant disorders. Current long-term survival rates for some of the more commonly treated disorders are summarized in Table 9–1.

TABLE 9–1. LONG-TERM RESULTS OF BONE MARROW TRANSPLANTATION

Disease	Survival Rate (%)[1]
Nonmalignant diseases	
Immunologic deficiency disease	50–90
Aplastic anemia, transfused	50–70
Aplastic anemia, untransfused	80–90
Thalassemia major	
Without liver damage	85–95
With liver damage	60–85
Malignant diseases	
Acute leukemia in relapse	10–30
Acute lymphoblastic leukemia, first or second remission	30–60
Acute myeloid leukemia, first remission	45–70
Chronic myeloid leukemia, accelerated or blastic phase	10–30
Lymphoma, Hodgkin's disease	
After failure of first line therapy	40–60
After failure of second line therapy	10–30

[1]Five-year, disease-free survival rate.
(From Thomas ED (1992). Bone marrow transplantation: Past experiences and future prospects. Semin Oncol. *19 (Suppl 7):4. Copyright 1992 W. B. Saunders Co.)*

Malignant Disorders

Table 9–2 lists malignant diseases for which BMT is a treatment option.

Acute Lymphocytic Leukemia. Allogeneic BMT for adults in first remission remains controversial (Meyer, 1992). A lack of controlled, randomized studies comparing BMT with standard chemotherapy makes a superior treatment approach unclear. On the other hand, BMT for acute lymphocytic leukemia (ALL) in first remission may be indicated for adults with adverse prognostic factors such as high leukocyte counts at diagnosis, prolonged time to remission, selected phenotypes, and the presence of certain chromosomal abnormalities.

BMT is generally not recommended for children with ALL in first remission, because standard chemotherapy cures approximately two-thirds of children in this situation (Sallan & Billet, 1992). Exceptions include children with certain chromosomal translocations. BMT is accepted as the treatment for both children and adults with ALL in second remission. Allogeneic matched-sibling transplants are generally recommended. However, when a suitable allogeneic donor is not available, autologous, purged-marrow transplantation may be recommended.

Acute Myelogenous Leukemia. Both autologous and allogeneic BMT have been used with success in the post-remission treatment of acute myelogenous leukemia

TABLE 9–2. POTENTIAL USE OF BONE MARROW TRANSPLANTATION IN BOTH MALIGNANT AND NON-MALIGNANT DISORDERS

Malignant Disorders

Acute lymphocytic leukemia

Acute nonlymphocytic leukemia

Chronic myelogenous leukemia

Preleukemia

Hairy cell leukemia

Chronic lymphocytic leukemia

Hodgkin and non-Hodgkin lymphoma

Selected solid tumors
  Breast cancer
  Lung cancer
  Testicular and germ cell tumors
  Neuroblastoma and other pediatric tumors
  Primary brain tumors
  Melanoma
  Ovarian cancer
  Sarcoma

Nonmalignant Disorders (Acquired and Congenital)

Aplastic anemia

Severe combined immunodeficiency disorder

Myelofibrosis

Osteopetrosis

Hematologic disorders
  Wiskott–Aldrich syndrome
  Fanconi anemia
  Diamond–Blackfan anemia
  Gaucher disease
  Cyclic neutropenia
  Chediak–Higashi syndrome
  Chronic granulomatous disease
  Thalassemia

Mucopolysaccharide storage diseases

Lipid storage diseases

Lysosomal diseases

(AML). It is recommended that patients with AML in first remission who have poor-risk features undergo BMT; the optimal postremission therapy is not clear for patients without poor-risk features (Jones & Santos, 1991). Because the results of intensive chemotherapy in first remission and BMT appear to overlap, some investigators suggest that BMT be deferred and offered as a salvage procedure to eligible patients whose disease recurs (Stone & Mayer, 1992). For children with AML in first remission who have a matched sibling donor, BMT is considered the treatment of choice (Dahl, 1990).

When a patient with AML in first remission undergoes BMT, an allograft is preferred if the patient is younger than 50 years and has a histocompatible donor. A purged autograft may be used in the absence of a histocompatible donor; preliminary outcomes are similar to those seen after allogeneic BMT (Jones & Santos, 1991). BMT in subsequent remissions results in less than optimal outcomes. Some authors suggest that BMT be considered early in the overall treatment of patients with acute leukemia who do not achieve a complete remission with conventional chemotherapy (Forman et al, 1991).

Chronic Myelogenous Leukemia. Allogeneic BMT is the only known possible cure of chronic myelogenous leukemia (CML). It is recommended that BMT be performed within 1 year of diagnosis in the chronic phase of the disease (Champlin et al, 1988). It is also known that advanced age and BMT in the accelerated or blastic phase are associated with poor outcome (Champlin, 1992). Because a large number of patients do not have a matched-sibling donor, matched-unrelated transplants have been performed but yield lower survival rates than those seen with matched-sibling donors (Marks & Goldman, 1992). A report of 185 unrelated donors described a follow-up period of nearly 5 years and an overall disease-free survival rate of 31% (Beatty, 1992). Initial attempts at autologous BMT for this disease have largely been unsuccessful, but current techniques focused on selecting normal hematopoietic progenitors and eliminating leukemic cells from autologous marrow offer a new direction for future research (Champlin, 1992).

Hodgkin and Non-Hodgkin Lymphoma. Autologous BMT has been widely applied in the treatment of Hodgkin and non-Hodgkin lymphomas. Patients with Hodgkin disease who are most likely to benefit from BMT are those who are treated before chemotherapy resistance develops, have a good performance status, and have a small tumor burden (Vose et al, 1990). Results of autologous BMT in the treatment of non-Hodgkin lymphomas are also better for patients with less advanced disease, especially those who still respond to chemotherapy (Gale et al, 1991). In recent years allogeneic BMT has been used successfully in the treatment of Hodgkin and non-Hodgkin lymphoma, suggesting a graft-versus-lymphoma effect that protects allogeneic recipients against relapse (Jones et al, 1991).

Other Malignant Disorders. BMT has been used to treat a variety of other malignant disorders, including myelodysplasia, hairy cell leukemia, Burkitt lymphoma, multiple myeloma, and refractory solid tumors. By 1991, approximately 400 autografts were reported for multiple myeloma (Gale et al, 1991). As noted with BMT for other malignant lesions, response rates are the highest among patients with less advanced disease (Barlogie & Gahrton, 1991).

Breast cancer is one malignant solid tumor for which autologous BMT has generated considerable interest and scrutiny over the past several years. Studies have been done in women with refractory disease, previously untreated metastatic disease, and metastatic disease responding to induction chemotherapy (Sledge & Antman, 1992). Several uncontrolled Phase I and II studies in the metastatic setting have suggested that 15–20% of women treated with high-dose chemotherapy and autologous

BMT may have durable complete remissions lasting several years (Kennedy et al, 1991; Peters et al, 1988; Antman et al, 1992; Kennedy et al, 1994). New therapeutic stratgies in the transplant setting will attempt to improve current treatment outcomes in metastatic breast cancer (Kennedy et al, 1994). Randomized trials are also now underway in earlier stage high-risk patients (ie, Stage II–III patients who have 10 or more lymph nodes) to determine whether standard chemotherapy followed by high-dose chemotherapy with autologous BMT improves survival rates.

Intensive chemotherapy and BMT have also played a role in the treatment of several pediatric tumors, such as neuroblastoma, Ewing sarcoma, rhabdomyosarcoma, Wilms tumor, osteogenic sarcoma, and brain tumors (Abramovitz, 1991). Most studies reported, however, have been small and uncontrolled (Gale et al, 1991). More than 200 children with neuroblastoma have received autografts of purged marrow; a 20% 3-year survival rate has been reported (Gale et al, 1991).

Nonmalignant Disorders

BMT has been used for numerous nonmalignant disorders, both acquired and congenital in nature (see Table 9–2).

Aplastic Anemia. Allogeneic BMT from a matched sibling has proved to be effective treatment of severe aplastic anemia; the highest survival rates are seen among patients younger than 18 years (Storb & Champlin, 1990). The risk for graft rejection is increased among patients who have undergone transfusion of red blood cells before the transplant (Champlin, 1990). This theoretically occurs because the patient becomes sensitized to transplantation antigens on donor cells. The risk, however, decreases with the infusion of larger numbers of bone marrow cells (Niederwieser et al, 1988). Transplantation using HLA partially matched family and unrelated donors has been performed but with less success than with matched-sibling donors (Storb & Champlin, 1991). These types of transplants will continue to be a focus of clinical investigation.

Severe Combined Immunodeficiency Disorder. Severe combined immunodeficiency disorder (SCIDS) results in an absence of antigen-specific T- and B-lymphocyte immunity in affected infants. The first successful allogeneic transplants were performed in children with SCIDS; BMT for this disorder has been on the frontline of clinical research, including the first successful use of T-lymphocyte-depleted haploidentical bone marrow and matched-unrelated donors (Lenarsky & Parkman, 1990). The most recent data reveal an overall survival rate of 70% when histocompatible BMT is used (Lenarsky & Parkman, 1990). Posttransplant immunosuppression is not routinely used. When a matched sibling is not available, a parent's marrow may be processed to remove T lymphocytes; the success rate of haploidentical T-cell-depleted marrow transplants is comparable with that seen when histocompatible donors are used (Lenarsky et al, 1990).

Other Congenital Disorders. Wiskott–Aldrich syndrome is an X-linked recessive immunodeficiency disorder in which affected male patients suffer from infections, eczema, and thrombocytopenia. The first complete correction of the syndrome by allogeneic transplantation occurred in 1977. Today it is one of the genetic disorders most amenable to complete correction by allogeneic BMT (Lenarsky et al, 1990). Patients with thalessemia, an erythroid disorder, could benefit from BMT. Over 250 patients have undergone BMT in Europe using marrow from histocompatible donors; the survival rate has been more than 80% (Lenarsky et al, 1990). Examples of other immunodeficiency and genetic disorders in which BMT has been used include chronic granulomatous disease, Fanconi anemia, sickle cell anemia, cyclic neutropenia, Chediak–Higashi syndrome, Diamond–Blackfan anemia, osteopetrosis, Gaucher disease, mucopolysaccharide storage diseases, mucolipidoses, and lysosomal diseases.

PREPARATION FOR A TRANSPLANT

Eligibility for a Transplant

The wide application of BMT is the result of not only a refinement of technologies and supportive care but also the evolution of appropriate eligibility criteria. The type and extent of disease are the primary determinants of a patient's eligibility for any of the various types of BMT. The risk for relapse after transplantation is reduced by conducting transplants in patients whose disease is in complete remission or those who have minimal residual disease at the time of transplantation. In addition, it has become apparent that referring patients earlier in their treatment course, before they have received multiple courses of chemotherapy, reduces the morbidity and mortality associated with BMT conditioning regimens. Early referral of patients for BMT after disease stabilization or induction of remission is strongly encouraged because of the relatively limited time many of the diseases are amenable to treatment by transplantation. Additional eligibility criteria are based on patient age, the lack of preexisting organ toxicity, the lack of comorbidity, and the availability of a suitable source of marrow. Examples of such criteria are given in Table 9–3.

Allogeneic BMT is the only type of transplant appropriate for the standard treatment of aplastic anemia, chronic myelogenous leukemia, and various genetic storage diseases. In general, allogeneic BMT is preferred for the acute leukemias, multiple myeloma, Hodgkin disease, and high-risk non-Hodgkin lymphomas, whereas autologous BMT is preferred for standard-risk non-Hodgkin lymphomas and most solid tumors amenable to treatment by BMT. It is highly likely that in the near future results of autologous BMT for the acute leukemias will improve sufficiently to make it the preferred BMT option for this patient population.

Financing a Transplant

Once a patient has been deemed eligible for BMT the issue of financing must be considered. Economic factors are a major determinant in the decision to undergo BMT because of its high cost and the concern of third-party payers that its use will overburden available health care dollars (Smith et al, 1992). Direct medical-care costs of BMT, including physician fees, hospital charges, and medications, account for approximately 10% of all transplant-related expenses. Indirect costs, including days of work missed due to illness, income lost due to premature death, and costs associated with trans-

**TABLE 9–3. GENERAL PATIENT ELIGIBILITY CRITERIA
FOR BONE MARROW TRANSPLANTATION**

Factor	Criteria
Age (years)	Allogeneic ≤ 55 Autologous ≤ 65
Major organ functioning	Cardiac: LVEF > 45% Pulmonary: FEC & FVC > 50% Renal: Creatinine ≤ 2.0 mg/dL Hepatic: Bilirubin ≤ 2.0 mg/dL

Suitable marrow source	Autologous: aspirable marrow
	  WBC count ≥ 3000
	  Plts ≥ 100,000

	Related allogeneic: HLA identical or 1 anti-
	gen mismatch
	  sibling or 1 antigen
	  mismatch parent or
	  child if patient younger than 20 years

	Unrelated allogeneic: HLA identical
Comorbidity	No active infections No AIDS diagnosis

LVEF, left ventricular ejection fraction; FEC, forced expiratory capacity; FVC, forced vital capacity; WBC, white blood cell; Plts, platelets; HLA, human leukocyte antigen; AIDS, acquired immunodeficiency syndrome.

portation, lodging, and meals, can consume up to 30 to 40% of a family income and may account for as much as 60% of the direct cost of BMT (Smith et al, 1992). The limitations of hospital accounting systems make it difficult to define the true cost of BMT; however, one study estimated the charges for allogeneic BMT to be approximately $200,000 per patient (Welch & Larson, 1989). Most transplant programs require third-party payer approval or other assurance of ability to pay before accepting potential BMT candidates. Many insurers have begun programs to assure quality care and the control of costs by designating select transplant programs as those in which their beneficiaries must be treated based on minimum standards for staffing, volume of procedures, and outcome. In these Institutes of Quality programs, participating hospitals agree to be reimbursed at a predetermined fee, regardless of resource consumption (Koska, 1990).

It has been suggested that, as with some other highly technical surgical procedures, there is a direct correlation between the volume of BMT procedures done by a transplant center and the quality of outcomes (Horowitz et al, 1992). Once presented with the option of BMT, candidates should be encouraged to consider several BMT treatment centers before making their choice. Factors to be taken into consideration, in addition to insurance company preference, include the quality of outcomes associated with an individual center, availability of lodging and support services, level of medical and nursing staff experience with the procedure, and availability of BMT treat-

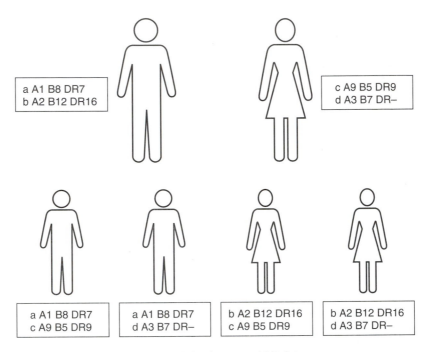

Figure 9–1. Inheritance of HLA types.

ment protocols for the management of the specific disease. With expansion of the number of treatment centers offering BMT, waiting lists for treatment have essentially been eliminated and centers have become highly competitive for patients.

Evaluation of Recipient and Donor

In the case of allogeneic transplants, HLA typing of the recipient and all potential donors is generally completed before the patient arrives at the BMT center. Full clarification of the patient's HLA type may require that his or her parents also be typed. The HLA loci of primary concern in BMT are HLA-A, HLA-B, and the HLA-DR loci. For each pair of antigens at these sites, one was inherited from the patient's mother and one was inherited from the patient's father (Figure 9–1). A full, or six-antigen, match is most desirable for allogeneic BMT. Although one-or-two-antigen-mismatched bone marrow transplants have been done, the greater the number of mismatched antigens, the greater are the incidence of GVHD and the transplant related mortality. Once a suitable donor has been identified through HLA typing, a mixed lymphocyte culture (MLC) must be conducted. Most transplant programs prefer that the donor accompany the patient to the BMT center for this test. A sample of the patient's lymphocytes is mixed with a sample of the donor lymphocytes and the culture is observed for evidence of adverse interactions. A negative MLC result allows the recipient to proceed with the preadmission evaluation.

Before and when the patient arrives at the transplant center, the BMT nurse co-ordinator is the primary patient contact and liaison. The nurse coordinator obtains from the referring physician the patient's past medical history, relevant chemother-apy treatment records, pathology slides, and all radiologic studies useful in the evalu-ation of the extent and stage of disease. Although some of the preliminary evaluation for eligibility may be conducted by the patient's referring physician, many studies may need to be repeated when the patient arrives at the transplant center.

Multiple members of the BMT team participate in the outpatient evaluation of prospective BMT recipients. In addition to medical and nursing evaluations, patients are evaluated by a dentist, nutritionist, social worker, and physical therapist. This is one of the most overwhelming periods in the BMT experience, and patients depend heavily on the BMT nurse-coordinator for education, guidance, explanations, and ad-vocacy. A healthy amount of ambivalence and anxiety is to be expected in BMT can-didates during this time. The nursing and social work staffs work closely at this point to assess patient and family coping skills and resources and to plan augmentation strategies if necessary. Profound ambivalence or anxiety should signal the need for a full psychiatric consultation and evaluation.

The final phase of the outpatient evaluation involves obtaining informed consent from both recipient and donor. Ideally, the patient and family should sit down with the BMT physician and nurse to discuss all potential risks and benefits of the planned BMT. Patients and their family should then be given sufficient time alone to absorb and discuss the information received and to identify any further questions they may have. Further discussion with the BMT team after the private family meeting should enable patient and donor to feel comfortable signing the requisite informed consent forms. As the transplant process moves forward, establishment of reliable venous ac-cess through placement of a multilumen right atrial central venous catheter may be done before admission to the inpatient unit.

Preparatory Regimens

BMT allows for highly intensive chemoradiotherapy regimens because it provides pro-tection against the dose-limiting toxicity of myelosuppression. When bone marrow support is provided through allogeneic, autologous, or peripheral stem cell products, the dose of chemotherapeutic agents used in BMT preparatory regimens reflects the new maximum tolerated dose based on nonhematopoietic dose-limiting toxicities (Herzig, 1992). The use of combination chemotherapy drug regimens is guided by the possibility of synergistic effects, the need to avoid overlapping toxicities, and the lack of mutual cross resistance (Herzig, 1992). Given all these factors, the selection of agents for use in BMT preparatory regimens is based primarily on antitumor activity for the specific disease. Commonly used agents are listed in Table 9-4. Alkylating agents are frequently used in BMT preparatory regimens because they exhibit little nonmyeloid toxicity, possess a steep dose-response curve, and lack cross resistance (Frei et al, 1989).

The use of total body irradiation (TBI) for conditioning of patients before BMT is a by-product of military research on radiation sickness conducted in response to the development and use of the atomic bomb during World War II (Yahalom & Fuks,

TABLE 9–4. CHEMOTHERAPEUTIC AGENTS COMMONLY USED IN BONE MARROW TRANSPLANTATION REGIMENS

Amsacrine
Busulfan
Carboplatin
Carmustine
Cyclophosphamide
Cytarabine
Etoposide
Ifosfamide
Melphalan
Nitrogen mustard
Thiotepa

1992). The dose-limiting toxicities of TBI in the setting of BMT are pulmonary and hepatic toxicity. Because of the relatively high toxicity of TBI, its use in BMT has been limited to those malignant tumors that exhibit a high sensitivity to irradiation, such as leukemias, lymphomas, and selected solid tumors. The importance of dose rate and fractionation schedules for TBI have been well demonstrated by studies that have shown a reduction in both pulmonary and mucosal toxicity when multiple fractions and lower dose rates have been used (Phillips et al, 1990; Yahalom & Fuks, 1992). In general the maximum dose of TBI in BMT is limited to 1000 cGy in a single fraction or 1500 cGy in fractionated dose schedules (Yahalom & Fuks, 1992).

The primary goals of all chemotherapy and chemoradiation BMT conditioning regimens are (1) the eradication of residual disease; (2) the formation of space for recipient marrow to allow for donor cell engraftment; and (3) in the case of allogeneic BMT, immunosuppression to prevent the rejection of donor marrow. Nurses must have strong knowledge of the principles and practices of cancer chemotherapy to provide effective patient and family education. This is especially important during administration of the preparatory regimen and during the period of marrow aplasia, when many toxicities related to the preparatory regimen may manifest themselves.

Marrow Harvesting

Viable bone marrow stem cells capable of engraftment can be obtained from peripheral blood, fetal liver, fetal umbilical cord blood, cadavers, or the sternum or pelvis of a live donor. The most commonly used bone marrow harvest procedure—harvesting from live donors—is essentially the same for both allogeneic and autologous bone marrow donation. The harvesting procedure itself has little risk associated with it other than the risks of anesthesia. Epidural anesthesia has been used increasingly in recent years for donations in which general anesthesia is contraindicated. In either case, the harvest is conducted under sterile conditions with the knowledge that the product is to be infused into a profoundly immunosuppressed recipient.

With heparinized syringes, marrow is removed by needle aspiration bilaterally from the posterior iliac crests by two harvesters working simultaneously. The goal is to obtain a minimum of approximately 2×10^8 nucleated cells per kilogram of body weight of the recipient of an allogeneic transplant or 1×10^8 cells for the recipient of an autologous graft (Barrett, 1991). Marrow processing or cryopreservation can result in the loss of as many as 30% of nucleated cells; consequently it is desirable to increase the total harvest volume when these techniques are used. Autologous donors who have been heavily pretreated often yield a smaller number of bone marrow stem cells in relation to the number of nucleated cells harvested and therefore also require harvesting of a greater number of nucleated cells per kilogram of body weight (Treleaven, 1991). Usually, only two skin punctures are required at each iliac crest harvest site. Skin elasticity allows the aspiration needle to be removed from the bone after each aspiration and reinserted into the bone at a different location without being removed from the skin entry site.

In the operating room, aspirated marrow is often filtered through successively smaller mesh stainless steel filters to remove fibrin clots and other debris. It has been suggested, however, that this filtration is unnecessary and that bone marrow can be placed directly after harvest into a dry, sterile blood bag containing preservative-free heparin (Treleaven, 1991). The latter method minimizes the potential for contamination.

Allogeneic donors usually have one to two units of red blood cells collected several weeks before harvesting for reinfusion after bone marrow harvesting. Autologous bone marrow donors are more likely to have received blood transfusions during earlier chemotherapy and will certainly receive them during the aplasia period after BMT. For this reason they do not require collection of autologous red cells before harvesting.

The morbidity and mortality associated with bone marrow harvesting has been minimal. Possible complications are listed in Table 9–5. A review of 3000 cases reported to the International Bone Marrow Transplant Registry found only two donor deaths, neither of which was a result of the harvest procedure itself (Bortin & Buckner, 1983). After harvesting, donors spend a brief period of time recovering from anesthesia and then are either discharged home or begin their BMT preparatory therapy.

TABLE 9–5. RISKS OF BONE MARROW HARVEST

Bruising
Bleeding
Pain at aspiration sites
Infection
Transient neuropathies
Hypotension secondary to volume loss
Psychologic maladjustment

Use of Peripheral Blood Progenitor Cells

Although hematopoietic stem cells are primarily found in the bone marrow, they can also be found in the peripheral circulation in smaller numbers. It is not clearly understood why peripheral blood contains progenitor cells or how they are regulated; circulating progenitors are quite immature, in a resting phase of the cell cycle, and do not actively contribute to hematopoiesis (Antman, 1992).

The use of peripheral blood progenitor cells (PBPCs) to facilitate engraftment in transplant patients, either alone or in combination with bone marrow, is an active area of research (Mazanet et al, 1991; Mason et al, 1991; Schwartzberg et al, 1991). Diseases for which this technology has been applied include acute leukemias, lymphomas, breast cancer, and other selected solid tumors (Whedon, 1991). Several studies of autologous transplantation have indicated that PBPCs, given either alone or in combination with bone marrow reinfusion, have resulted in earlier recovery of patients after dose-intensive therapy (Sledge & Antman, 1992).

The application of PBPC technology is an attractive one for several reasons. First, the use of PBPCs alone gives patients who might otherwise be ineligible for dose-intensive therapy the opportunity to undergo such a procedure. Secondly, PBPC harvests do not require general anesthesia; they are performed using an apheresis procedure. Thirdly, the reduced duration of aplasia associated with the use of PBPCs as support for high-dose chemotherapy with or without marrow or growth factors may significantly reduce the mortality, morbidity, and cost of high-dose therapy (Sledge & Antman, 1992). Ongoing studies will continue to address these issues in the transplant setting.

The methods for PBPC harvest involve the use of apheresis procedures, in which mononuclear cells can be collected for reinfusion. Once collected, these cells are cryopreserved in DMSO 10%. Traditionally, 7 to 10 leukaphereses were required to obtain adequate numbers of cells for transplantation, straining blood bank and related resources (Antman, 1992). More recently, methods have been used to deliberately increase the PBPC yield ("mobilization") and decrease the number of leukaphereses required to obtain these cells. These methods include the administration of cytotoxic chemotherapy to stimulate hematopoiesis during the recovery period, the use of specific cytokines, or a combination of both methods (Demetri & Antman, 1992; Rosenfeld & Nemunaitis, 1992; Rowe et al, 1994).

When peripheral blood progenitor cells are collected during steady-state hematopoiesis (in an unmobilized fashion), they appear to engraft at the same rate as bone marrow (Kessinger & Armitage, 1991). The recovery of blood counts can be accelerated when mobilized PBPCs are reinfused, although recommendations for the minimal number of these cells collected have not yet been determined (Rowe et al, 1994). The measurement of CD34+ cells (a type of differentiation antigen expressed by PBPCs) by flow cytometry is a promising technology which may help define whether an effective PBPC product has been obtained (Bender et al, 1992; Kessinger & Armitage, 1991).

Other unresolved issues in PBPC transplantation include whether these transplants are less likely to contain cancer cells than are bone marrow transplants or whether cancer cells in the blood have the same likelihood of causing relapse as

TABLE 9–6. COMMONLY USED BONE MARROW PURGING TECHNIQUES

Pharmacologic purging

Monoclonal antibodies + complement

Immunomagnetic purging: Monoclonal antibodies

+

Magnetic microspheres

Immunotoxin purging: Monoclonal antibodies

+

Immunotoxin

Lectin agglutination

Counterflow elutriation

CD34 positive selection

those in the bone marrow (Gale et al, 1991). Research will further clarify these issues and define the optimal application of PBPC technology to the treatment of malignant disease.

Manipulation of Autologous Bone Marrow

Graft engineering—the ex vivo manipulation of bone marrow before reinfusion—is conducted for one of two reasons. In the autologous setting, marrow is purged of residual tumor cells with proliferative potential. In the allogeneic setting, the goal of graft engineering is the modulation of GVHD. The first method used for the removal of residual tumor cells from the bone marrow graft was pharmacologic (Yeager et al, 1990). 4-Hydroperoxy-cyclophosphamide (4-HC), a synthetic analogue of the active metabolite of cyclophosphamide, is more toxic to tumor cells than to normal cells. Typically, marrow is incubated for 30 minutes in a proper concentration of 4-HC and tissue culture media then washed of any tumor cells and 4-HC and frozen for reinfusion at a later date. 4-HC purging has been found to prolong the period of aplasia after bone marrow infusion because of the loss of additional stem cells during the processing procedure (Davis et al, 1990).

Although controversy exists as to the place of purging in autologous BMT and its utility in prolonging disease-free survival of a patient who has undergone autologous BMT, the development of new methods for the ex vivo purging of bone innoculum has advanced rapidly. Additional single-agent and multidrug combinations have been developed for the pharmacologic purging of bone marrow. In addition, immunologic and physical techniques for marrow purging have been developed (Table 9–6). Most purging techniques rely on identification of tumor cells and their physical removal from the harvested marrow. Factors that complicate purging include the number of different tumor types for which specifically designed monoclonal antibodies are required and the high degree of heterogeneity that characterizes tumor cell populations. However, heterogeneity between normal hematopoietic cell populations is minimal. The most recent advance in marrow purging technology has been the development of positive selection techniques that help identify cells with stem cell characteristics.

CD34 is a cell surface marker found almost exclusively on normal, primitive hematopoietic cells. Reliable methods of identification and removal of CD34-positive cells should ultimately result in clean marrow (Lansdorp et al, 1992).

T-Cell Depletion of Allogeneic Bone Marrow

Upon identification of mature T lymphocytes as the causative agent in the development of GVHD, work on the development of mechanisms for the selective removal of T cells from the allogeneic graft began. It was soon discovered that full removal of all mature T cells resulted in an increase in the incidence of relapse after BMT, thought to be due to loss of a graft-versus-leukemia effect, and an increase in the risk for graft failure after BMT. Early T-cell-depletion techniques relied on the use of anti–T-cell monoclonal antibodies such as muromonab-CD3 (Barrett, 1991). Recent research has focused on the development of methods to quantitate the number of T cells reinfused, as is possible with counterflow elutriation, and the development of approaches that allow the selective removal of mature T cells while preventing the removal of natural killer (NK) cells (Noga et al, 1990). NK cells are thought to confer a degree of immunoprotection to a profoundly neutropenic host. Finally, the most exciting area of research has been the genetic manipulation of hematopoietic tissue. It is thought that the future of both allogeneic and autologous BMT lies in this direction of gene therapy.

Reinfusion of Marrow

The bone marrow reinfusion process is relatively uncomplicated and is technically similar in many ways to red blood cell transfusions. In the case of infusions of allogeneic ABO-incompatible bone marrow, autologous bone marrow, or PBPCs, the recipient should be well hydrated before and after marrow infusion with intravenous fluids containing sodium bicarbonate. This ensures adequate renal perfusion and urine alkalinization in the presence of intravascular red-cell lysis due to incompatibility or trauma. The volume of ABO-compatible allogeneic bone marrow infusions is 500–2000mL depending upon the harvest. In contrast, autologous and ABO incompatible allogeneic marrow volumes are only 200 to 600 mL because of volume reduction with processing to remove incompatible red cells and plasma or contaminating tumor cells. Volume reduction through the removal of red cells and plasma also may be indicated in the case of pediatric ABO-compatible bone marrow infusions.

Intravenous infusion of the cryoprotectant DMSO has been associated with a histamine release reaction consisting of flushing, a feeling of chest tightness, and abdominal cramping with or without nausea. In rare cases anaphylaxis and cardiac arrhythmias have occurred. Rapid infusion of DMSO has been associated with symptomatic bradycardia (Davis et al, 1990; Rapoport et al, 1991). Consequently autologous and PBPC infusions, which contain large amounts of DMSO, must be conducted slowly, and these bone marrow recipients are premedicated with antihistamines and connected to cardiac monitors for the duration of marrow infusion. Thawing of autologous and PBPC products is conducted at the patient's bedside by immersion in a warm-water bath. Thawed marrow is then drawn-up in a syringe and slowly administered through a central venous catheter. DMSO excretion is primarily through the lungs, producing a characteristic odor to the breath of the recipient for 2 to 12 hours after infusion.

Allogeneic marrows is administered in an intravenous infusion over 2 to 4 hours. Bone marrow products are never irradiated or administered through in-line filters or with intravenous infusion pumps. PBPC infusions are often conducted over several days because of their high volume and high DMSO content. All BMT recipients can expect a red tinge to their urine for up to 12 hours after marrow infusion because of mild intravascular red-cell lysis. Transfused marrow passes through the pulmonary capillary bed first and stays there for some time, producing a transient loss of pulmonary capacity. Stem cells then selectively migrate and nest in bone marrow microenvironmental niches (Tavassoli & Hardy, 1990).

POSTTRANSPLANT MANAGEMENT ISSUES

Clinically significant complications may occur during the first few weeks and months after bone marrow infusion. An interrelationship between these acute complications has been described by Ford and Ballard (1988) as follows.

1. The preparatory regimen would be fatal if the patient were not to undergo bone marrow infusion.
2. Complications are usually the result of the preparatory regimen or the marrow transplant not the disease.
3. Complications often occur simultaneously.
4. Clinical manifestations of different complications may be the same.
5. One complication may cause or exacerbate another.
6. The treatment of one complication may cause or exacerbate another.
7. The prophylaxis or treatment of one complication may need to be altered because of the development of another complication.

Not surprisingly, nursing assessment of, early intervention in, and management of these potentially life-threatening complications contributes significantly to patient outcome.

Hematopoietic Complications

As previously described, the preparatory regimen destroys a patient's bone marrow, leading to a profound aplasia that may last days or weeks until new progenitor cells are active. Even with the recovery of a normal neutrophil count, the humoral and cell-mediated immune responses of a patient who has undergone BMT remain abnormal for 1 year or more after the transplant. Consequently, the patient is at high risk for bacterial, fungal, and viral infections.

Infections. BMT centers practice a wide variety of infection control measures (Poe et al, 199X; Rogers, 1985). Isolation procedures range from single, hepa-filtered rooms and hand-washing requirements to strict laminar air flow environments. Housekeeping standards may be similar to those for other hospital units, or there may be elaborate disinfection procedures involving nurses as well as housekeepers. Modified diets or sterile food may be prescribed (Somerville, 1986). In addition, prophylactic anti-biotic, antiviral, and antifungal regimens are common. Very little research supports these practices, and there is a clear need for nursing research in these areas.

The person assessing a patient who has undergone BMT must be aware that the normal inflammatory response may be altered by both the lack of white blood cells (WBCs) and immunosuppressive medications. All possible sites of infection should be assessed at least once a day. Surveillance cultures are generally used to assist in making decisions about treatment choices. Broad-spectrum antibiotics should be initiated for any fever during neutropenia, and the patient should be carefully monitored for signs of sepsis (Klemm & Hubbard, 1990).

Bleeding. The megakaryocyte is generally the last cell to be produced as new marrow engrafts, and a patient who has undergone BMT may need months to achieve a normal platelet count (Caudell & Whedon, 1991). Bleeding is a common complication of BMT, but with rapid intervention it is fatal for only 1% of transplant patients (Ford & Ballard, 1988). Nursing care of a patient at risk for bleeding is summarized in Nursing Care Plan 9–1 (see p 278). Multiple platelet transfusions may be needed to maintain platelet counts of at least 20,000 to 30,000, leading in some instances to alloimmunization and platelet refractoriness. Hepatic dysfunction and uremia may contribute to bleeding tendencies, and replacement of clotting factors with fresh frozen plasma and cryoprecipitate may be necessary. Disseminated intravascular coagulation (DIC) may complicate the management of bleeding (Gobel, 1990).

Blood Product Support. Blood products transfused into an immunosuppressed BMT patient should be irradiated to prevent engraftment of transfused lymphocytes and the possible development of GVHD (Wujcik & Downs, 1992). For cytomegalo-vivus (CMV)-negative patients who undergo allogeneic BMT support with CMV-negative blood products decreases the risk of CMV pneumonitis (Ford & Eisenberg, 1990). This risk is much lower (2%) in autologous BMT (Wingard et al, 1988). Red cell transfusions are required to treat anemia. Although sometimes controversial, granulocyte transfusions may have benefit for neutropenic patients with severe infections (Dutcher, 1989).

Gastrointestinal Complications

A variety of gastrointestinal complications are seen after BMT. These complications can be mild to life-threatening in nature and are generally attributable to one or more of the following causes: direct effects of the conditioning regimen, infection of the gastrointestinal tract, acute or chronic GVHD, or side effects of other medications or treatments used during the transplant process (Vanacek, 1991; Wolford & McDonald, 1988).

Oral and Esophageal Mucositis. Severe oral complications occur in approximately 75% of recipients of allogeneic BMT and in a smaller percentage of recipients of autologous or syngeneic BMT (Carl & Higby, 1985). Oropharyngeal mucositis typically results from conditioning regimens, particularly those that include TBI (Barrett, 1986; Kolbinson et al, 1988). Specific high-dose chemotherapeutic agents thought to be associated with severe mucositis include cytosine arabinoside, cyclophosphamide, etoposide, melphalan, and thiotepa (Carl & Higby, 1985; Deeg et al, 1988). Mucositis tends to worsen within the first 2 weeks after therapy but usually heals within 3 weeks (Champlin & Gale, 1984).

Treatment of mucositis includes appropriate antimicrobial therapy, meticulous oral hygiene, and pain control. Thorough oral assessment is critical, including culturing probable lesions as needed. Acyclovir may be used prophylactically to prevent reactivation of herpes simplex virus (HSV) infection (Saral et al, 1983). Topical anesthetics may be used for relief from discomfort caused by mild mucositis; for severe mucositis, parenteral analgesia is usually required to promote comfort. Oral suction should be readily available. Patients may not be able to swallow or mobilize secretions and are at risk for aspiration. In addition, parenteral nutrition may be required for patients with dysphagia.

Salivary Gland Changes and Taste Changes. Bilateral parotitis and partial xerostomia (dry mouth) are frequently reported after TBI (Dreizen et al, 1979; Carl & Higby, 1985). This mumps-like swelling generally resolves in 24 to 48 hours and may be treated with analgesics.

Xerostomia can be caused by several chemotherapeutic agents (eg, high-dose alkylating agents, methotrexate), chronic GVHD, or some supportive care medications (eg, antiemetics or diuretics) used for transplant patients (Barrett & Bilous, 1984; Kolbinson et al, 1988; Barrett, 1986). Management includes frequent oral rinses, artificial saliva products, modification of diet to include moist or liquid foods, and avoidance of mucosal irritants (ie, dry foods, hot or spicy foods, nicotine, alcohol, commercial mouthwashes). Taste changes such as abnormal or diminished taste, are frequently reported by patients who have undergone BMT, the causes include the preparatory regimen, oral candidiasis, and antibiotics. These changes may persist for several weeks after the transplant (Barale, 1982) and may contribute to the patient's nutritional difficulties. Taste changes can be managed by patience in helping patients select foods they find desirable and by suggesting ways to enhance flavor through seasonings, sauces, and gravies. Patients can be reassured by learning that these taste changes usually improve over time.

Nausea and Vomiting. Nausea and vomiting can occur because of the conditioning regimen, organ damage, acute GVHD, infection, adverse side effects of other supportive medications, or psychologic causes. This problem can be much worse and more protracted for patients who undergo BMT than for most patients who receive chemotherapy (Schryber et al, 1987, Ford & Ballard, 1988). Medications such as cyclosporine, methotrexate, antibiotics, and narcotics may contribute to the problem (Cunningham et al, 1983; Wolford & McDonald, 1988). The sequelae of unremitting nausea and vomiting include electrolyte imbalances, Mallory–Weiss tears, major nutritional deficits, aspiration, psychologic problems, and prolonged hospitalization (Hogan, 1990).

The management of nausea and vomiting in a transplant patient includes thorough assessment, intervention with pharmacologic and nonpharmacologic strategies, and evaluation of response. A multiplicity of standard antiemetics are available to manage nausea and vomiting. Nonpharmacologic interventions include a restful environment, simple distraction techniques, and relaxation exercises.

Diarrhea and Enteritis. Diarrhea in a BMT patient may be due to mucosal damage from the conditioning regimen, acute or chronic GVHD, intestinal infection, or an underlying gastrointestinal problem (eg, irritable colon). Concomitant thrombocytopenia may further exacerbate the problem, resulting in bleeding.

Both TBI and certain high-dose chemotherapeutic agents (thiotepa, etoposide, melphalan, cytosine arabinoside, and methotrexate) can cause diffuse mucosal changes along the gastrointestinal tract (Deeg et al, 1988). These changes may result in watery diarrhea, cramps, pain, and anorexia. Infectious diarrhea may be caused by bacterial, fungal, viral, or parasitic infections. Examples of pathogens include *Clostridium difficile,* CMV, HSV, adenovirus, rotavirus, coxsackievirus, *Candida,* and *Giardia lamblia.* Acute GVHD, depending on severity, may cause profuse, watery diarrhea and gastrointestinal bleeding. Medications that may contribute to diarrhea include metoclopramide, antibiotics, oral magnesium, and antacids (Gauvreau, 1985).

Treatment of diarrhea is directed at identifying the cause, controlling any fluid and electrolyte and acid-base imbalances, providing symptomatic relief to the patient, and protecting the skin in the rectal area from severe excoriation. Additional interventions include the cautious use of antidiarrheal medications; strict management of volume status based on intake and output measurements, weights, and cardiovascular measurements; monitoring and replacement of electrolytes; and sitz baths, barrier creams, and nutritional supplementation (Gauvreau et al, 1981).

Gastrointestinal Bleeding. BMT patients are at high risk for gastrointestinal bleeding because of the long periods of thrombocytopenia after treatment. Patients must be monitored closely for both occult and frank bleeding. Stools and emesis should be frequently tested for occult blood. Antacids, sulcrafate, and histamine receptor antagonists may be used to protect the gastrointestinal mucosa.

Frank gastrointestinal bleeding requires emergency intervention; it is managed by finding and treating the source of bleeding. Hemodynamic stability must be maintained. Transfusions of multiple blood products are required to replace losses. Endoscopic procedures, surgical intervention, or angiography may be used to manage bleeding sites depending on the medical team's appraisal of risk versus benefit for the patient (Wolford & McDonald, 1988).

Renal and Genitourinary Complications

Renal Failure. Alterations in renal function may be due to drug toxicity, infectious processes (such as disseminated candidiasis), or ischemia. More than half of BMT patients experience renal compromise evidenced by a doubling in serum creatinine concentration (Wujcik & Downs, 1992). Acute renal failure necessitating hemodialysis has been reported to occur in 1 to 21% of patients who undergo allogeneic BMT (Shivnan & Shelton, in press; O'Quin & Moravec, 1988). Nursing care of a BMT patient in acute renal failure includes preventing drug nephrotoxicity through monitoring of medication usage and blood levels, preventing infection, maintaining fluid and electrolyte balance, and providing emotional support to the patient and family (King et al, 1992).

Electrolyte Imbalances. A syndrome of inappropriate antidiuretic hormone (SIADH) is a possible side effect of high-dose cyclophosphamide. Frequent monitoring of urine output and the use of diuretics to maintain euvolemia during administration of cyclophosphamide may minimize the incidence of this syndrome. Other common electrolyte imbalances include hypokalemia (amphotericin B administration) and hypomagnesemia (cyclosporine administration). Renal diabetes insipidus may be seen as a consequence of amphotericin B administration.

Hemorrhagic Cystitis. Damage to the transitional epithelium of the bladder and ureters from acrolein, a toxic metabolite of cyclophosphamide, may result in hemorrhagic cystitis in up to 24% of patients who undergo BMT (Ballard, 1991). An association between adenovirus or BK virus and hemorrhagic cystitis has been noted (Arthur et al, 1986). Preventive measures include vigorous hydration and diuresis, continuous bladder irrigation, or the use of mesna, which binds and inactivates acrolein. Treatment of hemorrhagic cystitis includes transfusion of blood components, hydration and close monitoring of urinary output, continuous bladder irrigation, and the instillation of substances such as alum or silver nitrate into the bladder (Wujcik & Downs, 1992). Prostaglandins also may be used. In severe cases, formalin may be instilled, the bladder may be temporarily bypassed with ureteral stints, or a cystectomy may be required (DeVries & Freiha, 1990).

Hepatic Complications

Venoocclusive Disease. Hepatic venoocclusive disease (VOD) is a common complication of both allogeneic and autologous BMT. The reported incidence of VOD is approximately 20%, with an associated mortality as high as 50% (Ayash et al, 1990; Jones et al, 1987; McDonald et al, 1985). Various preparatory regimens have been implicated, including a variety of combination chemotherapy regimens and chemoradiation therapy (Jones et al, 1987). Several factors have been identified as placing patients at increased risk for the development of VOD. McDonald and co-workers (1984) found that age greater than 15 years, a history of viral or chemical hepatitis, and an elevated aspartate aminotransferase (AST[SGOT]) level before the transplant predisposed the patient to the development of VOD. Jones and co-workers (1987) found that there was no statistically significant difference in VOD risk associated with the actual degree of elevation of AST level. The intensity of cytotoxic therapy before BMT also is believed to be a primary risk factor for development of VOD (Jones et al, 1987).

Pathologically, VOD is a result of injury to the endothelial lining of hepatic sinusoids and terminal hepatic veins (McDonald et al, 1984). Fluid and cellular debris resulting from this injury become entrapped within the endothelial lining obstructing hepatic venous outflow and impairing sinusoidal circulation. Sinusoidal congestion and venous outflow obstruction result in centrilobular congestion and necrosis of centrilobular hepatocytes. Outflow obstruction manifests as a rise in total bilirubin level, whereas hepatocyte necrosis results in elevation of serum alkaline phosphatase and AST levels.

VOD has been characterized as a distinct clinical syndrome, the onset of symptoms usually occurring between days 7 to 21 after BMT. The early onset of VOD within the post-BMT recovery period and the unique clinical features of VOD distinguish it from other hepatic problems, such as hepatic GVHD, which usually occur later in the posttransplant period. The early clinical symptoms of VOD are weight gain of 5% or more over baseline, lack of response to diuretics, right upper quadrant pain, and hyperbilirubinemia of 2 mg/dL or more. Following these symptoms by 3 to 10 days are hepatomegaly, elevated alkaline phosphatase and AST levels and ascites. With progressive, unrelenting disease, azotemia, encephalopathy, and coagulopathies usually develop. Although it has been associated with VOD, platelet transfusion refractoriness is believed to be a nonspecific sign of clinical deterioration after BMT rather than a characteristic element of VOD (Jones et al, 1987). Definitive, histologic confirmation of VOD by liver biopsy is difficult to obtain because of thrombocytopenia, coagulopathy due to the liver disease, and ascites. Jones and co-workers (1987) have shown that using the clinical criteria of hyperbilirubinemia of 2 mg/dL or more in association with two of the three other findings of ascites, painful hepatomegaly, and weight gain of 5% or more over baseline obviates the need for, and risks of, histologic confirmation of VOD.

Hyperbilirubinemia persistently greater than 15 mg/dL or hepatic encephalopathy is strongly predictive of fatal VOD. Mild cases of VOD gradually resolve a median of 20 days after the onset of symptoms (Jones et al, 1987). Once clinically apparent, VOD has proved to be highly resistant to therapeutic intervention. Consequently, research has focused on prophylaxis. Busulfan is an oral alkylating agent used frequently as part of BMT-conditioning regimens. Busulfan is rapidly absorbed in the gastrointestinal tract and has a plasma half-life of only 2 to 3 hours (Rohaly, 1989). Hepatic toxicity is the primary dose-limiting toxicity of high-dose busulfan. Therapeutic monitoring and dose adjustment of busulfan based on individual patient pharmacokinetics has proved to be highly effective in decreasing VOD-associated morbidity and mortality (Grochow et al, 1992). Because the endothelial damage of VOD induces the deposition of coagulation factors that contribute to the obstruction of hepatic venous outflow, continuous low-dose heparin (100 U/kg/per day) has been used to prevent development of VOD (Attal et al, 1992). Attal and co-workers (1992) in their series of 161 patients undergoing BMT were able to considerably reduce the incidence of VOD using continuous low-dose heparin from day 8 before BMT through day 30 after BMT without increasing the risk of bleeding or the requirement for blood product support. The use of pentoxifylline, a hemorrheologic agent administered orally on day 10 be-

fore BMT through day 100 posttransplant also has been shown to be effective in decreasing the incidence of VOD (Bianco et al, 1991).

Nursing care includes assessment and early detection of VOD and supportive
care. The goals of nursing care of a patient with VOD are (1) maintenance of intravascular volume and renal perfusion while minimizing extravascular fluid accumulation; (2) preventing additional insult to the liver; and (3) management of pain and
provision of comfort measures (Grandt, 1989). Blood products and plasma expanders
such as albumin are used to maintain intravascular volume and renal perfusion. Concentration of nutrition solutions and antibiotics helps minimize extravascular fluid accumulation. Spironolactone is the diuretic of choice in the clinical setting of VOD.
Frequent patient weight and abdominal girth measurements, orthostatic blood pressure, and central venous pressure (CVP) measurements as well as careful monitoring of
total fluid intake and output are important nursing assessments in the setting of VOD.
Management of pain and agitation associated with encephalopathy are complicated
by hepatic metabolism of many analgesics and sedatives. Morphine is the analgesic of
choice; *meperidine should be avoided* because accumulation of the by-product of its
metabolism, normeperidine, causes central nervous system irritability. Renally ex-
creted benzodiazepines are preferred for sedation. Patients and families require considerable emotional support when VOD presents as a complication of BMT.

Neurologic Complications

Central and peripheral nervous system toxicity may be due to infections, the side effects of medications, disturbances in metabolism, GVHD, or relapse. These complications occur in as many as 70% of patients (Meriney, 1991). Neurologic toxicity is most
often manifest as neuropathies, somnolence, confusion or disorientation, and
seizures, encephalopathy, or coma (Furlong & Galucci, 1992). Causes of neurologic
toxicity are summarized in Table 9–7.

Nursing care of a BMT patient experiencing neurologic toxicity should focus on
early detection of changes in mental status and central nervous system function, protection from injury, and support of the person's adaptation to neurologic impairment
(Wujcik & Downs, 1992).

Cardiopulmonary Complications

In spite of screening for adequate cardiac and pulmonary function, cardiac complications occur in as many as 25% of all patients who undergo BMT and pulmonary complications occur in about half of patients who undergo allogeneic BMT (Wikle, 1991).
Cardiopulmonary complications contribute considerably to the morbidity and mortality associated with BMT. Ventilator support, for example, has been reported as necessary for 16 to 26% of patients who undergo allogeneic BMT (O'Quin & Moravec,
1988; Shivnan & Shelton, in press). More than half of patients who have pulmonary
complications die; interstitial pneumonitis alone accounts for 40% of all BMT-related
deaths (Denardo et al, 1989; Wujcik & Downs, 1992).

Pulmonary Complications. Pulmonary infections may complicate the early posttransplant course or appear later, particularly in patients with chronic GVHD. Although some infections are bacterial, an immunocompromised host may be infected

TABLE 9–7. CAUSES OF NEUROLOGIC TOXICITY AFTER BONE MARROW TRANSPLANTATION

Infections

Meningitis due to infection with organisms such as *Listeria, Streptococcus, Klebsiella,* and *Escherichia coli*

Brain abscesses due to infection with *Aspergillus, Candida,* or *Cryptococcus*

Viral encephalitis due to infection with or reactivation of cytomegalovirus, varicella-zoster or adenovirus infection

Encephalopathy or brain abscesses due to infection with or reactivation of *Toxoplasma* infection

Preparatory regimen

Leukoencephalopathy, particularly after irradiation and high doses of methotrexate

Cerebellar dysfunction and other neurotoxicity from high-dose cytosine arabinoside

Peripheral neuropathies from etoposide

Medications

Ototoxicity from aminoglycosides

Neurotoxicity and seizures from ticarcillin and piperacillin

Tremors, parasthesias, and seizures from cyclosporine

Aseptic meningitis, sedation, and other neurotoxicities from intrathecal or systemic methotrexate

Euphoria, depression, or psychosis from corticosteroids

Bleeding

Cerebrovascular accidents and subarachnoid hemorrhages related to injury or spontaneously in thrombocytopenia

---

by a wide variety of other organisms, including fungi such as *Aspergillus* or *Candida* species, protozoa such as *Pneumocystis carinii,* or viruses such as CMV, HSV, or varicella-zoster (VZV). Infections with *Legionella pneumophila, Mycobacterium tuberculosis, Chlamydia trachomitis,* and *Toxoplasma gondii* also may be seen (Krowka et al, 1985). Chest radiographs and computed tomographic scans may be difficult to interpret if the patient has neutropenia, and therapy is often empiric. Bronchoalveolar lavage is often helpful, particularly in the diagnosis of CMV infections.

In spite of efforts such as the use of CMV-screened blood products, reactivation of CMV is a serious problem in BMT (Zaia, 1990). CMV remains the most common cause of interstitial pneumonitis in patients who undergo allogeneic BMT (Shivnan & Shelton, in press). Risk factors for the development of CMV interstitial pneumonitis include time since the transplant with peak incidence 30 to 90 days, the presence of acute GVHD, pretransplant CMV seropositivity, and intensity of treatment (Wingard et al, 1988). Current research into both the prophylaxis and the treatment of CMV interstitial pneumonitis includes the use of immune globulin, particularly preparations containing high titres of CMV antibody, foscarnet, and ganciclovir (Wikle, 1991; Zaia, 1990).

BMT patients also experience noninfectious pulmonary complications, often characterized as idiopathic interstitial pneumonitis or adult respiratory distress syndrome (ARDS). Particularly for patients who have undergone allogeneic BMT, the early posttransplant course may be complicated by a capillary leak or aseptic shock syndrome now thought to be due to the release of cytokines. This syndrome has been described as including shock in association with a high fever, renal insufficiency, hepatic damage, encephalopathy, hypoxia or pulmonary infiltrates, weight gain despite diuresis, and erythroderma (Miller et al, under review). Without careful management of fluid status, cardiac output, and oxygenation, the condition of such patients may rapidly deteriorate.

Other pulmonary complications include drug- or radiation-induced pulmonary damage and fibrosis, bronchiolitis obliterans associated with chronic GVHD, and pulmonary hemorrhage (Wikle, 1991). Nursing care of a BMT patient with worsening respiratory function must balance emotional support for the patient and family with the use of intensive care such as mechanical ventilation and hemodynamic monitoring. Advance directives such as living wills may be useful in guiding the care of such seriously ill patients.

Cardiac Complications. Cardiac damage may be caused by medications used in preparatory regimens, particularly the anthracyclines and cyclophosphamide. High doses of anthracyclines may result in cellular degeneration and necrosis of cardiac fibers. Such damage is cumulative and usually irreversible. High-dose cyclophosphamide may cause hemorrhagic myocardial necrosis, serosanguineous pericardial effusions, and pericarditis (Wujcik & Downs, 1992). Cardiac damage may also occur with TBI, particularly in patients who have received previous thoracic irradiation.

Infections of the valves, endocardium or myocardium are rare. Causative organisms include bacteria such as *Streptococcus* or *Staphylococcus,* fungi such as *Aspergillus,* protozoa such as *Toxoplasma,* and viruses such as adenovirus or coxsackievirus (Wikle, 1991).

Graft-Versus-Host Disease

Acute Graft-Versus-Host Disease. Acute GVHD is a major complication of BMT. It occurs in 40 to 60% of allogeneic transplants and as many as 10% of autologous transplants. This syndrome is a consequence of the immunologic reaction of donor T lymphocytes against host cells, the mirror image of rejection in solid-organ transplants (Freedman et al, 1990). Biologic mediators, or cytokines, may also be involved (Parkman, 1988). The sites most frequently affected are the skin, gastrointestinal tract, and liver. Risk factors include increased age and transplantation from female donors (Bross et al, 1984; Vogelsang et al, 1988).

Prophylaxis against acute GVHD may include both immunosuppressive agents administered to the patient and manipulation of the donor bone marrow to remove lymphocytes. Immunosuppressive agents commonly used include methotrexate, cyclosporine, and corticosteroids (Caudell, 1991). Other agents, such as antithymocyte globulin (ATG) and monoclonal antibodies, have been tried.

Acute GVHD may be as mild as an erythematous rash limited to parts of the skin or as severe as widespread desquamation of the skin, gastrointestinal bleeding and voluminous diarrhea, and liver failure. The disease usually occurs within the first 3

TABLE 9–8. THE JOHNS HOPKINS STAGING CRITERIA FOR ACUTE GRAFT-VERSUS-HOST DISEASE (GVHD)

Organ Site	Skin Extent of Rash	Liver Total Bilirubin (mg/dL)	Intestines Volume of Diarrhea (mL)
I	Rash < 25%	2.0–3.5	500–1000
II	Rash 25–50%	3.5–8.0	1000–1500
III	Erythroderma	8.0–15.0	1500–2500
IV	Bullae, desquamation	>15.0	>2500

	Overall Clinical Stage
Stage	*Explanation*
Stage O	Stage I clinical skin GVHD with grade 2 histology.
Stage I	Stage II clinical skin GVHD with grade ≥ 2 histology.
Stage II	Stage II–III clinical skin GVHD with grade ≥ 2 histology and stage I clinical liver or intestinal GVHD.
Stage IIo	Stage I clinical liver or intestinal GVHD without skin acute GVHD.
Stage IIs	Stage IV clinical skin GVHD with grade ≥ 2 histology and without liver or intestinal acute GVHD.
Stage III	Stage II–IV clinical skin GVHD with grade ≥ 2 histology and stage II–IV clinical liver or intestinal GVHD.
Stage IV	Stage III–IV clinical skin GVHD with grade ≥ 2 histology and stage II–IV clinical liver or intestinal GVHD. Two or more systems stage III or greater.

(From Wagner JE, Santos GW, Noga SJ, et al (1990). Bone marrow graft engineering by counterflow centrifugal elutriation: Results of a phase I–II clinical trial. Blood. 75:1372.)

months of BMT; its median onset is approximately 25 days after the transplant (Caudell, 1991). The severity of GVHD is determined both histologically (grading) and clinically (staging) (Table 9–8).

The prognosis and treatment depend on the severity of the syndrome. Mild cases may require no treatment or topical treatment with steroid ointments. Severe cases are treated with immunosuppressive agents such as high doses of methylprednisolone, ATG, antilymphocyte globulin (ALG), cyclosporine, and anti-T-cell immunotoxins (Vogelsang et al, 1988). Acute GVHD contributes greatly to the morbidity and mortality of BMT; 30 to 60% of patients with moderate to severe GVHD die of GVHD and related infectious complications (Weisdorf et al, 1990). Severe pain may be associated with both skin and gastrointestinal involvement (Shivnan & Sheidler, 1992).

Nursing care of a patient with acute GVHD is based on the major goals of preventing and monitoring for infection, maintaining a balanced fluid and electrolyte status, and promoting patient comfort. A nursing care plan for impaired skin integrity addresses some of the most common nursing needs of these complex patients (see Nursing Care Plan 9–2, p 278).

TABLE 9–9. MANIFESTATIONS OF CHRONIC GRAFT-VERSUS-HOST DISEASE

Organ	Clinical manifestations
Skin	Erythema, pruritis, hypo- or hyperpigmentation, alopecia, loss of sweating, scleroderma
Neuromuscular	Joint contractures, serositis, myositis
Ocular	Dry eyes, grittiness and burning of eyes, corneal abrasions, uveitis, membranous conjunctivitis
Oral	Pain, lichenoid changes, erythema, stomatitis, xerostomia, dental caries
GI tract	Anorexia, difficulty swallowing, retrosternal pain
Vaginal	Inflammation, dryness, stricture formation
Liver	Jaundice, cirrhosis
Lungs	Bronchiolitis obliterans
Immune system	Thrombocytopenia, hypogammaglobulinemia

Chronic Graft-Versus-Host Disease. Chronic GVHD is a complex syndrome that usually appears 2 months to 1 year after transplantation in as many as one-third of patients who undergo allogeneic BMT (McGarigle, 1990). Immunologically mediated, it resembles autoimmune disorders such as scleroderma and systemic lupus erythematosus in its clinical manifestations. Most patients have skin manifestations, but many other organs may be affected (Deeg et al, 1984; McCann & Solomon, 1991). These manifestations are summarized in Table 9–9.

Treatment of chronic GVHD includes immunosuppression with agents such as corticosteroids and azathioprine. Thalidomide has immunosuppressive properties that have shown promise (Vogelsang et al, 1988). Phototherapy using ultraviolet light and psoralen (PUVA) has been used to treat oral and skin manifestations. Some preliminary research has also been done using PUVA directly to leukopheresed WBCs (McCann & Solomon, 1991). Patients with chronic GVHD are at risk for infections and should receive antibiotic prophylaxis (Caudell, 1991).

ENGRAFTMENT AND DISCHARGE ISSUES

Planning for discharge occurs long before the patient's actual exit from the hospital. Nursing education before discharge is key in assisting patients in managing the transition from hospital to home. Important components of discharge education of transplant patients include infection and bleeding precautions, care of the vascular access device, nutrition, activity restrictions, exercise, sexuality, and medication. Table 9–10 lists symptoms that should prompt transplant patients to report for emergency care.

Nurses should keep in mind that leaving the inpatient treatment facility after BMT can induce a separation anxiety in both the patient and the family. After several weeks of enduring the rigors of treatment and close monitoring, patients and families may fear leaving the protective hospital environment.

TABLE 9–10. REPORTABLE SYMPTOMS

Temperature > 38°C, shaking chills, or dizziness

Temperature > 37.5°C with steroid therapy

Changes in the appearance of right atrial catheter
   insertion site (redness, pain, drainage, swelling)

Changes in the color or consistency of bowel movements
   (increasing volume or frequency)

Changes in the color of urine

Appearance of skin rash

Cough or shortness of breath

Nausea or vomiting

Anorexia

Inability to take prescribed medications

New onset of pain

Any noticeable bleeding, eg, bleeding gums, nosebleed

Decreasing energy level

Mouth sores or "cold sores"

(From Buchsel PC (1991). Ambulatory care: Before and after BMT. In: Whe-don MB, ed. Bone Marrow Transplantation: Principles, Practice and Nursing In-sights. Boston: Jones and Bartlett, 303. Copyright 1991 Jones & Bartlett Publishers, Inc.)

Examples of discharge criteria for transplant patients are outlined in Table 9–11. It is not unusual to see a wide spectrum of sophisticated parenteral therapies administered to transplant patients as needed in the ambulatory care setting. The expanding use of growth factors and PBPCs may shorten the length of hospitalization for selected transplant populations (Nimer and Champlin, 1990; Antman, 1992) and reduce transfusion requirements and morbidity due to infections, toxicity, and bleeding (Nimer & Champlin, 1990). These advances will certainly have an impact on outpatient care. Their potential contributions to an accelerated recovery for patients will continue to be investigated.

AMBULATORY CARE

Although BMT patients are usually seen in the outpatient department (OPD) for evaluation and screening before the transplant, it is the intensity and complexity of follow-up care that have the greatest impact on OPD resources. Initially the patient may visit daily for blood tests, intravenous hydration or parenteral nutrition, blood products, or amphotericin B (Buchsel, 1991). Each visit should include an assessment of the patient's physical status and adaptation to the outpatient role. During this time, the OPD nurse has a key role in assessment, prevention of complications, and symptom management (Buchsel, 1991). Comprehensive, individualized education is required to meet the informational needs of BMT patients and families. The transition

TABLE 9–11. ESTABLISHED DISCHARGE CRITERIA FOR BONE MARROW TRANSPLANTATION PATIENTS

Oral intake > 50% of baseline nutrient requirements

No more than 1500 mL of parenteral fluid within 24 hours is required

Nausea and vomiting controlled with oral medication

Diarrhea controlled at < 500 mL per day

Afebrile and off intravenous antibiotics for 48 hours

Platelet count > 15,000/mm^3

Granulocytes > 500/mm^3

Hematocrit > 30% for adults, > 25% for children

PO medications, for example, narcotics, antihypertensives, cyclosporine, and prednisone are tolerated for 48 hours

Family support within home

(From Buchsel PC (1991). Ambulatory care: Before and after BMT. In: Whedon MB, ed. Bone Marrow Transplantation: Principles, Practice and Nursing Insights. *Boston: Jones and Bartlett, 304. Copyright 1991 Jones & Bartlett Publishers, Inc.)*

from the protective environment of the inpatient unit to the OPD may be difficult for both the patient and family members (McGarigle, 1990). Problems such as depression, hypervigilance, and lack of compliance may surface.

Patients who undergo autologous BMT are usually discharged home to their primary care physician about 30 to 50 days after the transplant. Patients who undergo allogeneic BMT are usually under the care of the BMT OPD until 50 to 100 days after the transplant, being monitored for signs and symptoms of GVHD. All patients return for long-term follow-up appointments. At these visits, engraftment and disease status are assessed, as is organ function, hormone production, growth and development of children, and the presence of long-term complications of transplantation such as cataracts or chronic GVHD.

The possible long-term complications of BMT are summarized in Table 9–12 (Buchsel & Kelleher, 1989; Deeg et al, 1984; Freedman et al, 1990; Van der Wal et al, 1988). In addition, relapse of the original disease or secondary malignant neoplasms as a consequence of the intensive preparatory regimen may occur (Deeg et al, 1984). Sensitivity to the psychosocial aspects of these potentially devastating complications and support of the patient and family as they adapt to changes in their lives is an essential role of the BMT nurse.

THE PSYCHOSOCIAL IMPACT OF BMT

The psychosocial impact of BMT is felt before the transplant, during treatment, and a long time afterward by patients and their families and friends (Buchsel, 1990; Futterman & Wellisch, 1990; Patenaude, 1990). Haberman (1988) described six stages of

TABLE 9–12. LONG-TERM COMPLICATIONS OF BONE MARROW TRANSPLANTATION

Related to pretransplant regimen	Assess for	Nursing Interventions
Restrictive or obstructive lung disease	Increased effort	Teaching pulmonary toilet
	Decreased breath sounds	Sputum cultures
	Cough	
Leukoencephalopathy	Altered mental status	Careful neurologic assessment
	Cognitive dysfunction	
Peripheral neuropathies	Altered gait	Teaching safety measures
	Altered sensation	
Cataracts	Decreased visual acuity	Teaching safety measures
	Blurred vision	Teaching related to cataract removal and lens implant or contact lenses
Endocrine dysfunction	Hypo- or hyperthyroidism	Teaching related to replacement therapy
	Delayed growth in children	Sexual counseling
	Early menopause	
	Sterility	
Related to infections		
Varicella zoster	Unexplained persistent pain	Oral or IV acyclovir
	Tingling, itching	Pain management
	Vesicles	Skin care
	Fever, chills	Antipruritics
Other infections	Sinus congestion or pain	Preventive teaching
	Cough	Obtain specimens for culture
Related to engraftment		
Hemolytic anemia	Fatigue	Administer appropriate red blood cells
	Shortness of breath	
Graft failure	Decreased blood counts	Assess for infections
		Check for medications or other sources of marrow suppression
Related to chronic Graft Versus Host Disease		
Skin	Hypo- or hyperpigmentation	Skin care: sunscreen, hygiene, nonirritant lotions, cosmetics
	Pruritis	
	Dryness	
Mouth	Pain, soreness	Artificial saliva
	Decreased saliva	Nutritional supplements
	Difficulty swallowing	Soft diet
	Lichenoid changes	Dental hygiene education
Eyes	Burning, grittiness	Artificial tears
Gastrointestinal tract	Anorexia, weight loss	Nutritional supplements
	Persistent nausea, vomiting	Antiemetics
Vagina	Dryness	Water-soluble lubricants
	Adhesions, strictures	Sexual counseling
Liver	Cirrhosis	

TABLE 9–13. PSYCHOSOCIAL IMPACT OF BONE MARROW TRANSPLANTATION

Treatment Phase	Patient	Family and Friends
Pretransplant	Hope for cure	Hope for cure
	Pressure to decide	Anticipating role changes
	Finishing business	Financial commitment
	Denial	Search for donor
	Fear of death	Fear of death
Transplant	Defenselessness	Need for information
	Reality of illness	Vigilance
	Anxiety	Anxiety
	Depression	Helplessness
Posttransplant	Separation anxiety	Readjustment of roles
	Survivor guilt	Protectiveness
	Body image changes	

BMT and their evolving psychosocial implications: decision-making, preadmission, conditioning regime, immunosuppression, awaiting engraftment, and discharge.

Common themes emerging during the BMT process are summarized in Table 9–13. Although many of these concerns are faced by all people with cancer, their impact during BMT is heightened by the fact that the patient and family made a choice to undergo BMT. In addition, the unique experience of bone marrow donors may sometimes cause additional psychologic sequelae such as disturbances in mood and self-esteem (Ruggiero, 1988).

Patients and families need support and assistance in dealing with these multiple stressors. Psychologic support can be enhanced through access to mental health specialists such as psychiatrists, psychologists, and psychiatric liaison nurses. Behavioral interventions such as relaxation training, imagery, hypnosis, and biofeedback may be used and have proved helpful in other oncology settings (Ahles & Shedd, 1991). Support groups for both patients and families are provided in many institutions during and after transplantation.

Long term, the experience of BMT patients and families has been placed in the context of concepts of survivorship (Nims & Strom, 1988; Buchsel, 1990). A growing body of research suggests that most BMT survivors rate their quality of life as good to excellent, but some problems lessen the quality of life for a small percentage of survivors (Andrykowski et al, 1990; Ferrell et al, 1992a, 1992b; Wingard et al, 1991). Relationships with self, family, friends, employers, and often with a higher power are altered irreversibly, but this can be a positive or a negative experience. Social discrimination in areas such as employment and health insurance may be a problem for some survivors (Welch-McCaffrey et al, 1990; Wingard et al, 1991). Nursing plays a key role in providing information, understanding, and supporting the BMT survivor and family.

FUTURE TRENDS IN BMT

BMT has developed in a relatively short period of time from an experimental attempt at treating end-stage leukemia to a highly intensive, complex, and potentially curative treatment for patients with a wide variety of malignant and nonmalignant disorders. The nurse is essential in assessing the multiple levels of needs of BMT patients, coordinating and managing their care, and preparing and educating them and their families for the process of BMT. In addition, the BMT nurse may be called upon to collect nursing or medical research data, respond to an emergency, advocate for the patient or donor, identify ethical dilemmas, support a grieving family, or promote the concept of survivorship, possibly all in the same day.

As this specialized field evolves, current work in genetic engineering, bone marrow manipulation, GVHD prophylaxis and treatment, and the use of unrelated or mismatched donors will undoubtedly be expanded. Examples of areas for future research include further refinement of HLA typing and the use of oligotyping to better define matched transplants; the use of new immunosuppressive therapies in GVHD prophylaxis and treatment; the induction of GVHD in autologous BMT for its graft-versus-neoplasm effect; and the further definition and modulation of the role of tumor necrosis factor in GVHD and other complications of BMT. As supportive therapy such as the use of growth factors and improved prophylaxis against infectious complications decreases morbidity and mortality, new diseases (such as sickle cell anemia or cystic fibrosis) may be treated by BMT. In addition, second transplants may become more common when a relapse or a secondary malignant neoplasm occurs.

The BMT nurse will continue to be crucial to the quality of the BMT experience for both patient and family. Whether the outcome of BMT is a successful return to normal life, adaptation to an altered quality of life as a result of long-term complications, or loss of a loved one to a BMT-related complication, the nurse provides the continuity of care that helps and supports the BMT patient and family. This continuity will become even more crucial as societal and financial pressures move more of the transplant process to ambulatory care settings. BMT nurses are first and foremost oncology nurses, although their specialized expertise draws on both transplantation nursing and critical care nursing knowledge and skills. As new diseases are treated and new techniques are used, additional areas of nursing knowledge will be needed, such as the care of children with genetic diseases such as sickle cell anemia. The challenge to nurse educators, nurse researchers, clinical nurse specialists, and nurse managers and administrators will be to support and enhance the role of the staff nurse who chooses to make this exciting but difficult field his or her own.

REFERENCES

Abramovitz LZ (1991). Perspectives on pediatric bone marrow transplantation. In: Whedon MB, ed. *Bone Marrow Transplantation: Principles, Practice, and Nursing Insights.* Boston: Jones and Bartlett, 70–104.

Ahles TA, Shedd P. (1991). Psychosocial impact of bone marrow transplantation in adult patients. In Whedon MB, ed. *Bone Marrow Transplantation: Principles, Practice, and Nursing Insights.* Boston: Jones and Bartlett, 280–292.

Andrykowski MA, Altmaier EM, Barnett RL, et al (1990). The quality of life in adult survivors of allogeneic bone marrow transplantation. *Transplantation.* 50:399–406.

Antman K (1992). Hematopoietic stem cells: Clinical implications. *Marrow Transplant Rev.* 2:27–29.

Antman K, Ayash L, Elias A, et al (1992). A phase II study of high-dose cyclophosphamide, thiotepa, and carboplatin in women with measurable advanced breast cancer responding to standard-dose therapy. *J Clin Oncol.* 10:102–110.

Arthur RR, Shah KV, Baust SJ, et al (1986). Association of BK viruria with hemorrhagic cystitis in recipients of bone marrow transplants. *N Engl J Med.* 315:230–234.

Attal M, Huguet F, Rubie H, et al (1992). Prevention of hepatic veno-occlusive disease after bone marrow transplantation by continuous infusion of low-dose heparin: A prospective, randomized trial. *Blood.* 79:2834–2840.

Ayash LJ, Hunt M, Antman K, et al (1990). Hepatic venoocclusive disease in autologous bone marrow transplantation of solid tumors and lymphomas. *J Clin Oncol.* 8:1699–1706.

Ballard B (1991). Renal and hepatic complications. In: Whedon MB, ed. *Bone Marrow Transplantation: Principles, Practice, and Nursing Insights.* Boston: Jones and Bartlett, 240–261.

Barale KV, Aker SN, Martinsen CS (1982). Primary taste thresholds in children with leukemia undergoing marrow transplantation. *J Par E N.* 6:287–290.

Barlogie B, Gahrton G (1991). Bone marrow transplantation in multiple myeloma. *Bone Marrow Transplant.* 7:71–79.

Barrett AP (1986). Oral complications of bone marrow transplantation. *Aust NZ J Med.* 16:239–240.

Barrett AP, Bilous AM (1984). Oral patterns of acute and chronic graft-versus-host disease. *Arch Dermatol.* 120:1461–1465.

Barrett JA (1991). An introduction to bone marrow transplantation and processing. In: Gee AP, ed. *Bone Marrow Processing and Purging.* Boca Raton: CRC, 3–16.

Beatty P (1992). Results of allogeneic bone marrow transplantation with unrelated or mismatched donors. *Semin Oncol.* 19(Suppl 7):13–19.

Bender JG, To LB, Williams S, Schwartzberg LS (1992). Defining a therapeutic dose of peripheral blood stem cells. *J Hematother.* 1:329–341.

Bianco JA, Appelbaum FR, Nemunaitis J, et al (1991). Phase I-II trial of pentoxifylline for the prevention of transplant-related toxicities following bone marrow transplantation. *Blood.* 78:1205–1211.

Bortin MM, Buckner CD (1983). Major complications of marrow harvesting for transplantation. *Exp Hematol.* 11:916–919.

Bortin MM, Horowitz MM, Rimm AA (1992). Increasing utilization of allogeneic bone marrow transplantation. *Ann Intern Med.* 116:505–512.

Bortin MM, Rimm AA (1989). Increasing utilization of bone marrow transplantation. 2. Results of the 1985–1987 survey. *Transplantation.* 48:453–458.

Bross DS, Tutschka PJ, Farmer ER, et al. (1984). Predictive factors for acute graft-verus-host disease in patients transplanted with HLA-identical bone marrow. *Blood.* 63:1265–1270.

Buchsel PC (1990). Bone marrow transplantation. In: Groenwald SL, et al, eds. *Cancer Nursing: Principles and Practice,* 2nd ed. Boston: Jones & Bartlett, 307–337.

Buchsel PC (1991). Ambulatory care: Before and after BMT. In Whedon MB, ed. *Bone Marrow Transplantation: Principles, Practice, and Nursing Insights.* Boston: Jones and Bartlett, 295–311.

Carl W, Higby D (1985). Oral manifestations of bone marrow transplantation. *Am J Clin Oncol.* 8:81-87.

Caudell KA (1991). Graft-versus-host disease. In Whedon MB, ed. *Bone Marrow Transplantation: Principles, Practice, and Nursing Insights.* Boston: Jones and Bartlett, 160-181.

Caudell KA, Whedon MB (1991). Hematopoietic complications. In: Whedon MB, ed. *Bone Marrow Transplantation: Principles, Practice, and Nursing Insights.* Boston: Jones and Bartlett, 135-159.

Champlin R (1990). Bone marrow transplantation for aplastic anemia: Recent advances and comparisons with alternative therapies. In: Champlin R, ed. *Bone Marrow Transplantation.* Boston: Kluwer, 185-197.

Champlin R (1992). Marrow transplantation for CML: New questions. *Marrow Transplant Rev.* 2:21-22.

Champlin R, Gale R (1984). The early complications of bone marrow transplantation. *Semin Hematol.* 21:101-108.

Champlin R, Goldman J, Gale R (1988). Bone marrow transplantation in chronic myelogenous leukemia. *Semin Hematol.* 25:74-80.

Cunningham BA, Lenssen P, Aker SN, et al (1983). Nutritional considerations during marrow transplantation. *Nurs Clin North Am.* 18:585-595.

Dahl G (1990). Allogeneic bone marrow transplantation in a program of intensive sequential chemotherapy for children and young adults with acute nonlymphocytic leukemia in first remission. *J Clin Oncol.* 8:295-303.

Davis JM, Rowley SD, Braine HG, et al (1990). Clinical toxicity of cryopreserved bone marrow graft infusion. *Blood.* 75:781-786.

Deeg HJ, Klingemann HG, Phillips GL (1988). *A Guide to Bone Marrow Transplantation.* Berlin: Springer-Verlag.

Deeg HJ, Storb R, Thomas ED (1984). Bone marrow transplantation: A review of delayed complications. *Br J Haematol.* 57:185-208.

Demetri GD, Antman KH (1992). Granulocyte-macrophage colony-stimulating factors (GM-CSF): Preclinical and clinical investigations. *Semin Oncol.* 19:362-385.

Denardo SJ, Oye RK, Bellamy PE (1989). Efficacy of intensive care for bone marrow transplant patients with respiratory failure. *Crit Care Med.* 17:4-6.

DeVries CR, Freiha FS (1990). Hemorrhagic cystitis: A review. *J Urol.* 143:1-9.

Dreizen S, McCretie K, Dicke K, et al (1979). Oral complications of bone marrow transplantation. *Postgrad Med.* 66:187-193, 196.

Dutcher JP (1989). The potential benefit of granulocyte transfusion therapy. *Cancer Invest.* 7:457-462.

Ferrell B, Grant M, Schmidt GM, et al (1992a). The meaning of quality of life for bone marrow transplant survivors. 1. The impact of bone marrow transplant on quality of life. *Cancer Nurs.* 15:153-160.

Ferrell B, Grant M, Schmidt GM, et al (1992b). The meaning of quality of life for bone marrow transplant survivors. 2. Improving quality of life for bone marrow transplant survivors. *Cancer Nurs.* 15:247-253.

Ford R, Ballard B (1988). Acute complications after bone marrow transplantation. *Semin Oncol Nurs.* 4:15-24.

Ford R, Eisenberg S (1990). Bone marrow transplant: Recent advances and nursing implications. *Nurs Clin North Am.* 25:405-422.

Forman SJ, Schmidt GM, Nadamanee AP, et al (1991). Allogeneic bone marrow transplantation as therapy for primary induction failure for patients with acute leukemia. *J Clin Oncol.* 9:1570-1574.

Freedman S, Shivnan J, Tilles J, Klemm P (1990). Bone marrow transplantation: Overview and nursing implications. *Crit Care Nursing Q.* 13:51-62.

Frei E, Antman K, Teicher B, et al (1989). Bone marrow transplantation for solid tumors: Prospects. *J Clin Oncol.* 7:515-526.

Furlong TG, Galucci BB (1992). Neurological complications in bone marrow transplant patients. *Oncol Nurs Forum.* 19:320.

Futterman AD, Wellisch DK (1990). Psychodynamic themes of bone marrow transplantation: When I becomes thou. *Hematol Oncol Clin North Am.* 4:699-709.

Gale RP, Armitrage JO, Dicke KA (1991). Autotransplants now and in the future. *Bone Marrow Transplant.* 7:153-157.

Gauvreau JM (1985). Drug-induced interactions. In: Lensenn P, Aker SN, eds. *Nutritional Assessment and Management During Marrow Transplantation: A Resource Manual.* Seattle: Fred Hutchinson Cancer Center, 15-29.

Gauvreau JM, Lensenn P, Cheney C, et al (1981). Nutritional management of patients with graft-versus-host disease. *J Am Diet Assoc.* 79:673-677.

Gobel BH (1990). Bleeding. In: Groenwald SL, et al eds. *Cancer Nursing: Principles and Practice,* 2nd ed. Boston: Jones and Bartlett, 467-484.

Grandt D (1989). Hepatic veno-occlusive disease following bone marrow transplantation. *Oncol Nurs Forum.* 16:813-817.

Grochow LB, Piantadosi S, Santos G, Jones R. Busulfan dose adjustment decreases the risk of hepatic veno-occlusive disease in patients undergoing bone marrow transplantation (under review).

Haberman MR (1988). Psychosocial aspects of bone marrow transplantation. *Semin Oncol Nurs.* 4 (1):55-59.

Herzig, RH (1992). The role of autologous bone marrow transplantation in the treatment of solid tumors. *Semin Oncol.* 19 (Suppl 7):7-12.

Hogan CM (1990). Advances in the management of nausea and vomiting. *Nurs Clin North Am.* 25:480.

Horowitz MM, Przepiorka D, Champlin RE, et al (1992). Should HLA-identical sibling bone marrow transplants for leukemia be restricted to large centers? *Blood.* 79:2771-2774.

Jones R, Santos G (1991). Bone marrow transplantation in acute leukemia. *Marrow Transplant Rev.* 1:39-41, 48.

Jones RJ, Ambinder RF, Piantadosi S, Santos GW (1991). Evidence of a graft-versus-lymphoma effect associated with allogeneic bone marrow transplantation. *Blood.* 77:649-653.

Jones RM, Lee KS, Beschorner WE, et al (1987). Venoocclusive disease of the liver following bone marrow transplantation. *Transplantation.* 44:778-783.

Kennedy MJ, Vogelsang GB, Jones RJ, et al (1994). Phase I trial of interferon gamma to potentiate cyclosporine-induced graft-versus-host diseases in women undergoing autologous bone marrow transplantation for breast cancer. *J Clin Oncol.* 12:149-257.

Kennedy MJ, Beveridge RA, Rowley SD, et al (1991). High-dose chemotherapy with reinfusion of purged autologous bone marrow as initial therapy for metastatic breast cancer. *J Nat Cancer Inst.* 83:920-926.

Kessinger A, Armitage JO (1991). The evolving role of autologous peripheral stem cell transplantation following high-dose therapy for malignancies. *Blood.* 77:311-213.

King CR, Hoffart N, Murray ME (1992). Acute renal failure in bone marrow transplantation. *Oncol Nurs Forum.* 19:1327-1335.

Klemm PR, Hubbard SM (1990). Infection. In: Groenwald SL, et al eds. *Cancer Nursing: Principles and Practice,* 2nd ed. Boston: Jones and Bartlett, 442-466.

Klingemann HG, Phillips GL (1991). Immunotherapy after bone marrow transplantation. *Bone Marrow Transplant.* 8:73-81.

Kolbinson DA, Schubert MM, Flournoy N, Truelove EL (1988). Early oral changes following bone marrow transplantation. *Oral Surg.* 66:130–138.

Koska MT (1990). Institutes of Quality experience uneven volume. *Hospitals.* 64:44, 46–48.

Krowka MJ, Rosenow EC, Hoagland HC (1985). Pulmonary complications of bone marrow transplantation. *Chest.* 87:237–245.

Lansdorp PM, Thomas TE, Schmitt CR, Eaves CJ (1992). Marrow contamination: Positive selection. In: Armitage JO, Antman KH, eds. *High-Dose Cancer Therapy.* Baltimore: Williams & Wilkins, 127–139.

Lenarsky C, Kohn D, Parkman R (1990). Bone marrow transplantation for immunodeficiency and genetic diseases. In: Champlin R, ed. *Bone Marrow Transplantation.* Boston: Kluwer, 167–181.

Lenarsky C, Parkman R (1990). Bone marrow transplantation for the treatment of immune deficiency states. *Bone Marrow Transplantation.* 6:361–369.

Marks D, Goldman J (1992). Bone marrow transplantation in chronic myelogenous leukemia. *Marrow Transplant Rev.* 2:21–22.

Mason JR, Mullen M, Bessent E, et al (1991). Peripheral blood stem cells (PBSC) in patients receiving multiple cycles of high dose carboplatin (CBDCA) and granulocyte-macrophage colony stimulating factors (GM-CSF; Leukomax, Sandoz/Schering). *Proc Am Soc Clin Oncol.* 10:108.

Mazanet R, Elias A, Hunt M, et al (1991). Peripheral blood progenitor cells (PBPC)s added to bone marrow (BM) for hemopoietic rescue following high dose chemotherapy for solid tumors reduces morbidity and length of hospitalization. *Proc Am Soc Clin Oncol.* 10:324.

McCann S, Solomon R (1991). Chronic graft-versus host disease: Dermatological manifestations, nursing management, and research with extracorporeal chemophotopheresis. *Dermatol Nurs.* 3:221–228.

McDonald GB, Sharma P, Matthews DE, et al (1984). Venocclusive disease of the liver after bone marrow transplantation: Diagnosis, incidence and predisposing factors. *Hepatology.* 4:116–120.

McDonald GB, Sharma P, Matthews DE, et al (1985). The clinical course of 53 patients with venocclusive disease of the liver after marrow transplantation. *Transplantation.* 39:603–608.

McGarigle CJ (1990). Long-term follow-up of bone marrow transplant patients. *Yale J Biol Med.* 63:503–508.

Meriney DK (1991). Neurologic and neuromuscular complications of bone marrow transplantation. In: Whedon MB, ed. *Bone Marrow Transplantation: Principles, Practice, and Nursing Insights,* Boston: Jones and Bartlett, 262–279.

Meyer RM (1992). Acute lymphoblastic leukemia in adults. In: Brain M, Carbone P, eds. *Current Therapy in Hematology-Oncology,* 4th ed. Philadelphia: Decker, 54–63.

Miller CB, Hayashi RJ, Vogelsang GB, et al. "Aseptic shock syndrome" after bone marrow transplantation (under review).

Niederwieser D, Pepe M, Storb R, et al (1988). Improvement in rejection, engraftment rate, and survival without increase in graft-versus-host disease by high marrow cell dose in patients transplanted for aplastic anemia. *Br J Haematol.* 69:23–28.

Nimer SD, Champlin RE (1990). Therapeutic use of hemapoietic growth factors in bone marrow transplantation. In: Champlin R, ed. *Bone Marrow Transplantation.* Boston: Kluwer, 141–160.

Nims, JW, Strom S (1988). Late complications of bone marrow transplant recipients: Nursing care issues. *Semin Oncol Nurs.* 4:47–54.

Noga SJ, Wagner JE, Rowley SD, et al (1990). Using elutriation to engineer bone marrow allografts. *Prog Clin Biol Res.* 333:345–361.

O'Quin T, Moravec C (1988). The critically ill bone marrow transplant patient. *Semin Oncol Nurs.* 4:25–30.

Parkman R (1988). Cyclosporine: GVHD and beyond. *N Engl J Med.* 319:110–111.

Patenaude AF (1990). Psychological impact of bone marrow transplantation: Current perspectives. *Yale J Biol Med.* 63:515–519.

Peters WP, Shpall EJ, Jones RB, et al (1988). High-dose combination alkylating agent with bone marrow support as initial treatment for metastatic breast cancer. *J Clin Oncol.* 6: 1368–1376.

Phillips GL, Fay JW, Herzig RH, et al (1990). The treatment of progressive non-Hodgkin's lymphoma with intensive chemoradiotherapy and autologous marrow transplantation. *Blood.* 75:831–838.

Poe S, Larson E, McGuire D, Krumm S. Infection prevention practices in bone marrow transplant units. *Onc Nurs Forum* (in press).

Rappoport AP, Rowe JM, Packman CH, Ginsberg SJ (1991). Cardiac arrest after autologous marrow infusion. *Bone Marrow Transplant.* 7:401–403.

Rogers TR (1985). Prevention of infection in neutropenic bone marrow transplant patients. *Antibiot Chemother.* 33:90–113.

Rohaly J (1989). The use of busulfan therapy in bone marrow transplantation. *Cancer Nurs.* 12:144–152.

Rosenfeld C, Neumanitis J (1991). The role of granulocyte-macrophage stimulating factor-stimulated progenitor cells in oncology. *Semin Hematol.* 29:19–26.

Rowe JM, Ciobanu N, Ascensao J, et al (1994). Recommended guidelines for the management of autologous and allogeneic bone marrow transplantation. A report from the Eastern Cooperative Oncology Group (ECOG). *Ann Intern Med.* 120:143–158.

Ruggiero MR (1988). The donor in bone marrow transplantation. *Semin Oncol Nurs.* 4:9–14.

Sallan S, Billet A (1992). Acute leukemia in childhood. In: Brain M, Carbone P, eds. *Current Therapy in Hematology-Oncology,* 4th ed. Philadelphia: Decker, 68–73.

Santos G (1983). History of bone marrow transplantation. *Clin Haematol.* 12:611–639.

Saral R, Ambinder R, Burns W, et al (1983). Acyclovir prophylaxis against herpes simplex infection in patients with leukemia. *Ann Intern Med.* 99:773–776.

Schryber S, LaCasse CR, Barton-Burke M (1987). Autologous bone marrow transplantation. *Oncol Nurs Forum.* 14:74–80.

Schwartzberg L, West W, Birch R, et al (1991). Mobilized peripheral blood stem cells (PBSC) alone for hematologic reconstitution after high-dose chemotherapy for advanced malignancy. *Proc Am Soc Clin Oncol* 10:322.

Shivnan J, Shelton B. Bone marrow transplantation: Issues for critical care nurses. *Crit Care Nurse.* (in press).

Shivnan JC, Sheidler VR (1992). Pain associated with bone marrow transplantation: Unique features and treatments. *Oncol Nurs Forum.* 19:319.

Sledge GW, Antman KH (1992). Progress in chemotherapy for metastatic breast cancer. *Semin Oncol.* 19:317–332.

Smith TJ, Desch CE, Hillner BE (1992). Analysis of economic issues. In: Armitage JO, Antman KH, eds. *High-Dose Cancer Therapy.* Baltimore: Williams & Wilkins, 127–139.

Somerville ET (1986). Special diets for neutropenic patients: Do they make a difference? *Semin Oncol Nurs.* 2:55–58.

Stone R, Mayer R (1992). Acute myeloid leukemia. In: Brain M, Carbone P, eds. *Current Therapy in Hematology-Oncology,* 4th ed. Philadelphia: Decker, 63–68.

Storb R, Champlin R (1991). Bone marrow transplantation for severe aplastic anemia. *Bone Marrow Transplant.* 8:69–72.

Tavassoli M, Hardy CL (1990). Molecular basis of homing of intravenously transplanted stem cells to the marrow. *Blood.* 76:1059-1070.

Thomas ED, Storr R, Clift RA, et al (1975). Bone marrow transplantation. *N Engl J Med.* 292:832-843, 895-902.

Thomas ED (1992). Bone marrow transplantation: Past experiences and future prospects. *Semin Oncol.* 19 (Suppl 7):3-6.

Thomas ED, Ashley CA, Lochte HL, et al (1959). Homografts of bone marrow in dogs after lethal total-body radiation. *Blood.* 14:720-736.

Treleaven JG (1991). Bone marrow harvesting and reinfusion. In: Gee AP, ed. *Bone Marrow Processing and Purging.* Boca Raton: CRC Press, 31-38.

Vanacek KS (1991). Gastrointestinal complications of bone marrow transplantation. In: Whedon MB, ed. *Bone Marrow Transplantation: Principles, Practice, and Nursing Insights.* Boston: Jones and Bartlett, 206-239.

Van der Wal R, Nims J, Davies B (1988). Bone marrow transplantation in children: Nursing management of late effects. *Cancer Nurs.* 11:132-143.

Vogelsang G (1990). Acute graft-versus-host disease. In: Champlin R, ed. *Bone Marrow Transplantation.* Boston: Kluwer, 69.

Vogelsang GB, Hess AD, Santos GW (1988). Acute graft-versus-host disease: Clinical characteristics in the cyclosporine era. *Medicine.* 67:163-174.

Vose J, Armitrage J, Bierman P (1990). Bone marrow transplantation for Hodgkins disease, non-Hodgkins lymphoma and multiple myeloma. In: Champlin R, ed. *Bone Marrow Transplantation.* Kluwer, 259-275.

Weinberg P (1991). The human leukocyte antigen (HLA) system, the search for a matching donor, National Marrow Donor program development, and marrow donor issues. In: Whedon MB, ed. *Bone Marrow Transplantation. Principles, Practice, and Nursing Insights.* Boston: Jones and Bartlett, 105-131.

Weisdorf D, Haake R, Blazar B, et al (1990). Treatment of moderate/severe acute graft-versus-host disease after allogeneic bone marrow transplantation: An analysis of clinical risk features and outcome. *Blood.* 75:(4), 1024-1030.

Welch GH, Larson EB (1989). Cost effectiveness of bone marrow transplantation in acute non-lymphocytic leukemia. *N Engl J Med.* 321:807-812.

Welch-McCaffrey D, Leigh S, Loescher LJ, Hoffman B (1990). Psychosocial dimensions: Issues in survivorship. In: Groenwald SL, et al, eds. *Cancer Nursing: Principles and Practice,* 2nd ed. Boston: Jones and Bartlett, 373-382.

Whedon MB (1991). Autologous bone marrow transplantation: Clinical indications, treatment process, and outcomes. In: Whedon MB, ed. *Bone Marrow Transplantation: Principles, Practice, and Nursing Insights.* Boston: Jones and Bartlett, 49-69.

Wikle TJ (1991). Pulmonary and cardiac complications of bone marrow transplantation. In: Whedon MB, ed. *Bone Marrow Transplantation: Principles, Practice, and Nursing Insights.* Boston: Jones and Bartlett, 182-205.

Wingard JR (1991). Historical perspectives and future directions. In: Whedon MB, ed. *Bone Marrow Transplantation: Principles, Practice, and Nursing Insights.* Boston: Jones and Bartlett, 3-19.

Wingard JR, Curbow B, Baker F, Piantadosi S (1991). Health, functional status, and employment of adult survivors of bone marrow transplantation. *Ann Intern Med.* 114:113-118.

Wingard JR, Mellits ED, Sostrin MB, et al (1988). Interstitial pneumonitis after allogeneic bone marrow transplantation. *Transplantation.* 67:175-186.

Wingard JR, Sostrin MB, Vriesendorp HM, et al (1988). Interstitial pneumonitis following autologous bone marrow transplantation. *Transplantation.* 46:61-65.

Wolford JL, McDonald GB (1988). A problem-oriented approach to intestinal and liver disease after marrow transplantation. *J Clin Gastroenterol.* 10:419–433.

Wujcik D, Downs S (1992). Bone marrow transplantation. *Crit Care Nurs Clin North Am.* 4:149–166.

Yahalom J, Fuks ZY (1992). Strategies for the use of total body irradiation as systemic therapy in leukemia and lymphoma. In: Armitage JO, Antman KH, eds. *High-Dose Cancer Therapy.* Baltimore: Williams & Wilkins, 61–83.

Yeager AM, Rowley SD, Kaizer H, Santos GW (1990). Ex vivo chemopurging of autologous bone marrow with 4-hydroperoxycyclophosphamide to eliminate occult leukemic cells. *Am J Pediatr Hematol.* 12:245–256.

Zaia JA (1990). Viral infections associated with bone marrow transplantation. *Hematol Oncol Clin North Am.* 4:603–623.

NURSING CARE PLAN 9–1. THROMBOCYTOPENIA

Nursing Diagnosis	Expected Outcomes	Nursing Interventions
High Risk for Injury	• Patient remains free from injury.	• Assess skin and mouth every day for presence and extent of bruises, petechiae, purpura.
Related to	• Bleeding is controlled.	
• Low platelet count (<50,000/mm³)	• Patient describes self-care activities that protect against injury and maintain integrity of skin and mucous membranes.	• Assess sites of procedures and catheter insertion sites every day for oozing or bleeding.
• Dysfunctional platelets		
• Decreased clotting factors	• Intravascular fluid volume is maintained.	• Test urine, stool, emesis for occult or frank blood.
• Uremia		
		• Keep intact skin clean and moisturized by having patient take a shower daily and use bath oil or other lubricants.
Defining Characteristics		
• Bruises, petechiae		
• Oozing from venipuncture sites, procedure sites		• Instruct patient to avoid soaps, deodorants, perfumes, cosmetics, and other potential irritants and to use an electric razor if shaving is necessary.
• Subconjunctival hemorrhage		
• Epistaxis		
• Oral petechiae or bleeding		• Avoid invasive procedures whenever possible, including rectal temperatures, suppositories, and intramuscular injections. Protect against falls by maintaining safe, well-lit environment. Keep call bell in reach. Keep side rails up when appropriate. Ensure that patient wears appropriate footwear.
• Hemoptysis		
• Hematemesis		
• Melena or frank blood in stool		
• Hematuria		
• Painful or swollen joints		
• Altered mental status		

- Monitor vaginal bleeding and administer medications as ordered to suppress menses. Institute oral care regimen that incorporates use of mouth swabs and nonirritating mouthwash.
- Control epistaxis by applying pressure, ice, topical clotting or vasoconstrictive agents as ordered.
- Administer blood products as ordered.
- Implement patient teaching plan to assist patient in assuming self-care.

NURSING CARE PLAN 9–2. ACUTE GRAFT-VERSUS-HOST DISEASE OF THE SKIN

Nursing Diagnosis	Expected Outcomes	Nursing Interventions
Impaired Skin Integrity	• Skin remains intact, clean, and free from infection.	• Assess skin every day for presence and extent of erythema, blisters, and skin loss.
Related to	• Patient relates relief of itching, burning, and pain.	• Assess sites of infection every day for erythema, pain, swelling, and exudate. (Possible sites of infection include the oropharynx, perirectal and perineal skin, sites of central and peripheral lines, and procedure sites.) Assess breath sounds and bowel sounds and check for abdominal tenderness.
• Lymphocyte destruction of epidermis	• Patient describes self-care activities that protect and maintain integrity of skin.	
• Scratching due to pruritus		
Defining Characteristics		• Culture suspicious sites for bacteriologic and mycologic testing.
• Erythematous maculopapular rash		• Assess for systemic signs of infection every 4 hours (temperature, pulse, respiration, blood pressure).
• Bullae		
• Desquamation		• Assess for pain using age-appropriate pain assessment tool.
• Subjective complaints of itching, burning, and pain		• Assess for itching.
		• Keep intact skin clean and moisturized by having patient take a shower daily and use bath oil or other lubricants.
		• Instruct patient to avoid soaps, deodorants, perfumes, cosmetics, and other potential irritants.

- Clean and protect broken areas using sterile technique and antiseptic or antibacterial ointments or barriers as appropriate.
- Assess need for specialized bed therapy.
- Administer antipruritic and analgesic medications as ordered and indicated.
- Instruct patient to protect skin from sun by using appropriate clothing and sunscreen.
- Implement patient teaching plan to assist patient in assuming self-care.

NURSING CARE PLAN 9–3. ALTERED NUTRITION

Nursing Diagnosis	Expected Outcomes	Nursing Interventions

Altered Nutrition: Less Than Body Requirements
 	
Related to
• Mucositis
• Xerostomia
• Taste changes
• Nausea and vomiting
• Diarrhea, enteritis
 	
Defining Characteristics
• Poor oral intake
• Episodes of nausea and vomiting
• Caloric and protein intake less than requirements
• Weight loss
• Fatigue
• Complaints of xerostomia and taste changes
• Anorexia
• Oral pain
• Breakdown of oral or esophageal mucosa
• Episodes of diarrhea
• Malabsorption
• Abnormal laboratory values that reflect nutritional status
	• Patient maintains adequate nutritional status during transplant process, especially during times of poor oral intake and gastrointestinal complications.
	• Patient reports improvement in or relief of nausea and vomiting.
	• Patient reports improvement in or relief of diarrhea and eventually returns to normal bowel pattern.
	• Patient reports methods found to be useful in overcoming xerostomia or taste changes.
	• Fluid and electrolyte status is maintained within normal limits. Patient reports relief from oral pain.
	• Healing of mucositis becomes evident.
		• Administer anesthetics and analgesics as needed for mucositis.
		• Instruct patient to adjust diet as needed for mucositis:
		  Mild mucositis: soft, bland diet; avoidance of spicy, acidic or irritating foods; dessert ices, ice chips, or other cool foods as desired
		  Moderate to severe mucositis: consider total parenteral nutrition if patient unable to maintain adequate caloric and protein intake
		• Inspect oral cavity every shift; monitor for tissue breakdown or lesions. Culture possible lesions as needed.
		• Consider using artificial saliva as needed for xerostomia. Experiment with foods that have a high liquid content for management of xerostomia. Have patient avoid substances that dry the oral cavity, such as commercial mouthwashes, lemon glycerine swabs, alcohol, nicotine.
		• Promote and educate patient about good oral and dental care.
		• Consult with dietician regarding food preferences and food aversions; attempt to provide desired foods if possible. Offer small, frequent feedings. Experiment with flavors, seasonings, sauces, and gravies.

- Monitor degree and severity of dysphagia; help patient identify foods that are easy to swallow.
- Provide oral suction for patient unable to swallow or mobilize secretions.
- Administer antimicrobial therapy (topical, oral, or parenteral) as ordered.
- Administer antidiarrheal agents as ordered; auscultate abdomen for presence of bowel sounds.
- Collect stool cultures as needed and send them to the laboratory.
- Modify diet to low-residue for diarrhea; have patient avoid foods known to be intestinal irritants, such as lactose-containing products, high-fiber foods, caffeine.
- Consider allowing patient nothing by mouth for bowel rest during periods of severe enteritis (due to graft-versus-host disease [GVHD] or mucositis); oral foods or fluids can be reintroduced according to institutional procedure.
- Administer anti-GVHD medications as ordered.
- Monitor laboratory values, weights, hemodynamic values, intake and output for signs of dehydration, electrolyte depletion, or bleeding.

(*continued*)

NURSING CARE PLAN 9–3. ALTERED NUTRITION (*continued*)

Nursing Diagnosis	Expected Outcomes	Nursing Interventions
		• Administer fluids and electrolytes or blood products as ordered.
		• Assess history of nausea and vomiting, previous antiemetics used and patients response, and other measures that have been found to relieve symptoms.
		• Administer antiemetics as needed.
		• Facilitate use of nonpharmacologic interventions for management of nausea and vomiting, eg, rest, distraction, music, relaxation exercises.
		• Facilitate supportive interventions for patients experiencing emotional distress related to gastrointestinal complications (eg, consultation for counseling, behavioral intervention).

NURSING CARE PLAN 9–4. DISCHARGE AFTER BONE MARROW TRANSPLANTATION

Nursing Diagnosis	Expected Outcomes	Nursing Interventions

Knowledge Deficit (Self-Care After Discharge from Bone Marrow Transplantation Facility)	• Patient verbalizes self-care measures related to prevention of infection after discharge.	• Teach about infection prevention according to institutional procedure
		
		  Avoidance of people with infectious diseases
		
		  Use of good hand-washing techniques
		
		  Wearing of a mask, if applicable
		
		  Avoidance of crowds, swimming, hot tubs
		
		  Avoidance of live viral vaccinations for 1 year
		
		  Restricted contact with pets and gardening, if applicable
		
		  Good oral and dental care

Defining Characteristics	• Patient verbalizes self-care measures related to prevention of bleeding after discharge.	
• Patient or family questions about treatment and follow-up care	• Patient states conditions to report to physician or nurse after discharge that require emergency evaluation or care.	• Teach about prevention of bleeding if patient has thrombocytopenia at discharge
• Inability to perform self-care activities proficiently	• Patient relates appropriate nutritional strategies to be used after discharge.	
	• Patient outlines guidelines for safe sexual practices after discharge.	• Give safety precautions: wearing of slippers or shoes; removal of obstacles from path of ambulation; careful handling of sharp objects; avoidance of hard-bristled toothbrush and flossing; avoidance of rectal thermometers and suppositories; avoidance of straining during bowel movements (stool softeners may be necessary); avoidance of
	• Patient outlines activity guidelines for resumption of activity and exercise after discharge.	
	• Patient outlines prescribed discharge medications, including reason for use, schedule, and side effects to report.	
	• Patient states understanding of outpatient follow-up schedule.	
	• Patient demonstrates safe, aseptic technique in caring for vascular access device upon discharge (if applicable).	

(continued)

NURSING CARE PLAN 9–4. DISCHARGE AFTER BONE MARROW TRANSPLANTATION (*continued*)

Nursing Diagnosis	Expected Outcomes	Nursing Interventions
Knowledge Deficit (continued)		forceful nose-blowing; avoidance of rigorous exercise during which injury might occur. Inform patient about possible need for continued outpatient platelet therapy
		• Educate patient about reportable symptoms; provide patient with emergency telephone number and name of person to contact
		Fever of 100.4°F (38°C) or higher
		Shaking chills
		New cough, shortness of breath, pain or difficulty breathing
		Chest pain, heart palpitations
		Headaches, dizziness, blurred vision or changes in vision, stiff neck, new difficulty with walking or balance
		New onset of nausea and vomiting or diarrhea; increased difficulty eating or keeping liquids down; inability to keep medications down
		New oral lesions, plaques, ulcers, or soreness
		Pain, burning, frequency, or bleeding on urination; low-back pain; foul odor to urine

Any new rash, itching, sores, redness of skin

Any joint or muscle pain, stiffness when walking

New onset of pain

Vaginal or penile discharge

Any signs of bleeding, such as a nosebleed, new unusual bruising, bleeding gums, blood in stool or urine

Any swelling, tenderness, or irritation of eyes

Redness, tenderness, swelling, or drainage from vascular access catheter exit site

- Promote good nutrition after bone marrow transplant; collaborate with dietician as needed to develop, implement, and evaluate strategies to enhance oral intake

High protein and calorie intake after transplant; specific meal items that provide high intake and are tolerated

Symptom management of gastrointestinal complications as needed (see Nursing Care Plan 9–3)

Adequate oral fluid intake

Avoidance of raw or undercooked eggs, fish, meat

(continued)

NURSING CARE PLAN 9–4. DISCHARGE AFTER BONE MARROW TRANSPLANTATION (*continued*)

Nursing Diagnosis	Expected Outcomes	Nursing Interventions
Knowledge Deficit (continued)		Thorough washing of all fruits and vegetables
		Defrosting frozen foods in refrigerator
		Refrigerating leftover food promptly
		• Outline sexual self-care after transplant
		Avoidance of multiple partners
		Use of devices and practices to prevent sexually transmitted diseases
		Postponing intercourse until platelet count is 50,000/mm^3 or higher
		Appropriate contraception
		Good hygiene
		Use of water-soluble lubricant to alleviate vaginal dryness; alerting physician or nurse if intercourse is painful
		Awareness that stress of hospitalization or continued treatment may decrease libido
		• Outline posttransplant activity and exercise guidelines; collaborate with physical therapist if specialized intervention is needed
		Walking, stair-climbing, stationary bicycling; gradual resumption of physical activity

Avoidance of rigorous activities in which injury is a risk, particularly during thrombocytopenia

Reporting decline in energy level to nurse or physician

Planning to return to work, school, driving contingent on energy level and physical status; discussion with physician before resumption

Use of adequate sunscreen

- Review discharge medication with patient, including reason for use, schedule and side effects to report. Discourage use of over-the-counter medications until approved by physician. Instruct patient to avoid aspirin, aspirin-containing products, or ibuprofen-containing products because they may enhance risk of bleeding.

- Provide follow-up schedule and information about whom to call in an emergency.

- Incorporate family member into teaching.

10

Corneal Transplantation

Victoria B. Navarro
Frances M. Tolley

"Who would believe that so small a space could contain the images of the universe?"

Leonardo da Vinci (1452–1519)

The search for the treatment of corneal scarring dates back to ancient Egyptian times. Interest in corneal pathology gained momentum in the 18th century. Scientists were searching for ways and means to replace an opaque cornea with a transparent material to restore sight. Work with experimental grafts eventually led to corneal transplantation. Penetrating keratoplasty (PK) is the transplant procedure discussed in this chapter.

HISTORY

The first corneal transplant was reported by Pelliere de Quengsy in 1789 (Thomas, 1955). In that operation, a portion of glass cut to specification was used to replace a scarred cornea. Although the results were unsuccessful, this crude operation triggered much interest in the concept and initiated vast investigation and experimentation in the field of corneal transplantation.

During the 19th century, experimentation with transplantation was confined mainly to animals. A variety of tissue substitutes were tried, including glass, heterografts or xenografts (grafts from different species), and homografts (grafts from same species). A few attempts at heterotransplantation, from animal donors to human recipients, were unsuccessful in obtaining a clear graft. However, results did indicate that grafted tissue could remain healed to the host cornea.

291

The first successful human corneal transplant was reported by Zirm in 1906 (Thomas, 1955). The donor graft was human tissue. Ortin's research in 1914 (Thomas, 1955) confirmed that homografts were second only to autografts (donor from same individual) in results achieved. Because autografts are rarely an option, homografts became the graft of choice. Autografts may be contralateral (right eye to left eye or left eye to right eye) or rotating ipsilateral (autograft rotated in the same eye). Isografts are transplants between homozygotic twins (Buxton et al, 1993).

The 1950s ushered in the modern era of corneal transplantation with improved understanding of the pathophysiologic features of the cornea; improved microsurgical instrumentation and surgical techniques; the development of fine, nonreactive suture materials; and the introduction of eye banking techniques. In addition, anti-inflammatory and immunosuppressive drugs have reduced the incidence of graft rejection. By 1990, more than 40,631 grafts had been performed in the United States (Buxton et al, 1993). PK is the most frequently and successfully performed transplantation procedure. The 2-year survival rate is more than 90% for initial grafts into avascular corneas (Collaborative Corneal Transplantation Studies [CCTS] Research Group, 1992).

ANATOMY AND PHYSIOLOGY

The cornea is the main refracting surface of the eye (Fig. 10-1). This unique tissue is transparent because of its lack of vascularity. The transparent surface allows light rays to be focused onto the retina. The cornea is made up of five distinct layers, each having specific characteristics (Fig. 10-2). The preocular tear film, which covers the corneal surface, produces an environment essential for corneal structure and function (Lemp, 1993). The tear film fills in and smooths out spaces caused by irregularities on the epithelial surface and acts as the anterior refracting surface of the eye. Blinking the upper lid distributes the tear film and provides a shearing force against the corneal surface. If blinking is prevented or incomplete, the tear film thins and evaporates, leaving dry spots in the tear film and subsequently the epithelium. The prognosis for a successful graft decreases in conditions associated with abnormalities of the tear film (Lemp, 1993).

The corneal epithelium provides an optical interface with the tear film and a barrier to the external environment. This layer contains most nerve fibers, the exposure of which causes severe pain. Damage to this layer results in an epithelial defect that can be a single acute episode or a chronic condition that leads to infection, thinning, and corneal perforation (Vaughan & Asbury, 1983).

The corneal stroma represents 90% of the corneal thickness. Its principle component is collagen, which arranged in layers (lamellae) gives tensile strength to the cornea (McDermott, 1993). The Bowman layer, the anterior surface of this structure, is highly resistant to trauma. The posterior border of the stroma, the Descemet membrane, thickens with age. Damage to the Descemet membrane by disease or injury exposes the most posterior layer, the endothelium, to damage. The endothelium maintains hydration of the cornea. Endothelial cells do not regenerate. Endothelial cell loss

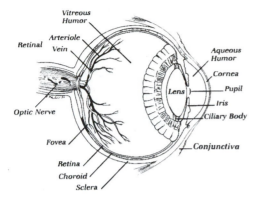

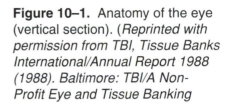

Figure 10–1. Anatomy of the eye (vertical section). (*Reprinted with permission from TBI, Tissue Banks International/Annual Report 1988 (1988). Baltimore: TBI/A Non-Profit Eye and Tissue Banking*

or trauma leads to a disruption of normal fluid balance in corneal tissue with eventual corneal edema and opacity (Fig. 10-3).

One last structural area of the cornea is the limbus, the junction between the cornea and the conjunctiva and sclera. The limbus is the location of the capillary bed that along with the tear film and aqueous humor, nourishes the cornea, which contains no vascular structures (Stein et al, 1988).

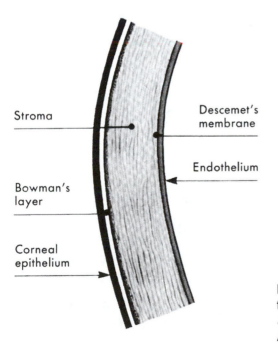

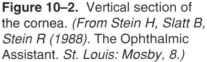

Figure 10–2. Vertical section of the cornea. (*From Stein H, Slatt B, Stein R (1988).* The Ophthalmic Assistant. *St. Louis: Mosby, 8.)*

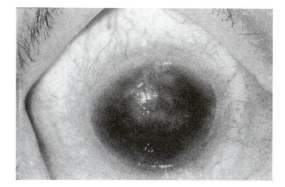

Figure 10–3. Corneal edema. (*Reprinted with permission from Brightbill FS (1986). Corneal Surgery, Theory, Technique & Tissue. St. Louis: Mosby, 135.)*

INDICATIONS FOR PENETRATING KERATOPLASTY

Keratoconus

Keratoconus is a condition in which the cornea assumes a conical shape with progressive thinning and protrusion (Fig. 10–4). The marked irregular surface and thinning cause mild to profound visual impairment. The condition is usually bilateral and affects all races. Women show a higher incidence of keratoconus than men, 50 to 65% of documented cases. The onset of the condition typically occurs at puberty with thinning of the central cornea and the development of irregular astigmatism. The disease may progress for 20 years. Heredity in some instances can be identified as the leading causative factor, and there is documented association with other systemic and ocular diseases (Feder, 1993). It is of interest that a history of eye rubbing has been identi-

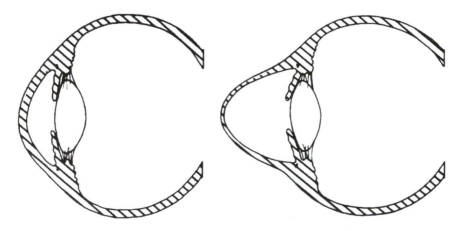

Figure 10–4. (Left) side view of cornea. (Right) keratoconus. *(Reprinted with permission from Vaughan D, Asbury T (1983). General Ophthalmology. Los Altos, California: Lange, 98.)*

fied in 66–70% of keratoconus patients. This may be a link between other ocular diseases that cause itching and irritation. Nineteen to twenty-six percent of these patients have a history of contact lens wear prior to diagnosis (Feder, 1993). Symptoms include visual blurring and distortion, photophobia, glare, and ocular irritation. PK has a 90% success rate in keratoconus, the highest success rate among other disease conditions (Vaughn & Asbury, 1983).

Fuch Dystrophy

Fuch dystrophy is a degenerative process that is most common in postmenopausal women. Gradual decompensation of the endothelium leads to disruption of fluid balance in the cornea and endothelial excrescences (an abnormal protuberance or growth of tissue) referred to as *guttata.* Corneal endothelial decompensation leads to corneal edema and thickening (Vaughn & Asbury, 1983).

Herpes Simplex Keratitis

Herpes simplex virus (HSV) infection is one of the most common causes of infectious blindness in the United States (Lanier, 1993). Infections of this type range from mild with a single episode to recurrent stromal keratitis, which is sight-threatening and lasts up to 12 months with residual scarring. PK may be performed in an effort to save the patient's vision when medical therapy is unsuccessful. The success rate is lower than in other diagnoses because of the amount of inflammation and vascularization in the recipient cornea. These patients are also subject to recurrent HSV infection in the donor graft and to homograft reaction. Lanier (1993) reported the incidences of homograft reaction to be as high as 79%. Despite these unfavorable odds, successful grafts can be achieved when the operation is performed on noninflamed eyes and when postoperative complications are anticipated and treated (Lanier, 1993).

Pseudophakic Bullous Keratopathy

Pseudophakic bullous keratopathy (PBK) has been the most common condition leading to PK since the late 1970s. During the late 1970s and the early 1980s, cataract surgeries were performed using intraocular lenses that came into contact with the corneal endothelium. These lenses implanted in the anterior chamber caused endothelial cell loss and irreversible corneal edema. The incidence of PBK has declined with improved lens design. If detected early, PBK can be treated by careful control of intraocular pressure and inflammation along with surgical exchange of the intraocular lens when necessary (Buxton et al, 1993).

Chemical Burns

Chemical burns are severe injuries that often occur bilaterally. The alkaline or acidic nature of the chemical, its concentration, and the length of exposure determine the severity of injury (Kinoshita & Manabe, 1993). The effects of chemical injury range from faint haziness of the cornea with no loss of epithelial cells to complete epithelial loss and corneal opacity with potential for scarring, ulceration, and perforation (American Academy of Ophthalmology, 1985). If the injured eye does not perforate, the ocular surface heals in a few years with varying degrees of scarring and vascularization.

PK is deferred until scarring has occurred, sometimes years after the initial injury. The prognosis for the restoration of vision for these patients is uncertain because there is often considerable scarring and vascularization in the host cornea. Other surgical interventions include conjunctival transplantation for less severe injuries in which sections of conjunctiva from the healthy eye are sutured onto the damaged limbus. Another surgical procedure uses donor corneal epithelium to resurface the damaged cornea (Kinoshita & Manabe, 1993).

Regraft

Graft failure continues to be a leading indication for PK. At one institution, 10% of PKs performed were regrafts (Rapriano, et al, 1990). Primary graft failure, allograft reaction, and recurrent host disease are the main indications for regraft. Twenty-three to thirty percent of patients with herpes keratitis require regrafts. Historically, the prognosis for regrafts has been considered grim. It is now considered a relatively successful procedure in part because of improved management of graft rejection and improved antiviral medical therapy.

DEVELOPMENT OF SURGICAL EQUIPMENT AND TECHNIQUE

In 1886, von Hipple constructed the first trephine with a circular cutting edge (Thomas, 1955). This corneal trephine (Fig. 10–5), improved through the years, has helped ophthalmic surgeons achieve the most accurate cut to approximate a perfect fit for the donor button (excised circular corneal graft tissue) and its recipient bed (Tanne, 1986).

   The development of microsurgical techniques has dramatically increased the success rate of corneal transplantation. Microsurgical technique involves magnification of the operative field, adaptation of functions and dimensions of surgical instruments, and refinement of suture materials to minimize surgical trauma to tissues.

   The operating microscope introduced in the 1970s is the principal part of microsurgical instrumentation. It allows visualization of structures previously left unseen. To complement this visual magnification, ophthalmic instruments have been

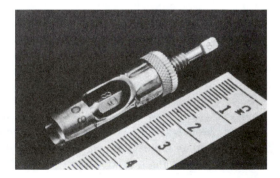

Figure 10–5. Corneal trephine. *(Reprinted with permission from Vaughan D, Asbury T (1983).* General Ophthalmology. *Los Altos, California: Lange, 104.)*

reduced in size and weight (Draeger & Klein, 1987). The finer 10–0 monofilament nylon suture has replaced silk and absorbable sutures. Its low reactive properties decrease postoperative inflammation and vascularization of the operative site, and its tensile strength and elasticity reduce the incidence of wound leak and dehiscense (Hutz & Ullerich, 1987). In the first successful corneal transplant, in 1906, the donor graft was held by only two sutures passed through the conjunctiva and sclera (Thomas, 1955).

Viscoelastic materials (such as sodium hyaluronate) have maximized the survival of the donor graft endothelium. The viscoelastic material is injected into the anterior chamber to firm the globe, coat and protect surfaces, and separate tissue spaces. Adhesions are also avoided postoperatively. Viscoelastic materials are used in the preparation of the donor corneal button and in the trephination of the recipient eye. Because the most important complication of the use of viscoelastic material is the development of glaucoma or increased intraocular pressure, the smallest amount of a viscoelastic material as possible, consistent with clinical objectives, should be used (Levenson & Imperia, 1993). The viscoelastic material is removed at the end of the operation.

PENETRATING KERATOPLASTY

Preoperative Evaluation

The decision to perform PK should be a joint agreement between the surgeon and an informed patient. The expected visual outcome must be evaluated, and the impact of other ocular conditions must be considered preoperatively. The patient's history should include accurate information on the best visual acuity before corneal opacity. Other conditions such as strabismus, amblyopia, retinal disease, or glaucoma can influence the visual prognosis. Previous operations such as cataract extraction should be explored with specific information about postoperative visual acuity, surgical technique, and intraocular lenses used. Ruling out other causes of vision loss can validate the decision to perform PK. Lid or tear film abnormalities such as dry-eye syndrome should be treated before the operation. Compliance with glaucoma therapy has serious implications for postoperative control of intraocular pressure to prevent damage to the corneal graft.

Other patient factors such as age, vision in the eye not operated on, availability of support for immediate and long-term follow-up care, and the patient's ability to comprehend and comply with care requirements are important factors in the decision-making process (Buxton et al, 1993).

A complete examination of all ocular structures is performed to determine any existing conditions that will have an impact on graft survival. The lids and facial skin are examined for scarring from trauma, infection, or previous operations. Improper lid closure can cause exposure keratitis and graft destruction (Forstot, 1993). The tear film and conjunctiva are evaluated because they are the environment of the donor graft. The corneal examination includes evaluation of vascularization, size of opacity, and location and assessment of corneal thickness. Extensive thinning has an impact on the type of graft performed. Irregularities in the corneal surface indicate astigmatism and may have implications for the severity of postoperative astigmatism (Forstot, 1993).

Penetrating Keratoplasty Procedure

PK is a surgical procedure in which abnormal full-thickness corneal tissue is removed from a host and replaced with full-thickness corneal tissue. Lamellar keratoplasty is a partial-thickness graft (Fig. 10-6).

The operation may be performed with general endotracheal anesthesia or with retrobulbar and seventh-nerve regional anesthesia combined with intravenous analgesics and hypnotic medication. After the patient's head is positioned and the eye being operated on draped, a wire or solid-blade lid speculum is inserted between the lids; care is taken to make sure there is no pressure on the globe. A scleral support or fixation ring is sutured to the sclera to stabilize the globe during trephination. Because unequal placement of fixation sutures can cause irregularity in the graft recipient bed and considerable astigmatism, some corneal surgeons use a larger ring so that the sutured ring is farther from the limbus. Many surgeons have discontinued the use of the fixation ring, although bridle sutures are placed beneath the superior and inferior rectus muscles (Fig. 10-7). The surgeon then inspects the status of the cornea using a microscope. The appropriate graft size is marked on the surface of the cornea with a trephine. The surgeon then prepares the donor cornea. The donor cornea with the scleral rim is removed from the storage vial and placed on a polytetrafluoroethylene (PTFE) cutting block with the epithelial surface facing down. The corneal button is cut using a trephine slightly larger than the recipient graft bed (0.20–0.50 mm). Balanced salt solution, viscoelastic material, or donor storage medium is placed on the endothelial surface to keep it moist. A moist chamber is made for temporary storage of the donor button.

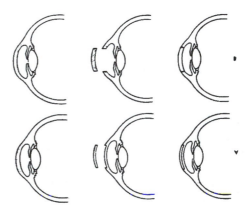

Figure 10–6. (A) Lamellar, or partial penetrating, corneal transplant. (B) Penetrating, or full-thickness, corneal transplant. *(Reprinted with permission from Stein H, Slatt B, Stein R (1988).* The Ophthalmic Assistant. *St. Louis: Mosby Year Book, 589.)*

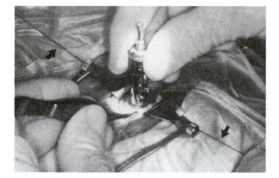

Figure 10–7. Bridle sutures (arrows) placed beneath superior and inferior vectus muscles. *(Reprinted with permission from Brightbill FS (1993).* Corneal Surgery: Theory, Technique & Tissue, *2nd ed. St. Louis: Mosby Year Book, 211.)*

The surgeon then prepares the recipient bed. The surgeon places a trephine of the preferred diameter perpendicular to the corneal tissue (Fig. 10-8). The surgeon rotates the trephine in a circular motion until the uniform depth is obtained. The depth is usually three-fourths of the way or completely through the anterior chamber. The surgeon completes the cutting by using scissors to remove the damaged host cornea (Fig. 10-9). Additional surgical procedures, such as cataract extraction and implantation of the intraocular lens, are then performed. The donor cornea is then placed on the recipient bed and sutured (Danneffel, 1990). To anchor the donor button in position, cardinal sutures are placed at the 12, 6, 3 and 9 o'clock positions.

Suturing technique distorts corneal curvature and influences the degree of postoperative astigmatism (refractive error). Suturing techniques include continuous (single or double) (Fig. 10-10A), interrupted (Fig. 10-10B) or a combination of suturing techniques and is based on the surgeon's preference. The surgeon chooses the suture pattern that works best for obtaining secure anatomic closure, minimal astigmatism, and average corneal curvature. The advantages of a continuous suture include ease of placement and removal, fewer knots that stimulate vascularization, and the ability to adjust loop tension under intraoperative keratometric control and postoperatively during a slit-lamp examination. The disadvantage is the potential for loss of wound in-

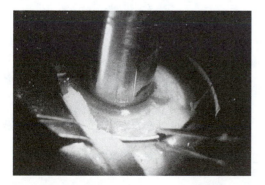

Figure 10–8. Trephination of the host cornea. *(Reprinted with permission from Brightbill FS (1993).* Corneal Surgery: Theory, Technique & Tissue, *2nd ed. St. Louis: Mosby, 107.)*

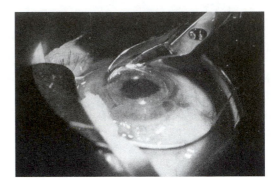

Figure 10–9. Removal of damaged host cornea with scissors. *(Reprinted with permission from Brightbill FS (1993).* Corneal Surgery: Theory, Technique & Tissue, *2nd ed. St. Louis: Mosby*

tegrity if the suture breaks inadvertently (during suture adjustment postoperatively) (Troutman et al, 1993). Adjustment of suture tension during the operation is more easily accomplished with continuous suturing. In addition, continuous suturing also lessens tissue reaction at suture sites (Casey & Mayer, 1984) and is recommended in operations on highly vascularized corneas (Gottsch et al, 1993). Sutures are left in place for 12 to 18 months depending on the clinical condition of the damaged host cornea. In children, because of faster healing and the possibility of vascularity, sutures are removed sooner than in adults. Interrupted suturing allows selective suture removal, increasing control of astigmatism postoperatively. Postoperative suture removal may take 6 weeks to 18 months (Troutman et al, 1993). At the end of the procedure, antibiotics and corticosteroids are administered by subconjunctival injection or topically. A patch and shield are applied (Abbott, 1993).

Intraoperative complications specific to the keratoplasty procedure are problems arising from trephination (eg, disparity of donor–recipient buttons or trauma to the iris or lens) and from flattening of the anterior chamber that does not adequately reform because of loose or inadequate sutures, resulting in wound leakage (Danneffel,

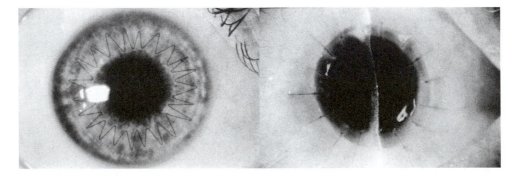

Figure 10–10. (**A**) Continuous suturing technique in penetrating keratoplasty. (**B**) Interrupted suturing technique in penetrating keratoplasty.

1990). Other intraoperative complications are similar to those of other ocular procedures (eg, hemorrhage from the retrobulbar block, expulsive hemorrhage, loss of vitreous humor from the eye).

Penetrating Keratoplasty in Pediatric Patients

Children and infants who undergo PK present unique problems for the surgeon and nursing staff working with them. The indications, surgical techniques, postoperative medical care, and nursing management are specific to pediatric patients. In the recent past, corneal transplantation was considered futile in children. The prognosis is not equal to that among adults, but studies show that clear grafts can be achieved (Stulting, 1993). Indications for PK in children can be divided into three categories: congenital (Peter anomaly, glaucoma, multiple anterior segment anomalies); acquired nontraumatic (herpes simplex keratitis, bacterial keratitis, keratoconus); and acquired traumatic (corneal laceration, blood stain, nonpenetrating injury with a scar). Within these categories, patients with congenital opacities fare the worst (Stulting, 1993).

Other factors influence the prognosis of pediatric grafts. Surgically the eye is smaller, more elastic, and less rigid than the eye of an adult. There is a possibility that the eye will collapse during the operation. The eyes of children heal rapidly, and sutures may loosen. Inflammatory responses are severe and are difficult to detect. Infants and children cannot describe symptoms of graft rejection. At times a poor visual outcome is attributed to amblyopia, a degenerative retinal condition that develops when light and visual images to the retina have been blocked by an opaque cornea (Stulting, 1993).

The decision to perform PK must be considered carefully by the surgeon and the parents of the child, particularly if the ocular condition is congenital. Both parent and surgeon must commit to a long-term partnership to achieve graft clarity and visual rehabilitation. Parents should be aware of the success rate for pediatric PK and that because of other factors, the visual outcome may be limited despite a successful operation. Frequent visits to the ophthalmologist and repeated examinations under anesthesia become integral to maintaining the graft. The nurse should reinforce the information provided by the physician while assessing the family's response to the child's ocular condition and treatment demands. The nurse should assess the home environment and work with the family to ensure that home care needs are met. Follow-up visits, administration of medication, safety measures, ocular protection, and signs and symptoms of graft failure are the essential components of the postoperative teaching plan. The financial impact of the child's condition should be discussed and appropriate referrals made to social workers or other supportive services. The nursing staff acts as emotional support for the family, allowing them to verbalize fears and feelings of guilt or anguish over the child's condition. Support can be offered by uniting parents with other families whose child has a similar condition or by referral to local or national support groups for parents of visually impaired children, such as the Parents of Blind Children, a division of the National Federation of the Blind. The increased success of PK can be attributed to good collaboration between the child's family and the health care team.

EYE BANKING

Increased interest in PK between 1950 and 1970 was the impetus for the rapid proliferation of eye banks throughout the United States. In 1935, Filatov of Odessa, Russia pioneered the use of cadaver tissue for donor material in PK. He advocated studies of methods of preservation and sought assistance from the government to facilitate obtaining cadavers' eyes (Payne, 1980).

In the early 1940s, Paton (1950) obtained permission to use eye tissue obtained from executed prisoners (Farge, 1989). He suggested that living people could agree to give their eyes upon death, and next-of-kin could be approached by hospital staff to donate a deceased relative's eyes.

In 1944, through the efforts of Paton, eye banks founded in New York began as organized entities, known as Eye Bank for Sight Restoration, Inc. The primary aims were to provide donor materials to qualified ophthalmic surgeons, not only for grafting but also for teaching of surgical technique, and to scientists for research in the causes of blindness, particularly from ocular disease or injury (TBI Eye Research Program, 1988).

In 1961, The American Academy of Ophthalmology and Otolaryngology supported the formation of the Eye Bank Association of America (EBAA) to give medical and ethical guidance and attempt standardization of procedures. EBAA is recognized as the standard-setting agency in the United States and is focused on ensuring quality donor tissue and eliminating the possibility of disease transmission by keratoplasty.

In 1968 the Medical Eye Bank of Maryland initiated the establishment of Tissue Banks International (TBI), a not-for-profit network of 12 eye banks across the United States. By 1990, TBI processed more than 8000 transplantable corneas. In every city with a TBI-affiliated eye bank, patient waiting lists have been virtually eliminated, and corneal graft operations are performed on a scheduled basis (Griffith & Sterner, 1993). TBI continues to monitor quality control of the tissue processed and to inform eye banks of technical innovations, particularly storage media. To facilitate sharing of surplus corneas with countries without a productive eye-banking system, TBI formed the International Federation of Eye Banks (IFEB) in 1989. IFEB helps establish eye banks and monitors the quality of facilities and eye tissue for its member eye banks. It also serves as an information network (Griffith & Valmadrid, 1993).

Removal of Corneal Tissue

Corneal tissue is retrieved from the donor eye by enucleation (complete surgical removal of the globe) and subsequent corneal excision or by in situ removal of the cornea. Enucleation is performed under aseptic technique; care is taken that there is no damage to the corneal endothelium. The cornea should not be touched or physically distorted, and the fragile tissues surrounding the eye should not be excessively manipulated while the globe is being removed. Endothelial cell loss must be minimized during excision of the corneoscleral rim. An in situ excision of the corneoscleral rim is performed when the legal consent dictates that only the cornea may be removed from the donor (Lisitza, 1993).

Suitability of Donor Material

The corneal endothelium of an enucleated eye survives in vitro for 6 hours at 37°C. Optimum tissue quality is retained within this time. Endothelial survival in a cadaver depends on ambient temperature. Therefore, if donor tissue is to remain viable, it is mandatory that ice packs be placed over the lids of the cadaver if there is delay in enucleation. Enucleated eyes can be preserved more effectively because tissues of small mass cool rapidly and temperature control is more accurate (Casey & Mayer, 1984). Therefore, enucleation should be performed as soon as possible. Beyond 6 hours, the supply of glucose in the aqueous humor and endothelium is exhausted and necrosis occurs (Casey & Mayer, 1984). The risk for contamination by bacteria and fungi increases as the interval between death and enucleation lengthens (Dhanda & Kalevar, 1972). Prolonged retention of the eye in the cadaver makes the eye hypotonic (Ehrlich & Abel, 1972). Ocular hypotony causes folds in the Descemet membrane, which leads to circumscribed loss of endothelial cells (Kaufman, et al, 1987).

The status of the endothelium is of crucial importance. It is recognized that as many as 70% of the cells may eventually be lost. As the cell count falls below 1000 per mm^2 the likelihood of corneal edema increases progressively. It is therefore desirable to use donor corneas with a minimum of 2000 cells per mm^2 (O'Day, 1993). The endothelial cell count decreases with age. Because normal cell loss occurs during the operation because of tissue trauma and because accelerated loss is associated with wound healing, it is best to use the freshest, youngest eyes available. Most surgeons prefer to use tissue from people younger than 65 years. Eyes from infants younger than 3 months are soft, flaccid, and technically difficult to manipulate, thus many surgeons prefer not to use them. O'Day (1993) suggested that the use of young donor tissue be limited to donors older than 2 years because of myopic shift induced by steep transplantation curvatures. Studies, however, have not demonstrated a definitive relation between donor age and graft clarity (Kaufman et al, 1987; O'Day, 1993).

The EBAA medical standards have identified contraindications to the use of donor tissue (Table 10–1). Transmission of donor disease to the recipient is rare because of the refined tissue evaluation techniques that are now routinely practiced by eye banks. Nevertheless, infections, neoplastic diseases, and corneal disorders may be acquired by corneal transplantation. Very serious are viral infections, but only rabies, Creutzfeldt–Jakob disease, and hepatitis B have had documented transmission (O'Day, 1989). There has been no documented transmission of the acquired immunodeficiency syndrome (AIDS).

Tissue assessment is performed if the cornea is acceptable for transplantation. A gross examination of the globe is performed to look at the general transparency of the cornea and for foreign bodies. In addition, a slit-lamp examination evaluates the epithelium for abrasions and foreign bodies and for the presence of corneal disease. If the cornea is determined to be of surgical quality, the cornea with its scleral rim is removed from the rest of the globe. A slit-lamp examination is again performed to describe the quality of the four corneal layers. For borderline cases (ie, when corneas from older donors or from donors who have been dead for more than 12 hours are used) the tissue is examined under a specular microscope to determine the density

TABLE 10–1. CONTRAINDICATIONS TO THE USE OF DONOR TISSUE FOR PENETRATING KERATOPLASY

Systemic Disorders

Death of unknown cause

Death of central nervous system diseases of unknown cause

Creutzfeldt–Jacob disease

Subacute sclerosing panendophthalmitis

Progressive multifocal leukoencephalopathy

Congenital rubella

Reye syndrome

Active viral encephalitis or encephalitis of unknown origin

Active septicemia (bacteremia, fungemia, viremia)

Active bacteria or fungal endophthalmitis

Rabies

Active syphilis

Active leukemia

Active disseminated lymphoma

Hepatitis B surface antigen–positive donors

Hepatitis C–seropositive donors

Receipt of human pituitary-derived growth hormone during the years 1963 to 1985.

HIV-seropositivity of donor

Acquired immunodeficiency syndrome (AIDS)

Children (younger than 13 years) or infant of mother with AIDS or at high risk for HIV infection

High risk for HIV infection

   People with clinical or laboratory evidence of HIV infection

   Men who have had sex with another man one or more times since 1977

   Past or present intravenous drug abusers

People immigrating since 1977 from pattern II countries where heterosexual activity is reported as the predominant means of transmission of HIV (such as Haiti, central Africa)

People with hemophilia who have received clotting factor concentrates

Sexual partners of any of the foregoing

Men or women who have engaged in prostitution since 1977 and people who have been their heterosexual partners within the past 6 months.

HTLV-1 or HTLV-II infection

Intrinsic Eye Disease

Retinoblastoma

Malignant tumors of the anterior ocular segment

Active ocular or intraocular inflammation: conjunctivitis, scleritis, iritis, uveitis, vitritis, choroiditis, retinitis, congenital or acquired disorders of the eye that would preclude a successful outcome for the intended use, such as central donor corneal scar for an intended penetrating keratoplasty, keratoconus, and keratoglobus

Pterygia or other superficial disorders of the conjunctiva or corneal surface involving the central optical area of the corneal button

Prior Intraocular or Anterior Segment Operation

Refractive corneal procedures, such as radial keratotomy, lamellar inserts

Laser photoablation operation

Anterior segment operation such as cataract operation, intraocular lens implant, glaucoma filtration

HIV, human immunodeficiency virus; HTLV, human T-cell lymphotropic virus.

(Reprinted with permission from Eye Bank Association of America. EBAA Medical Standards. Washington, D.C.: EBAA: September 20, 1990, 4–5.)

and morphology of the endothelium. The recent development of the computerized morphometric analysis system accelerates the entire process of specular microscopic evaluation of the endothelium and provides information not available by traditional manual methods of evaluation. The system has the ability to receive direct image input from specular microscopes (Laing, 1993). Surface antigen testing is done for the presence of hepatitis B and human immunodeficiency virus (HIV) antibodies.

Storage and Preservation

The simplest storage method is placing the cornea in a moist chamber at 4°C at the time of enucleation. The tissue must be used within 24 hours (Casey & Mayer, 1984). McCarey–Kaufmann medium allows storage of corneas for 5 to 7 days. Chondroitin sulfate dextran corneal storage medium can keep the cornea viable for at least 2 weeks. Using tissue culture medium at a storage temperature of 31 to 37°C allows preservation for up to 35 days without remarkable loss of endothelial cells and ultrastructural defects (Pels & Schuchard, 1993).

Corneal cryopreservation and cryoconservation theoretically allow the longest period of preservation. However, the technique is quite complicated and must be carefully controlled. The freezing and thawing may cause tissue damage and cell destruction (Kaufman et al, 1987). This method is indicated for prolonged storage of corneas with high cell density and rare human leukocyte antigen (HLA)-matching and as a source for emergency grafts.

Legislation on Procurement of Corneal Tissue

The Medical Examiner Law, first passed in Maryland in 1975 and copied in 15 states, permits a medical examiner or justice of the peace to authorize the removal of corneas, leaving the globe within the socket, while the cause of death is being determined (Maryland Anatomical Gift Act, 1974). This can be done without the consent of next of kin except in cases of known family disapproval (Payne, 1980). Either the medical examiner or the justice of the peace then becomes the legal donor. This allows removal of the cornea in a timely manner when a family member cannot be located. To increase the percentage of actual donors from the pool of potential donors, the Omnibus Budget Reconciliation Act of 1986 (Public Law No. 99–509) implemented the recommendations of the Task Force on Organ Procurement and Transplantation by adding Section 1138 to the Social Security Act (Stevens, 1993). Hospitals maintain their eligibility to participate in Medicare or Medicaid by institutionalizing a required request policy. Written protocols require hospital personnel to make routine inquiries of family members to identify potential organ donors and to notify an organ procurement agency of the potential donor.

COMPLICATIONS

Early Graft Failure

Although advances in microsurgery and eye banking have decreased the incidence of primary or early graft failure to a minimal level, complications may still occur in the immediately postoperative period. Poor quality of donor tissue, surgical trauma, or acute infection can result in decreased endothelial function, corneal edema, and graft failure. Efforts must be made to ensure that the donor material is of surgical quality, and meticulous surgical technique must be used to protect the donor endothelium. Persistent increased intraocular pressure (IOP) can cause irreversible damage in the early postoperative period.

Rejection

Corneal graft rejection remains the primary cause of graft failure (Coster, 1989). The failure rate is documented as being 5 to 10%, but for patients with a history of previous graft rejection or extensive vascularization, the incidence is as high as 50% (Stern, 1988). Many graft rejections can be treated medically with topical corticosteroids when discovered in the early stages of the process (Fig. 10-11). Corneal graft rejection has been described since 1948; physicians report sudden clouding of a previously clear graft (Shapiro et al, 1993). Allograft reaction is a complex immune process. It can be summarized as sensitization of the host immune system to foreign antigens followed by localization of the foreign graft cells. This is followed by destruction of the donor endothelium with subsequent edema and loss of graft clarity (Shapiro et al, 1993). Graft rejection is defined in three descriptive categories in Table 10-2 (Shapiro et al, 1993).

Several host factors seem to increase the risk of graft rejection. The primary factor identified is the presence of corneal vascularization in the recipient. Other important risk factors include a history of prior grafts, bilateral grafts, patient age (with younger recipients being at a higher risk) and the presence of scarring (synechiae)

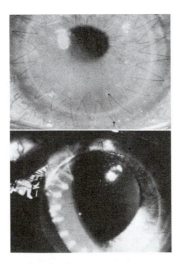

Figure 10–11. (**A**) Endothelial rejection with corneal edema 6 months after keratoplasty. (**B**) Improvement after 4 days of intensive corticosteroid therapy. *(Reprinted with permission from Brightbill FS (1993). Corneal Surgery: Theory, Technique & Tissue. St. Louis: Mosby, 258.)*

TABLE 10–2. GRAFT REJECTION

	Epithelial Rejection	Subepithelial Infiltrates	Endothelial Rejection
Characteristics	Elevated line of rejection visible on fluorescein staining Rejection line starts in periphery and moves toward central graft	White deposits beneath Bowman layer randomly positioned in donor cornea, visible by slit-lamp examination may appear in conjunction with epithelial or endothelial rejection lines	Graft edema Precipitates donor tissue form chain like configurations Endothelial rejection line starts in peripheral area of vascularization and moves centrally Stromal edema and folds in Descemet membrane Lymphocytes found free floating or between endothelial cells
Patient complaint	Asymptomatic	Asymptomatic	Decreased vision, pain, redness
Postoperative onset	Range: 1–13 months Average: 3 months	Range: 6 weeks to 21 months Average: 10 months	Range: 2 weeks to 29 months, longest onset recorded as 35 years Average: 8 months
Patient age	More common in patients younger than 50 years	More common in patients younger than 50 years	Most common in patients younger than 50 years
Treatment	Aggressive topical steroids Close monitoring by physician	Aggressive topical steroids Close monitoring by physicians	Mild reaction Topical steroids every hour while awake Steroid ointment hour of sleep Frequent exams by physician Severe rejection Subconjunctival injection of 12–24 mg dexamethosone Oral prednisone (80 mg) daily or single dose of IV methylprednisone
Consequences	Does not destroy graft or reduce vision but may be present before other forms of rejection	Does not destroy graft or reduce vision but suggests smoldering host reaction May leave subepithelial scars	Graft destruction Decreased vision Corneal edema

or inflammation (Holland & Olsen, 1993). Much effort is being directed at preventing immune corneal graft rejection by four methods. One approach is to reduce the antigenic difference between host and donor through tissue matching. Some investigations are studying ways to decrease host immune response by irradiation of the recipient graft bed with ultraviolet beams. Other investigators are exploring methods of decreasing host response, including suppression of wound healing to prevent revascularization and repopulation of the graft by accessory cells of the recipient. Inflammatory responses are also controlled by topical steroids. The final preventive measure is the use of pharmacologic immunosuppressants to interfere with the immune response. Agents used are corticosteroids, azathioprine and cyclosporine (Coster, 1989).

Elevated Intraocular Pressure

Chronic elevated IOP or glaucoma has been shown to cause endothelial cell loss after PK. The incidence reported ranges from 13 to 89% in aphakic eyes; the overall rate is 33.6% (Newton & Burk, 1993). Postoperative glaucoma can be caused by inflammation, poor suturing technique, and by medications used intra- and postoperatively. The incidence is also higher when the patient has a history of glaucoma and when PK is combined with cataract extraction. Monitoring of the patient postoperatively for moderate to severely elevated IOP is critical. The IOP can be measured accurately with an electronic applanation tonometer, a pneumatic applanation tonometer, or a Tonopen handheld digital electronic device (Newton & Burk, 1993). Once established, the condition can be treated with pharmacologic agents currently used to treat chronic glaucoma. Other forms of treatment can be considered if the patient does not respond to medical therapy. Surgical intervention is often necessary, although risks to the graft exist with any intraocular procedure (Newton & Burk, 1993).

Postkeratoplasty Infection

Postoperative infections have a low incidence and usually occur within 6 months of the operation. Early postoperative infections such as infectious keratitis can result from intraoperative contamination, recurrent host disease such as HSV infection, use of contaminated donor material, or loose, ruptured or exposed sutures that trap debris or errode the epithelial surface (Robinson & Hyndiuk, 1993). Later infections can be associated with contact lens use and with epithelial defects that result from pre-existing conditions such as dry-eye syndromes. The overall prognosis for postoperative graft infections is very grim; many patients require regrafts (Robinson & Hyndiuk, 1993).

Endophthalmitis, an infection that involves the entire eye, can occur in the early or late postoperative period. It can be attributed to use of contaminated donor material, intraoperative contamination, or an infection that originates in the graft and eventually invades the posterior chamber of the eye. Efforts to prevent this devastating complication include postoperative administration of antibiotics, routine cultures of donor material, and research to identify alternative antibiotics to add to donor storage media (Robinson & Hyndiuk, 1993).

IMPLICATIONS FOR OPHTHALMIC NURSING PRACTICE

For many years the goal of nursing care was to keep patients immobile to prevent wound dehiscence and any systemic complications resulting from general anesthesia and immobility. The length of stay for these patients as late as 1985 was 5 to 8 days. Improvement in suturing material and technique has reduced the incidence of complications of wound closure and healing. Most patients have local anesthesia with or without sedation and are out of bed within hours of the completion of the operation. Most patients are admitted on the day of surgery and leave 1 to 2 days postoperatively; some operations are performed on an outpatient basis. Consequently, the goal of nursing care is to monitor patients for acute postoperative complications and to plan for self-care in the home environment.

Alteration in comfort may be expected after any surgical procedure. Patients who have undergone corneal transplants typically describe a sensation of postoperative eye discomfort rather than acute pain. The scientific rationale is that most nerve fibers are located centrally in the corneal epithelium and decrease along the periphery, where a circular incision is made using a trephine to remove the diseased cornea and to prepare the recipient bed. The nurse administers acetaminophen for eye discomfort or pain and evaluates the patient's response. Eye pain not relieved by a mild analgesic may be a symptom of increased IOP.

The risk for increased IOP is present in the early and long-term postoperative periods. This condition is evidenced by eye pain that radiates to the head accompanied by nausea and vomiting. Acetazolamide is usually given orally to prevent or reduce increased IOP. In addition, an ophthalmic beta blocker, betaxolol may be administered. Ophthalmic corticosteroids administered postoperatively twice a day and sometimes at bedtime may induce increased IOP. Corticosteroids reduce inflammation and promote graft acceptance but also delay wound healing. The steroid therapy is maintained for 3 months and is then tapered.

Risk for injury and self-care deficit are related to the sensory-perceptual alteration caused by postoperative patching of the eye. The nurse makes an assessment of the patient's proprioception, ability to adapt to unfamiliar hospital surroundings, and ability to perform activities of daily living (ADL). The nurse orients the patient to the room, maintains a safe environment, and assists the patient in maximizing the performance of ADL. The eye patch is removed on the first or second postoperative visit. Eyeglasses are then worn during the day, and an eye shield is applied at bedtime. Patients must not bend from the waist for prolonged periods. This position may increase IOP and may also cause the patient to lose balance and fall. For 6 to 8 weeks after the operation, patients must avoid situations that expose the eye to blunt trauma, such as contact sports, and environmental contaminants, such as dust and chlorinated water in swimming pools. ADL can be resumed at the patient's comfort level.

The risk for infection exists, but symptoms may not be apparent until after the patient is discharged. The nurse makes an assessment of the patient's health management practices and demonstrates eye care and hygiene to the patient. Instruction should emphasize the importance of not touching or rubbing the eye that was operated on. The patient's ability to perform eye care and to administer medications after discharge should be carefully evaluated by the nurse.

Discharge planning is initiated preoperatively and is continued postoperatively. The nurse identifies the risk for noncompliance with long-term follow-up care. The cause may be knowledge deficit of graft failure and visual rehabilitation, physical or mental handicap, or lack of a support system. Prevention of graft rejection makes the care of the corneal-transplant recipient unique compared with the care of patients who have undergone other intraocular procedures. Because graft failure can occur in the early and late recovery periods, patients are taught to be aware of signs and symptoms of graft failure for their lifetime. The nurse instructs the patient to call the ophthalmologist immediately when any of the following occurs: redness; increased drainage; persistent eye pain with foreign body sensation (indicative of inflammation, infection, wound dehiscence); eye pain compatible with increased IOP; and decreased vision (indicative of corneal edema).

The media has promoted the myth that transplant recipients have 20/20 visual acuity after the eye patch is removed. Despite a technically successful corneal graft, the final visual acuity may be disappointing because of the new optical surface that has formed. The ophthalmologist waits for months to allow adequate wound healing before selectively removing sutures. Suturing technique and timing of selective suture removal affect the degree of corneal distortion and resultant astigmatism. Correction of this refractive error with eyeglasses or a contact lens determines the final visual outcome. It is important that the nurse assess the patient's expectations for visual improvement and educate the patient about visual rehabilitation.

Last, the nurse makes an assessment of the patient's ability to comply with frequent clinic visits for several months (for selective suture removal, tapering of ophthalmic corticosteroids, and evaluation of the graft site and visual acuity) and initiates referrals if indicated (see Nursing Care Plan 10-1, p 314).

INNOVATIONS IN CORNEAL TRANSPLANTATION

Several research projects are underway to advance eye-banking technology. The goal is improving the application and understanding of donor criteria by studying factors that directly affect tissue suitability, (such as age, timing, medical conditions, and enhanced preservation and storage techniques) (TBI, 1988).

A study (Sandoz Cyclosporin Trial) conducted by 13 eye centers tested the safety and efficacy of cyclosporine ophthalmic ointment for corneal transplant patients at high risk, that is, those with a history of a failed graft and those with increased vascularization of the graft site (Gottsch et al, 1993). The results indicated that the use of cyclosporine showed no benefit, and the study was subsequently discontinued.

The excimer laser, approved by the United States Food and Drug Administration for clinical tests, has the ability to excise corneal scar tissue (caused by infection or trauma and certain dystrophies involving the superficial third of the cornea) more accurately than the surgical or diamond knives currently available. Laser excision minimizes the deleterious effects on adjacent corneal cells. This procedure is an alternative to corneal transplantation in selected cases. Excimer laser phototherapeutic keratectomies have been performed on some patients with recurrent host disease and have obviated the need for repeat keratoplasty (Gottsch et al, 1993).

The AIDS/Hepatitis B and Corneal Transplantation Study is a project designed to determine if HIV and hepatitis B virus can be transmitted in corneal transplants. The preliminary findings in this project indicated that only a very low concentration of HIV can exist in corneal tissue. The study also demonstrated that current tests using cadaveric donor blood are effective in screening donors (TBI, 1988).

The Collaborative Corneal Transplant Study (CCTS), conducted by several eye centers researched the effectiveness of histocompatibility matching in high-risk corneal transplantation. The studies, completed in 1992, demonstrated that (1) neither HLA-A or HLA-DR antigen matching substantially reduces the likelihood of corneal graft failure; (2) a positive donor-recipient crossmatch does not dramatically increase the risk of corneal failure; and (3) ABO blood group matching, which can be achieved with relatively little effort and expense, may be effective in reducing the risk of graft failure. The most important conclusion is that high-dose postoperative steroid therapy, good compliance, and close follow-up care are the keys to successful corneal transplantation in recipients at high risk (CCTS Research Group, 1992).

In summary, the incidence of blindness due to corneal disease continues to be prevalent in the United States and to a greater extent in nonindustrialized nations. With increasing public acceptance of tissue donation, advances in ophthalmology, and the growth of eye-banking and its international networking system, corneal transplantation may be the only transplant procedure available to all health care consumers regardless of medical condition and epidemiologic factors such as age, socioeconomic status, and nationality.

REFERENCES

Abbott RL (1993). Aphakic and pseudophakic keratoplasty. In: Brightbill FS, ed. *Corneal Surgery: Theory, Technique and Tissue,* 2nd ed. St Louis: Mosby Year Book, 141–151.

American Academy of Ophthalmology Staff (1985). External disease and cornea. *Ophthalmology Basic and Clinical Science Course,* 7. San Francisco: American Academy of Ophthalmology.

Buxton JN, Buxton DF, Westphalen JA (1993). Indications and contraindications. In: Brightbill FS, ed. *Corneal Surgery: Theory, Technique and Tissue,* 2nd ed. St. Louis: Mosby Year Book, 77.

Casey TA, Mayer DJ (1984). *Corneal Grafting, Principles and Practice.* Philadelphia: Saunders, 49–95.

The Collaborative Corneal Transplantation Studies Research Group (1992). The collaborative corneal transplantation studies (CCTS). *Arch Ophthalmol.* 110: 1392–1403.

Coster DJ (1989). Mechanisms of corneal graft failure: The erosion of corneal privilege. *Eye* 2:251–261.

Danneffel MB (1990). Corneal transplantation. In: Sigardson-Poor KM, Haggerty LM, eds. *Nursing Care of the Transplant Recipient.* Philadelphia: Saunders, 259–279.

Dhanda RP, Kalevar V (1972). Eye banks, sources of donor material and the law. *Int JP Ophthalmol Clin.* 12:71.

Draeger J, Klein L (1987). Microsurgical instruments. In: Draeger J, ed. *Ophthalmic Microsurgery.* Basel: Karger, 61–87.

Ehrlich D, Abel PA Jr (1978). Simplified collection of corneal donor material. *Ann Ophthalmol.* 10:362–364.

Farge E (1989). Eye banking: 1944 to the present. In: Albert D, ed. History of ophthalmology. *Surv Ophthalmol.* 33:260–263.

Feder RS (1993). Recipient diseases. In: Brightbill FS, ed. *Corneal Surgery: Theory, Technique and Tissue,* 2nd ed. St. Louis: Mosby Year Book, 111–113.

Forstot SL (1993). Preoperative evaluation. In: Brightbill FS, ed. *Corneal Surgery: Theory, Technique and Tissue,* 2nd ed. St. Louis: Mosby Year Book 97–100.

Gottsch J, Sulewski M, Stark W (1993). Regrafting. In: Brightbill FS, ed. *Corneal Surgery: Theory, Technique and Tissue,* 2nd ed. St. Louis: Mosby Year Book 317–321.

Griffith FN, Sterner KD (1993). Distribution: The Tissue Banks International system. In: Brightbill FS, ed. *Corneal Surgery: Theory, Technique and Tissue,* 2nd ed. St. Louis: Mosby Year Book, 705–706.

Griffith FN, Valmadrid CT (1993). International supply of corneal surgery. In: Brightbill FS, ed. *Corneal Surgery: Theory, Technique and Tissue,* 2nd ed. St. Louis: Mosby Year Book, 734–743.

Holland E, Olsen T (1993). Immunosuppression in high-risk corneal transplantation. In: Brightbill FS, ed. *Corneal Surgery: Theory, Technique and Tissue,* 2nd ed. St. Louis: Mosby Year Book, 260–264.

Hutz W, Ullerich K (1987). Microsurgical suture material. In: Draeger J, ed. *Ophthalmic Microsurgery.* Basel: Karger, 135–148.

Kaufman H, Winter R, Draeger J (1987). Eye banking in corneal microsurgery. In: Draeger J, ed. *Ophthalmic Microsurgery.* Basel: Karger, 170–180.

Kinoshita S, Manabe R (1993). Chemical burns. In: Brightbill FS, ed. *Corneal Surgery: Theory, Technique and Tissue,* 2nd ed. St. Louis: Mosby Year Book, 309–315.

Laing RA (1993) Secular microscopy of donor corneas. In: Brightbill FS, ed. *Corneal Surgery: Theory, Technique and Tissue,* 2nd ed. St. Louis: Mosby Year Book, 580.

Lanier JD (1993). Herpes simplex leukoma. In: Brightbill FS, ed. *Corneal Surgery: Theory, Technique and Tissue,* 2nd ed. St. Louis, Missouri: Mosby Year Book, 132–136.

Lemp M. (1993). The preocular tear film in corneal grafting. In: Brightbill FS, ed. *Corneal Surgery: Theory, Technique and Tissue,* 2nd ed. St. Louis: Mosby Year Book, 3–7.

Levenson JD, Imperia PS (1993). Viscoelastic materials. In: Brightbill FS, ed. *Corneal Surgery: Theory, Technique and Tissue,* 2nd ed. St. Louis: Mosby Year Book, 212–219.

Lisitza MA (1993). Tissue removal. In: Brightbill FS, ed. *Corneal Surgery: Theory, Technique and Tissue,* 2nd ed. St. Louis: Mosby Year Book, 563–569.

McDermott M (1993). Stromal wound healing. In: Brightbill FS, ed. *Corneal Surgery: Theory, Technique and Tissue,* 2nd ed. St. Louis: Mosby Year Book, 44.

Newton C, Burk L (1993). Glaucoma. In: Brightbill FS, ed. *Corneal Surgery: Theory, Technique and Tissue,* 2nd ed. St. Louis: Mosby Year Book, 247–250.

O'Day M (1989). Diseases potentially transmitted through corneal transplantation. *Ophthalmology.* 96:1133–1136.

O'Day M (1993). Donor selection. In: Brightbill FS, ed. *Corneal Surgery: Theory, Technique and Tissue,* 2nd ed. St. Louis: Mosby Year Book, 549–555.

Paton R (1950). Corneal transplants. *Am J Ophthalmol.* 33:3–5.

Payne J (1980). New directions in eyebanking. *Trans Am Ophthalmol Soc.* 78:983–1022.

Pels L, Schuchard, Y (1993). Organ culture in the Netherlands. In: Brightbill FS, ed. *Corneal Surgery: Theory, Technique and Tissue,* 2nd ed. St. Louis: Mosby Year Book, 622-631.

Rapriano CJ, Cohen E, Brady S, et al (1990). Indications for and outcomes of repeat penetrating keratoplasty. *Am J Ophthalmol.* 109:689-695.

Robinson J, Hyndiuk R (1993). Post keratoplasty infections. In: Brightbill FS, ed. *Corneal Surgery: Theory, Technique and Tissue,* 2nd ed. St. Louis: Mosby Year Book, 270-272.

Shapiro M, Mandel M, Krachmer J (1993). Rejection. In: Brightbill FS, ed. *Corneal Surgery: Theory, Technique and Tissue,* 2nd ed. St. Louis: Mosby Year Book, 254-265.

Stein H, Slatt B, Stein R (1988). *The Ophthalmic Assistant.* St. Louis: Mosby.

Stern GA (1988). Update on the medical management of corneal and external eye diseases, corneal transplantation and keratorefractive surgery. *Ophthalmology.* 95:842-854.

Stevens MJ (1993). Evolution of required request and routine referral laws. In: Brightbill FS, ed. *Corneal Surgery: Theory, Technique and Tissue,* 2nd ed. St. Louis: Mosby Year Book, 688-691.

Stulting RD (1993). Penetrating keratoplasty in children. In: Brightbill FS, ed. *Corneal Surgery: Theory, Technique and Tissue,* 2nd ed. St. Louis: Mosby Year Book, 374-384.

Tanne E (1986). Corneal trephines and cutting blocks. In: Brightbill FS, ed. *Corneal Surgery: Theory, Technique and Tissue.* St. Louis: Mosby, 258.

TBI Eye Research Program (1988). Baltimore: TBI, 1-3.

Thomas C (1955). *The Cornea.* Springfield, Ill: Thomas.

Troutman R, Haight D, Belmont B (1993). Suture materials and techniques. In: Brightbill FS, ed. *Corneal Surgery: Theory, Technique and Tissue,* 2nd ed. St. Louis: Mosby, 199-211.

Vaughan D, Asbury T (1983). *General Ophthalmology.* Los Altos, California: Lange.

NURSING CARE PLAN 10–1. PENETRATING KERATOPLASTY

Nursing Diagnosis	Expected Outcomes	Nursing Interventions
Sensory/Perceptual Alteration (*Visual*) *Related to* • Disease process, operation, and eye covering	• Patient demonstrates ability to perform activities of daily living (ADL) at pre-admission level during hospitalization	• Encourage patient to maximize abilities in performing ADL • Allow patient sufficient time to perform ADL • Provide assistance as needed. • Use verbal interaction and visual aids.

Anxiety *Related to*
 	
• Visual improvement and prognosis
• Surgical procedure
• Quality and source of donor tissue
• Potential for organisms in donor tissue, eg, hepatitis, human immunodeficiency virus (HIV)
• Long-term follow-up care
• graft failure
• Refractive error (astigmatism) even after successful operation
	• Patient verbalizes concerns related to vision, outcome, operation, donor tissue.	• Provide opportunities for patient and family members to share feelings.
		   Correct misinformation.
		   Answer questions.
		   Refer to appropriate resources.
		• Identify patient's support system.

High Risk for Injury *Related to*
 	
• Visual impairment
	• Patient
	   States safety precautions
	   Patient is free from injury.
	   Patient appropriately requests assistance for (ADL) and ambulation during hospitalization.
		• Orient patient to surroundings, equipment and safety measures.
		   Implement safety precautions.
		   Assist patient as needed.
		• Assess patient's self-care, independent functions, home environment, support system.
		• Reinforce importance of safety measures.

High Risk for Infection

Related to

- Postoperative ocular incision

- Eye is free of corneal wound infection and endophthalmitis postoperatively

- Use clean technique when cleansing eyelids and performing dressing changes. Teach the patient this technique, and emphasize the importance of cleansing eyelids only when necessary.
- Teach patient and family members to watch continually for and promptly report signs and symptoms of infection

Altered Health Maintenance

Related to

- Knowledge deficit of eye care
- Resumption of activities
- Medications
- Signs and symptoms of complications
- Long-term follow-up care
- Visual rehabilitation

- Patient and family are able to comply with postdischarge regimen.
- Patient and family use available resources for assistance with home care and transportation to follow-up appointments.

- Explain and demonstrate proper cleansing of the eyelids; emphasize the need for hand washing.
- Consult with the physician for care instructions for complicated wounds.
- Reinforce postoperative activity instructions as indicated
  - Avoidance of strenuous activities such as contact sports, diving, racket sports, and skiing.
  - Avoidance of dusty environments, swimming and other situations that increase the risk of eye contamination until the epithelium is completely healed.

(continued)

NURSING CARE PLAN 10–1. PENETRATING KERATOPLASTY *(continued)*

Nursing Diagnosis	Expected Outcomes	Nursing Interventions
Altered Health Maintenance (continued)		Resumption of activities such as hair washing, reading, and driving as soon as comfort and vision permit.
		Avoidance of bending over at the waist for several months after the operation.
		Avoidance of touching, rubbing, or scratching the eye operated on.
		• Review the purpose, action, dosage, and possible side effects of prescribed medications, which may include corticosteroids or antibiotics.
		• Review proper administration of eye drops. For a client with poor vision, review ways of distinguishing eye drop containers, eg, by size, shape, or color.
		• Explain the purpose and use of an eye patch and shield. Reinforce wearing them until the first postoperative follow-up visit and wearing eye protection such as glasses for at least 2 weeks after the operation.
		• Teach patient to watch for and promptly report signs and symptoms of complications

Redness and swelling

Pain

Altered vision

Increased tearing and drainage

- Validate understanding of the physician's explanations of long-term follow-up care

  Schedule of postoperative visits

  First operative day

  1 postoperatively

  3–4 weeks postoperatively

  4–6 weeks postoperatively

  8–12 weeks postoperatively

  6, 9, and 12 months postoperatively then every 6 months until all sutures are removed. Sequential suture removal is done for as long as 2 years.

- Explain routine procedures during follow-up visit.

  Review signs and symptoms of graft failure with patient; review current medications, dosage, frequency of use, any difficulties with eye drop administration or side effects of medication.

  Assess visual acuity, distance and near vision.

  Evaluate level of astigmatism.

(continued)

NURSING CARE PLAN 10–1. PENETRATING KERATOPLASTY

Nursing Diagnosis	Expected Outcomes	Nursing Interventions
Altered Health Maintenance (continued)		Measure corneal thickness.
		Perform slit-lamp examination of donor graft, sutures, signs of edema, inflammation or vascularization.
		Apply fluorescein to epithelium when indicated to highlight epithelial defects.
		Measure intraocular fluid pressure.
		Perform retinal examination.
		Review new treatment plans, medication changes, schedule for subsequent visits.
		• Explain and discuss visual rehabilitation process
		Corrective refraction for astigmatism begins about 2 months after the operation.
		Prescription for glasses or hard contact lenses is provided as soon as the refraction seems to be stabilizing, which may take as long as 6 months.
		Astigmatic keratotomy, a refractive operation to reduce astigmatism, has been performed in some cases.

11

Transplantation of the Small Intestine

Mimi Funovits,
Sandra M. Staschak-Chicko,
Judith A. Kovalak,
Kathy A. Altieri

The clinical care of a recipient of a small-intestinal transplant is one of the most difficult and complex nursing challenges. Human intestinal transplantation began in the United States in the early 1960s with poor results. Few developments occurred over the following two decades to warrant enthusiasm for continued trials. The rather late development of this field has been the result of several problems that only recently have been resolved. These include a determination of which segment of the gastrointestinal (GI) tract can be transplanted, the development of immunotherapy sufficiently powerful to prevent intestinal allograft rejection, and the development of methods that can be used to monitor graft function and detect allograft rejection before immunologic destruction of the graft or death of the patient. The resolution of these problems has developed gradually over the last several years. Major advances in immunosuppressant therapy, coupled with improvements in surgical technique, have reintroduced transplantation of the small intestine to clinical practice with increasing frequency and success. It is clear from our experience at the University of Pittsburgh Medical Center (UPMC), that patients with short-bowel syndrome can benefit from intestinal transplantation as evidenced by discontinuation of intravenous nutritional support and enjoyment of unrestricted oral diets. This chapter describes how the UPMC Transplant Institute approaches the series of related, but unique, clinical problems of recipients of small-intestinal transplants.

319

Essentially any part of the intestine can be transplanted, but a minimum of 70 cm of intestine is required for the recipient to be able to maintain adequate nutrition using the allograft as the sole source of absorption (Deltz et al, 1989). The distal small intestine, because of its adaptive potential and selective absorptive function (bile acids and vitamin B_{12}), is preferred over the proximal intestine but has been utilized less often because of its greater content of intestinal lymphoid tissue. With the development of immunosuppressive agents having the T-cell inhibitory activity of oral FK-506 (Prograf) and, to a lesser degree, intravenous cyclosporine, transplantation of the small intestine, including the distal small intestine with its large intrinsic lymphoid tissue is possible without the development of irreversible allograft rejection or graft-versus-host disease (GVHD).

The methods used to monitor graft function vary widely from center to center. The absorption of elements such as iron, simple sugars such as D-xylose, and complex disaccharides such as maltose and lipophilic vitamins have all been used to monitor graft function. None seems to be more valuable than the other. Typically several such substrates are used at a single center to monitor graft function.

The use of flexible fiberoptic endoscopy with directed multiple mucosal biopsies has revolutionized the clinical management of small-intestinal allografts. It makes possible the detection of intestinal graft rejection before a clinical crisis occurs and enables specific treatment to be instituted at the first evidence of rejection.

TREATMENT OPTIONS FOR SHORT-BOWEL SYNDROME

Historically, patients with intestinal failure treated with surgical resection of all or most of their small intestine were permanently dependent on total parenteral nutrition (TPN) for their existence. TPN dependency, limited venous access, multiple episodes of sepsis, and TPN-induced cholestatic liver disease resulting in liver failure are complications that initiated consideration of small-intestinal transplantation.

Transplantation of the small intestine at the UPMC is now considered a treatment modality for short-bowel syndrome. It enables patients to discontinue intravenous nutritional support and enjoy an unrestricted oral diet. Isolated small-intestinal transplantation is used when liver function is normal and in the absence of cirrhosis. If liver failure or cirrhosis is present, our approach entails combined liver and small-intestinal transplantation. We perform a multivisceral organ transplant when thrombosis of the celiac axis is present or severe dysmotility of the stomach to the large intestine is documented in disorders such as intestinal pseudoobstruction. A multivisceral graft may include stomach, duodenum, pancreas, liver, small intestine, and large intestine.

INDICATIONS FOR SMALL-INTESTINAL TRANSPLANTATION

The primary indication for small-intestinal transplantation is short-bowel syndrome or incorrectable intestinal disease (Todo et al, 1993). Causes of short-bowel syndrome may be classified as either structural or vascular in nature. Disorders that primarily affect adults include Crohn disease, Gardner syndrome, radiation enteritis, superior mesenteric artery or vein thrombosis, and trauma to the intestinal vasculature. Intestinal atresia, gastroschisis, volvulus, necrotizing enterocolitis (NEC), microvillous atrophy, and pseudoobstruction are causes most frequently diagnosed in the pediatric population (Edes, 1990; Grosfeld et al, 1986; Lennard-Jones, 1990; Wood, 1990). The definition, causation, and clinical presentations of the aforementioned disorders are summarized in Table 11–1.

RECIPIENT EVALUATION AND SELECTION PROCESS

Patients being considered for a small-intestinal transplant must meet certain basic criteria before undergoing the evaluation process. Absolute need for permanent intravenous nutritional support, age, and general medical condition are factors to be considered. Ideally, patients who are 50 years of age or younger who do not exhibit other major underlying medical illnesses are considered suitable candidates. Table 11–2 outlines the current exclusion criteria for small-intestinal transplantation. Local or systemic infection (sepsis) is a relative contraindication, as it is with all organ transplants.

The pretransplant evaluation process consists of tests and procedures designed to assess the patient's suitability for small-intestinal transplantation. Testing may vary for each patient depending on the patient's original diagnosis and current medical conditions; therefore, each patient must undergo an initial evaluation by the transplant team. Additional testing, if necessary, can be performed by the patient's local physician or at the transplant center. The main goal of the evaluation process is to determine the technical feasibility of the surgical procedure and to identify any associated risk factors that may alter the nature and course of the operation or subsequent postoperative care. Such evaluation includes thorough nutritional and biochemical assessment, endoscopic and radiologic studies, metabolic assessment, and neuro-psychiatric and social service assessments. Table 11–3 outlines the guidelines for preoperative evaluation of intestinal-transplant recipients.

Patient selection for a small-intestinal transplant is determined by the transplant team, pending satisfactory review of the results of the evaluation (Funovits et al, 1993). Once selected, patients are placed on the active waiting list for an intestinal graft according to the criteria established by the United Network for Organ Sharing (UNOS), the federal agency responsible for national allocation of donor organs and tissues.

PREOPERATIVE PREPARATION

Potential donors are identified by the organ procurement agency and are referred to the transplant team for consideration. Acceptable donors of small intestine should meet the following criteria: ABO compatibility; body size equal to or 25% smaller than

TABLE 11–1. CAUSES OF SHORT-BOWEL SYNDROME

Cause	Definition	Etiologic Theories	Clinical Presentations
Structural			
Intestinal atresia	Complete obliteration of the intestinal lumen due to occlusion or total absence of segment	Vascular insufficiency during intrauterine life, failure of recanalization of duodenum during 12th week of intrauterine life, or autosomal recessive trait	Colicky abdominal pain; bilious vomiting; abdominal distention; constipation in neonatal period
Gastroschisis	Failure of the anterior abdominal wall to fuse in the midline between 2 and 4 weeks of embryonic development, resulting in anterior abdominal wall hernia. The extruded intestine is never covered by a membrane.	Unclear. Occurs 1 in 50,000 births.	Apparent at birth. Prematurity in 50% of cases. Operation required. Short-bowel syndrome results when excessive amount of intestine is resected.
Necrotizing enterocolitis	Diffuse area of patchy necrosis of mucosa of small or large intestine	Conditions associated with prematurity; may be manifestation of either hypoxia or infection or poor perfusion of intestinal tissue during the prenatal period	Sudden onset of abdominal distention; vomiting; bloody diarrhea. Radiography reveals small-intestinal distention, sometimes with a feathery appearance indicative of mucosal ulceration
Microvillus atrophy	Severely abnormal exposed surface epithelium with the appearance of short and depleted microvilli by light microscopy.	Abnormality of cytoskeleton myosin causing accumulation of secretory granules and involution of microvilli. Diagnosis made by biopsy. Congenital.	Intractable diarrhea, which may lead to severe dehydration. Presents early in life.
Pseudoobstruction	Rare clinical condition in which impaired intestinal propulsion causes recurrent symptoms of obstruction in the absence of mechanical obstruction. May involve either segments of or the entire gastrointestinal tract and may involve the urinary bladder. Categorized into either neuropathic or myopathic forms.	Autosomal recessive inheritance, although spontaneous mutations and prenatal or postnatal acquired disease cannot be excluded.	Abdominal distention; constipation; bilious and nonbilious vomiting; failure to gain weight; vomiting; diarrhea; failure to void; urinary tract infections. Symptoms may be present at birth or begin during infancy or later in life.

TABLE 11–1. CAUSES OF SHORT-BOWEL SYNDROME (*continued*)

Cause	Definition	Etiologic Theories	Clinical Presentations
Crohn Disease	Indolent chronic inflammation capable of involving entire alimentary tract from mouth to anus. Inflammation extends through all layers of intestinal wall and involves the adjacent mesentery and lymph nodes.	Unknown	Nausea; vomiting; fever; abdominal pain; intestinal obstruction; systemic manifestations including arthritis, arthralgia, liver disease, pruritis and skin lesions.
Gardner syndrome familial polyposis, desmoid tumor	Multiple adenamatous polyps that can be flat (sessile) or on a stalk (pedunculate) that arise from the mucosal surface anywhere in the small intestine or colon	Autosomal dominant disease in which approximately 20% of people affected do not have a family history.	Gastrointestinal bleeding; diarrhea; abdominal pain; epidermoid cysts on face, back, upper and lower extremities; dental abnormalities (unerupted or supemomery teeth). Onset of symptoms occurs 10 years after development of polyps.
Radiation enteritis	Radiation-induced intestinal-cell injury.	Inhibition of DNA synthesis of intestinal tissue cells (epithelial, vascular, and connective tissue components)	Colicky abdominal pain; nausea; vomiting; intestinal obstruction; fistulas involving intestine, pelvic, and abdominal organs; malabsorption. Occurs in patients with a history of intraabdominal, often pelvic, malignant tumors.
Vascular			
Superior mesenteric artery or vein thrombosis	Thrombolytic occlusion of blood supply to intestine.	Inborn; coagulation deficiency in the liver	Abdominal cramping; vomiting; profuse sweating; decreased bowel sounds; stupor; weakness; fatigue
Trauma to intestinal vasculature (superior mesenteric artery, superior mesenteric vein)	Interruption of blood supply to intestine. Obstruction of blood supply leads to gangrene and peritonitis.	Abdominal trauma (operation, gunshot wound, blunt abdominal injury)	Abdominal pain; abdominal distention; vomiting. Intestinal resection required.
Midgut volvulus	Disordered movement of the intestine around the superior mesenteric artery during course of embryologic development.	Unknown	Abdominal pain; abdominal distention; vomiting; obstruction of blood supply, which if complete leads to extensive gangrene and peritonitis. Operation required. Presents early in life.

TABLE 11–2. EXCLUSION CRITERIA FOR SMALL-INTESTINAL TRANSPLANTATION

No need for permanent intravenous nutritional support
Incurable malignant tumor
Severe cardiopulmonary insufficiency
Extensive atherosclerosis
Active drug addiction
Advanced neurologic dysfunction

the recipient (to facilitate surgical feasibility), absence of infection; absence of manifestations of atherosclerosis (from which anastomotic complications may arise); and normal liver function and injury studies, especially when a combined liver–small intestine or a multivisceral graft is necessary.

Donor preparation requires decontamination of the intestine and is carried out to eliminate microorganisms present in the intestinal tract before transplantation. Currently, intestinal decontamination is accomplished by administering 2 to 3 L of GoLytely through a nasogastric tube along with a combination of polymixin B (colistin), gentamycin, and nystatin. Systemic broad-spectrum antibiotics are administered intravenously for prophylaxis.

Recipient preparation is begun immediately upon notification that there is a suitable donor. Results of preoperative testing (ie, electrocardiogram [ECG], chest radiography, and blood tests) are obtained, and intestinal decontamination is administered according to the same formula as for the donor. Systemic broad-spectrum antibiotic therapy is also initiated.

The surgical recovery of the intestinal graft includes an en bloc segment from stomach to large intestine. The intestinal graft is flushed with cold University of Wisconsin (UW) solution for preservation during transport. One liter of UW solution is used for both aortic and portal infusion (Starzl et al, 1992; Todo et al, 1992). Selective infusion of the isolated small intestine has not yet been attempted. Currently, the longest cold preservation time is 13 hours.

OPERATIVE PROCEDURE

The surgical procedure starts with a midline incision that extends from the xiphoid process to the symphysis pubis. A midtransverse incision on one or both sides is usually performed when indicated. After the abdominal exposure, the diseased intestine is usually resected up to the third or fourth part of the duodenum and down to the ileocecal valve or previous ileocolic anastomosis. For vascular reconstruction of the intestinal graft, the superior mesenteric vein (SMV) is usually dissected up to its confluence with the splenic vein. If dissection of the SMV is not feasible, dissection of the recipient portal vein by mobilization of the second portion of the duodenum is usually performed for reconstruction of the venous outflow of the intestinal graft. After removal of the native intestine and proper hemostasis, the intestinal graft is brought

TABLE 11–3. PREOPERATIVE EVALUATION GUIDELINES FOR INTESTINAL-TRANSPLANT RECIPIENTS

Nutritional Assessment

To provide baseline information of the patient's pre-transplant nutritional status
    Complete dietary history
    Total parenteral nutrition (TPN) requirements
    Measurement of serum vitamins, minerals, trace elements
    Anthropometric measurements, skinfold thickness

Biochemical Assessment

To assess the function of the parenchymal organs and to detect the presence of underlying medical
    problems in patients with complicated medical histories
Basic Laboratory Tests
    Complete blood count with differential and platelet count
    Electrolytes, BUN, creatinine levels
    Glucose, calcium, magnesium, phosphorus, zinc, and uric acid levels
    Alkaline phosphatase, ALT, AST, GGTP, bilirubin (direct, indirect and total) levels
    Prothrombin time, partial thromboplastin time, protein C and S levels, and anti-thrombin III level
    Total protein, albumin, cholesterol, and triglyceride levels
    Serum B_{12}, folate, iron, and ferritin levels
    24-hour urine collection for creatinine clearance and protein excretion measures
Blood typing, HLA typing, quick PRA measurement
Virologic Testing
    Hepatitis, HIV, cytomegalovirus, Epstein–Barr virus, varicella-zoster virus, and toxoplasmosis

Endoscopic Assessment

To assess for the presence of esophageal or gastric varices
    Upper endoscopy

Radiologic Assessment

To assess the hepatic and mesenteric vascular systems
    Abdominal Doppler ultrasonography
    Abdominal computed tomography
    Angiography (performed as needed in cases of extensive thrombosis of the visceral vessels)
    Doppler ultrasonography of upper extremities performed as needed when occlusion of the sub-
        clavian veins is considered likely because of prolonged central line placement

Metabolic Assessment

To determine the type and severity of intestinal malabsorption
    D-xylose tolerance test
    Nitrogen excretion studies
    Fecal fat analysis

Neuropsychiatric and Social Services Assessment

To assess for patient compliance and emotional ability to undergo transplantation and to determine
    patient–family dynamics and support systems
    Interview with patient and family members by psychiatric nurse liaison and social worker
    Neurologic evaluation as indicated

BUN, blood urea nitrogen; ALT (SGPT), alanine aminotransferase; AST (SGOT), aspartate aminotransferase; GGTP, serum gamma-glutamyl transpeptidase; HLA, human leukocyte antigen; PRA, percent reactive antibody; HIV, human immunodeficiency virus; UGI, upper gastrointestinal series.

(Adapted with permission from Funovits M, Altieri KA, Kovalak, JA, Staschak-Chicko S (1993). Crit Care Nurs Clin North Am 5:203–213.)

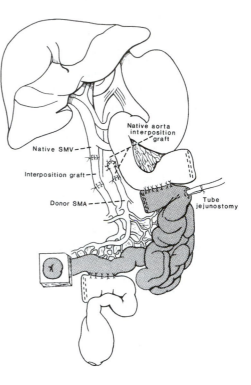

Figure 11–1. Surgical anastomoses of intestinal allograft. SMV, superior mesenteric vein; SMA, superior mesenteric artery. *(Adapted with permission from Funovits M, Altieri KA, Kovalak JA, Staschak-Chicko S (1994).* Crit Care Nurs Clin North Am, *5:203–213.*

to the operative field and the superior mesenteric artery (SMA) of the graft is usually anastomosed to the infrarenal aorta of the recipient. The SMV of the graft is usually anastomosed either to the SMV of the recipient (end-to-end) or to the side of the portal vein. Arterial or venous grafts are usually used as a vascular conduit if needed. After reperfusion of the intestinal graft by unclamping the SMA followed by the SMV, attention is usually paid to reestablishment of GI continuity. The first step is to anastomose the proximal jejunum of the graft to the proximal end of the remaining native intestine (duodenum or jejunum). The remaining part of the distal recipient intestine (colon or ileum), if present, is usually anastomosed to the side of the ileum 20 to 30 cm proximal to its end. The terminal end of the ileum is exteriorized through the abdominal wall as a temporary ileostomy for early graft decompression and monitoring of the intestinal graft. A proximal jejunostomy tube is placed for early decompression of the proximal intestine and for tube feeding in the early postoperative period. In our last six patients, recovery of the right colon (cecum, ascending colon, and part of the transverse colon) was performed to preserve the graft ileocecal valve. The rationale for this maneuver is to minimize the occurrence of diarrhea and bacterial colonization of the small intestine in these patients. The complexity of the recipient operation depends primarily on the number of previous operations and the nature of the intestinal disease. An average operative time is 8 hours.

NURSING DIAGNOSIS AND POSTOPERATIVE MANAGEMENT

Nursing care of an intestinal-transplant recipient should be aimed at astute observation, thorough assessment, timely intervention, and perceptive evaluation of the patient's response to the transplant process. Complications tend to occur suddenly, and rejection may mimic septic episodes, which require the clinician to remain vigilant for subtle changes in the patient. Care of these patients requires knowledge of the transplant process and a comprehensive understanding of the nursing management guidelines outlined in Nursing Care Plans 11-1, 11-2, and 11-3, see pp 322-335).

Acute Phase: The Intensive Care Unit

Critical to nursing assessment is recognition of potential postoperative complications and a thorough understanding of patient responses to nursing and medical interventions. The following discussion of nursing care focuses on prevention and treatment of the postoperative complications that commonly occur during the acute postoperative recovery phase.

   After the operation, the recipient is admitted directly to a transplant intensive care unit (ICU). At the UPMC, medical care is directed by the members of the intestinal transplant team in conjunction with the critical care medical staff. Nursing care is provided by staff specifically trained in the acute care of patients undergoing intestinal transplantation (Funovits et al, 1993).

High Risk for Alteration in Oxygenation.   The goals of nursing management of the respiratory system are to maintain adequate oxygenation and accurately measure for signs of hypoxemia and hypoventilation during weaning from mechanical ventilation (Staschak & Zamberlan, 1990). An endotracheal tube attached to a ventilator provides respiratory support and airway protection. Prolonged anesthesia, in conjunction with a debilitated physical status, necessitates short-term ventilatory support. Endotracheal tube cuff pressure is monitored every 2 hours to prevent aspiration and tracheal ischemia. Arterial blood gas (ABG) values are monitored on admission to the ICU and every 4 to 6 hours to maintain adequate oxygen levels. Pulse oximetry is used to identify decremental changes in oxygen saturation.

   Nursing management facilitates adequate oxygen delivery to the patient. Baseline respiratory status is assessed, chest radiographs are interpreted, and ABG values are determined. The continued consequences of operative hypothermia may include metabolic alkalosis, decreased anesthetic metabolism, and altered oxygen consumption. The nurse carefully evaluates the need for analgesics. Careful attention should be given to an aggressive pulmonary toilet regimen. Endotracheal suctioning should be performed every 2 hours and as needed. The lungs should be hyperoxygenated before endotracheal suctioning. The patient should be repositioned every 2 hours, and aggressive chest physical therapy is given to loosen and mobilize secretions. Persistent hypoventilation may be caused by incisional pain. Patients who are severely malnourished and debilitated may have generalized muscle weakness, necessitating prolonged mechanical ventilation. After extubation, patients are carefully monitored, and if difficulties are encountered with oxygenation or ventilation, prompt reintubation or a tracheostomy may be required (Staschak & Zamberlan, 1990).

High Risk for Alterations in Cardiovascular Status. The goals of nursing management of the cardiovascular system are to maintain adequate cardiac functioning and tissue perfusion while monitoring for complications. The most important cause of cardiovascular instability in the acute postoperative phase is hypovolemia. Intensive hemodynamic monitoring and assessment should be the focus of nursing management. Monitoring should include measurement of heart rate and rhythm, filling pressures of the right and left sides of the heart, cardiac output, and systemic and pulmonary vascular resistance. This allows for the necessary titration of fluids and vasoactive drugs.

Hypotension may occur as a result of hypovolemia. Hypovolemia occurs secondary to a massive shift of intravascular fluid to the interstitial spaces (third-space loss). The factors that contribute to this fluid shift are the abdominal surgical procedure, the physiologic stress of the operation, massive fluid resuscitation in the perioperative period, and hypoalbuminemia. In addition, hypothermia (core body temperature, 33 to 34°C) precipitates a pronounced hypovolemic state as the patient warms. Renal dose dopamine 2 µg/kg per minute may be used to optimize cardiac output and perfusion of vital organs.

Nursing management should be directed at strict monitoring for signs of decreased cardiac output, cardiac arrhythmias, and fluid loss. Adequate tissue perfusion is determined by assessment of urinary output, skin temperature, capillary refill (particularly in the extremities), and serum lactate levels.

High Risk for Loss of the Transplanted Organ Secondary to Ischemia and Technical Complications. The goals of nursing management are to recognize, report, and monitor for signs and symptoms of ischemic damage and technical complications. Initial graft dysfunction may result from ischemic injury to the organ during recovery. The severity of this phenomenon ranges from mild to severe. The problem can be identified endoscopically or histologically by mucosal ulcerations or a sloughing of the entire intestinal mucosa. Although the patient does not exhibit any specific clinical manifestations with mild ischemia, more severe ischemic injury may cause bleeding of the intestinal mucosa and an increase in watery, bloody stoma output and may precipitate a translocation episode. (An episode when bacteria normally colonizing the intestine become invasive and the patient's condition becomes septic with positive blood cultures.)

Vascular and anastomotic complications are uncommon. Vascular complications include stenosis or thrombosis of the arterial or venous vasculature. When vascular occlusion occurs, early surgical intervention may salvage the graft. Surgical intervention would include segmental resection for a partial blockage and retransplantation for patients with a total blockage. A pale-appearing intestinal stoma may indicate a vascular complication.

An intestinal anastomotic leak is another potential post-operative complication that may occur during the first postoperative week. The nurse should observe for abdominal distention with tenderness, an increased white blood cell (WBC) count, and fever. Surgical intervention is necessary to correct this complication, but risk for the development of a leak is minimized by decompression of the intestine with the proximal jejunostomy and distal ileostomy.

High Risk for Fluid and Electrolyte Imbalances Related to Operative Factors.

The goal of nursing management is to retain homeostatic fluid and electrolyte balance (Staschak & Zamberlan, 1990). When the patient arrives in the transplant ICU, the nurse should assess for fluid volume deficit or overload resulting from the surgical procedure. Fluid and electrolyte imbalance occurs secondary to large volume losses and intraoperative volume replacement. Nursing management includes strict hourly intake and output measurements. Patients usually arrive in the transplant ICU with a pulmonary artery catheter, two No. 8 Fr introducers used for rapid volume infusion, radial and femoral arterial lines, a nasogastric tube, an ileostomy, a jejunostomy, two to three Jackson–Pratt drains, and a Foley catheter.

The nurse must be aware of the continued risk for fluid volume deficit and electrolyte imbalances related to enteric losses and inadequate volume replacement; therefore, strict measurement (or quantification) of these losses is imperative. Enteric output through the ileostomy, nasogastric tube, jejunostomy tube, and rectum should be measured carefully. The expected ileostomy output in the first 24 to 48 hours should be 200 to 300 mL/24 hours of serosanguineous drainage, which should increase to 1 to 2 L/24 hours. Rectal losses can be measured in a rectal bag for patients with an ileosigmoid anastomosis (Funovits et al, 1993).

Altered Immune System—Risk for Organ Rejection and Infection During Graft Adaptation.

The nursing goal is monitoring the patient for potential signs of rejection and to administer appropriate therapy (Staschak & Zamberlan, 1990). Although rejection can occur at any time, the risk for rejection is greatest during the first 30 postoperative days and gradually declines during the third postoperative month. The isolated intestinal graft appears to be more vulnerable to rejection than the liver in patients with a combined liver and small-intestinal graft (Abu-Elmagd et al, 1993). The intestine is thought to induce graft rejection more vigorously than other organs, because it has abundant lymphoreticular cells in the Peyer's patches, lamina propria, and mesenteric lymph nodes (Todo et al, 1993).

Physical examination of a patient with intestinal rejection may reveal abdominal distention, diffuse abdominal pain, infrequent or absent bowel sounds, and an edematous, pale, or dusky stomal mucosa. A high stomal output accompanied by sluggish or absent intestinal motility also is an early clinical sign of graft dysfunction. Initially, ileostomy output begins slowly. The usual amount of enteric losses expected after the first postoperative day is 1 L/24 hours. A total of 2 to 3 L/24 hours can be expected after the second or third post-operative day. A sudden increase in enteric output (>3 L/24 hours) can signal an early rejection episode (Funovits et al, 1993). Table 11–4 details clinical signs of intestinal graft rejection and treatment.

Care of recipients is often difficult because severe rejection may have a fulminant presentation that closely mimics septic shock. This condition must be rapidly diag-

TABLE 11–4. CLINICAL SIGNS OF INTESTINAL GRAFT REJECTION AND TREATMENT

Rejection	Clinical Findings	Endoscopic Findings	Treatment
Acute			
Mild to Moderate	Fever Abdominal pain Vomiting Increase in stomal output Watery diarrhea	Ischemic, dusky mucosa Mucosal edema Hyperemia Loss of fine mucosal pattern Decrease of peristalsis	Increase of FK-506 dose Bolus of steroids Steroid recycle
Severe	Severe diarrhea Abdominal pain Abdominal distention Metabolic acidosis Positive blood culture Adult respiratory distress syndrome	Ulceration Mucosal sloughing Bleeding Loss of peristalsis	Increase of FK-506 dose Recycle of steroids Muromonab-CD3
Chronic			
	Chronic diarrhea Malabsorption Progressive weight loss	Pseudomembrane Hypoperistalsis Loss of mucosal fold Oily intestinal contents	Retransplantation

(Adapted with permission from Todo S, Tzakis AG, Abu-Elmagd K (1992). Intestinal transplantation in composite visceral grafts or alone: Monitoring of intestinal graft rejection and treatment. Ann Surg. 216:227.

nosed because rejection requires augmented immunosuppression, whereas septic shock (bacteremia) requires antibiotics and a reduction in immunosuppression. Intestinal biopsies are the principal method of diagnosing rejection in this setting.

Immunosuppressive therapy is initiated perioperatively and consists of FK-506 and steroids. The current success of intestinal transplantation can be attributed, in part, to the use of FK-506 (Hoffman et al, 1990; Lee et al, 1990). Ongoing clinical pharmacokinetic studies at the UPMC suggest that FK-506, unlike cyclosporine, is absorbed by the intestinal graft during the critical early postoperative phase of graft adaptation, reducing the incidence of rejection episodes.

FK-506. FK-506, a recently FDA approved immunosuppressive agent, is produced by the Fujisawa Pharmaceutical Company of Osaka, Japan (Staschak-Chicko et al, 1992). Multicenter prospective randomized trials in the United States, Europe, and Japan are evaluating the drug in comparison with cyclosporine as primary therapy for preventing transplant rejection. FK-506 has been used at the UPMC as the primary antirejection therapy in all intestinal-transplant recipients. It has clinical efficacy in the prevention and reversal of organ transplant rejection. FK-506 is well absorbed from the transplanted small intestine; the dosing regimen is similar to that used in liver transplant patients (Jain et al, 1992).

Although FK-506 is considerably more potent than cyclosporine, both drugs selectively inhibit T-lymphocyte activation and proliferation. FK-506 is a macrolide lactone antibiotic, similar in structure to erythromycin. It is isolated from the fermentation broth of *Streptomyces tsukibaensis,* a soil fungus found in Northern Japan (Kino et al, 1987; Thompson, 1990). In addition to prevention and reversal of organ rejection, the apparent benefits of FK-506 include minimization or elimination of steroids (particularly beneficial in children); the absence of bone marrow suppression, gingival hyperplasia and hirsutism; and a reduced incidence of antihypertensive therapy (Staschak-Chicko et al, 1992).

The principal side effects of FK-506 include nephrotoxicity, neurotoxicity, and diabetogenicity, similar to those of cyclosporine. The greatest risk of nephrotoxicity occurs in the early postoperative period, when high blood levels may result after intravenous administration. This complication may be overcome by continuous infusion of FK-506, as opposed to bolus injection. Serious neurotoxicity has been seen only in liver graft recipients with poor graft function and the highest perioperative plasma trough drug levels. Downward dose adjustment, guided by careful drug monitoring, must be considered if there is liver dysfunction. Moderate diabetogenic effects, comparable to those reported for conventional immunosuppressive regimens, have been ascribed to FK-506, both in animals and transplant patients.

Posttransplant lymphoproliferative disorders (PTLD) are complications of continuous immunosuppressive therapy and have been reported in recipients of small-intestinal transplants given FK-506 in combination with other immunosuppressants (Todo et al, 1993). The incidence of PTLD among all transplant patients receiving FK-506 at the UPMC has been reported to be 0.7%, which compares favorably with that among the general transplant population (Staschak et al, 1992).

Administration of FK-506 is initiated perioperatively. It is given intravenously, 0.1 to 0.15 mg/kg per day through either a central or a peripheral line. When enteral feedings are initiated 1 to 2 weeks postoperatively, oral FK-506 (capsules) 0.3 mg/kg per day is given in two divided doses. The dose adjustment of FK-506 is based on the quality of renal function, evidence of graft rejection, quality of graft function, and daily trough plasma levels of FK-506 (Funovits et al, 1993).

Nursing considerations for patients receiving FK-506 include monitoring for side effects, establishing a regular dosing regimen, and patient education and support during experimental therapy. The nurse must assess and safely monitor the patient to minimize nephrotoxicity and give appropriate support. Nurses must assess for side effects throughout continuous intravenous infusion. The greatest risk of side effects is during the early postoperative period, when high blood levels may occur. The first intravenous doses of FK-506 usually cause headaches, nausea, vomiting, anorexia, and burning or tingling of the lips, tongue, hands, and feet; however, these side effects are virtually eliminated once oral dosing is established. The most frequent side effects of intravenous administration, nausea and vomiting, are treated with antiemetics. Hyperkalemia due to low aldosterone and renin levels has been observed, and treatment with a potassium-restricted diet or fludrocortisone acetate (0.1 mg two times a day) can be instituted. Oral FK-506 is well tolerated, causing only transient nausea or vomiting and insomnia. At present, correlations between symptoms and plasma levels are poorly understood; however, a novel "artificial intelligence dosing system" is being used to help predict drug regimens.

At the UPMC, an accurate and simple computerized dosing algorithm for FK-506 and prednisone has been developed by the Pittsburgh Transplantation Institute informatics and clinical staff. The algorithm applied at the bedside or outpatient clinic facilitates standardization of patient management. A simple automated drug-dosing program includes minimizing the learning curve for the physician prescribing the drug, particularly for drugs with large pharmacokinetic variability and a narrow therapeutic index. It should also improve patient care by reducing toxicity and decreasing the length of hospital stay experienced by patients, both of which should result in a cost-to-benefit advantage (McMichael et al, 1991).

Steroids. Intravenous steroid therapy is initiated perioperatively with a 1-g bolus and is tapered in decrements of 40 mg (steroid recycle) over the first 5 days (200, 160, 120, 80, 40, and 20 mg). Maintenance steroid therapy consists of an oral dose of prednisone 20 mg daily. Complete steroid withdrawal may be attempted, but the time frame is highly variable. Low-dose azathioprine may be added to the immunosuppressive regimen in the presence of subtherapeutic levels of FK-506, evidence of renal toxicity, or persistent or recurrent episodes of rejection or if a strong positive crossmatch is identified (Funovits et al, 1993).

Intestinal-transplant recipients are at greatest risk for infectious complications during the first 3 months after transplantation. In the acute phase, the factors that predispose a patient to infectious complications are implantation of a "dirty" organ; surgical complications; bacteremia from multiple invasive lines, catheters, and drains; respiratory infections related to ventilatory support; incisions; and bacterial translocation in an immunocompromised patient.

To prevent bacterial overgrowth of the intestinal mucosa, patients undergo intestinal decontamination for 4 weeks postoperatively. Decontamination includes a combination of polymixin B (colistin), gentamicin, and nystatin, either orally or by nasogastric tube. If sepsis, persistent rejection, or the detection of pathogenic organisms in high concentration ($>10^9$) occurs after the initial period of decontamination, the same antibiotic mixture is resumed (Reyes et al, 1992). Weekly quantitative stool cultures are evaluated to detect the presence of pathogens. Nursing management goals are directed at identification of risk factors, daily assessment for clinical signs of infection, and adherence to strict aseptic technique.

Alteration in Kidney Function Related to Acute Renal Failure and Antibiotic or FK-506 Nephrotoxicities. Nursing management is directed at monitoring hourly urinary output and serum creatinine levels. Intraoperative and postoperative risk factors that contribute to renal insufficiency include intraoperative events such as hemorrhage and hypotension, postoperative hypovolemia, translocation, and nephrotoxic agents. One or several of these contributing factors may cause acute tubular necrosis. For most patients, this is a short-term problem, and resolution is observed within 3 to 4 weeks. During this time hemodialysis or hemoperfusion may be required. In addition to monitoring of renal function, careful assessment of serum drug levels of antibiotics and immunosuppressants is required. Acute tubular necrosis is more likely to resolve if the immunosuppressant dose is reduced and if nephrotoxic antibiotic drugs are eliminated or given in renal doses (Marsh et al, 1988).

Altered Nutrition: Less Than Body Requirements Related to Graft Adaptation and Preexisting Malnutrition.   Nursing management should be directed at providing adequate nutritional intake and promoting wound healing. Malnutrition in an intestinal-transplant patient can lead to weight loss, muscle wasting, negative nitrogen balance, impaired wound healing, and decreased resistance to infection. Additional postoperative factors that may increase the patient's nutritional needs are fever, infection, bacterial translocation, secondary surgical procedures, and mechanical ventilation.

TPN is required for at least 4 weeks after transplantation, during which time the graft begins to adapt but is still unable to absorb the necessary nutrients and calories to maintain adequate health and healing. Enteral feedings, through the jejunostomy tube, are usually initiated 1 to 2 weeks after transplantation as GI motility begins to recover. A dietary consultation should be obtained when the patient arrives in the ICU. Nurses should work closely with the dietician and clinical pharmacist to ensure delivery of adequate calories, monitor serum electrolytes, and obtain daily weights.

Intermediate Phase: The Surgical Unit

After stabilization in the ICU, the recipient is transferred to a transplant surgical unit. The potential for development of serious complications continues to remain high during this postoperative period and may necessitate more than one ICU stay. This section focuses on pertinent nursing diagnoses that relate to the postoperative recovery phase. Nursing care of intestinal-transplant recipients centers on detection of complications and collaboration with the transplant team for intervention.

Risk for Fluid Volume Deficit and Electrolyte Imbalances Related to Abnormal Fluid Losses.   The goals of nursing management are to maintain adequate fluid and electrolyte intake and balance. The risk for excessive fluid volume loss continues during the intermediate postoperative phase. Intestinal graft adaptation is a slow process, and ostomy output remains high (1.5 to 2 L/24 hours) during this period. Although individual enteric output is variable, abrupt changes from baseline may be important and should be reported. In addition, development of fever or infection, with an increase in metabolic rate, can place the patient at risk for the development of hypovolemia. Patients usually arrive in the surgical unit with a nasogastric tube, a triple-lumen central venous catheter, an ileostomy, a jejunostomy tube, and Jackson–Pratt drains. Nursing management includes strict and accurate measurement of enteric losses through the ileostomy, nasogastric tube, jejunostomy tube, and rectum. Additional losses through the abdominal Jackson–Pratt drains and dressings should be carefully measured. Observation of decreased urinary output, decreased central venous pressure (CVP) and blood pressure, and increased hemoglobin level and hematocrit can signal a hypovolemic episode and the need for additional hydration.

TPN continues for at least 4 weeks after the operation. In addition to TPN, patients may require fluids such as lactated Ringer or 0.9% normal saline solution (if hyperkalemic), to help maintain their homeostatic fluid balance. Even after discharge, high stomal output and resulting hypovolemic episodes may result in frequent readmissions to the hospital for rehydration.

Frequent metabolic and electrolyte imbalances can occur during this phase of the patient's recovery. The most important causative factor is continued high ostomy output. Hyponatremia, hypokalemia, and metabolic acidosis may occur secondary to hypovolemia. Serum sodium and potassium levels are monitored regularly, and supplements are given when indicated to minimize life-threatening complications. Hypomagnesemia is a frequent problem. Although many patients are hypomagnesemic from malnutrition before transplantation, this condition continues postoperatively and may be related to immunosuppressive therapy. Neuromuscular irritability and insomnia are frequent clinical manifestations of hypomagnesemia. Magnesium oxide or magnesium sulfate (in cases of hypophosphatemia or alkalosis) are titrated to assure optimal therapeutic levels. Magnesium should be administered at least 3 hours before or after the FK-506 dose to prevent FK-506 malabsorption (Steeves et al, 1991). Daily biochemical monitoring of all electrolytes is required for 2 to 4 weeks postoperatively, then two to three times a week until discharge from the hospital. Supplementation of electrolytes is administered by either the intravenous, oral, or jejunostomy route.

Risk for Impaired Skin Integrity Related to Chemical Destruction. The goals of nursing management are to assess the patient for risks of chemical tissue destruction, to monitor for epidermal erosion, and to participate in a treatment plan to promote tissue healing.

Poorly fitting ostomy appliances, uncontrolled fecal incontinence, and drainage from the jejunostomy tube site are contributing factors that place the patient at risk for damage to the epidermal and dermal tissue. A high ostomy output, particularly during a rejection episode, is an important concern and can cause peristomal excoriation. Correct measurement of the stoma is important to ensure proper fit of the pouch. Skin breakdown or infection is evidenced by redness, rash, itching, warmth, swelling, pain, and drainage. Frequent changes of the ostomy bag, the use of commercial products for skin preparation, and an ostomy nurse specialist consultation early in the postoperative course help prevent skin problems and assist in the management of any skin irritation and breakdown.

Altered Immune System: Risk for Organ Rejection During Graft Adaptation. The goals of nursing management are to monitor for potential signs of rejection and to administer appropriate therapy. There are no recognized specific biochemical measurements of intestinal graft rejection. Recovery of graft function or rejection is monitored by clinical, radiologic, endoscopic, histologic, and nutritional assessments. Physical examination of a patient with intestinal rejection may reveal abdominal distention, diffuse abdominal pain, infrequent or absent bowel sounds, and an edematous or dusky stomal mucosa. A high stomal output (>3 liters/24 hours) accompanied by sluggish or even absent intestinal motility also is an early clinical sign of graft dysfunction. Complete recovery of graft function generally occurs 4 to 6 weeks after transplantation with considerable reduction in stomal output and marked improvement of abdominal signs (Todo et al, 1992). The nurse must remain alert for the development of any clinical changes in the patient. An immediate intestinal biopsy is performed if there is evidence of rejection. Early detection of rejection is crucial to graft survival.

Gastric emptying time and intestinal transit time are the two radiologic markers used to assess graft function. Ideally, patients should exhibit a gastric emptying time of 30 minutes to 1 hour and a transit time of 2 to 4 hours. Endoscopic assessment is performed through the stoma until the stoma is reversed approximately 1 year after the transplant. Ileoscopy with biopsy is performed once a week during the early postoperative period to observe for signs of rejection. Because rejection may occur in only one segment of the transplanted intestine, biopsies are intermittently performed by upper endoscopy or colonoscopy. A graft that is dysfunctional, because of either preservation injury or a rejection episode, may show an edematous, flat mucosa, multiple ulcerative areas, and even complete sloughing of the intestinal mucosa (Todo et al, 1992; Abu-Elmagd et al, 1993).

Histologic monitoring of the intestinal allograft is performed with each endoscopic assessment. An immediate mucosal biopsy is performed when there is evidence of rejection to make an early diagnosis and initiate therapy. Biopsies are performed twice a week for 4 weeks, once a week for 2 months, then once a month for 6 months.

Nutritional assessment of a recipient of an intestine should include parenteral nutrition requirements, changes in weight, and absorption abilities of the allograft. Daily weights, accurate and complete daily caloric counts, and intake and output records should be carefully maintained. Anthropometric measurements, including skin-fold and midarm circumference are useful in determining the absorption function of the graft. Table 11-5 details nutritional considerations for the assessment of intestinal graft function. A sudden increase in enteric output (>3 liters/24 hours) may signal early graft rejection and should be reported immediately. Treatment of a rejection episode may consist of a steroid bolus or recycle, changing or increasing the immunosuppressive drugs, or the administration of monoclonal antibody.

Altered Nutrition: Less Than Body Requirements. Postoperatively, adaptation of the intestinal graft is a slow process, and the patient remains at risk for weight loss and inadequate caloric intake. Nutritional deficiencies generally occur secondary to poor absorptive ability of the graft and inadequate parenteral, enteral, or oral intake. In conjunction with the nutritional team, nurses provide daily nutritional assessment and management and facilitate optimal nutritional health. The nutritional care of this patient population is guided by calometric monitoring, nitrogen balance, metabolic status, and serial anthropometric measurements.

TPN is mandatory for at least 4 weeks after transplantation. Reinstitution of TPN is usually recommended during moderate to severe rejection episodes or when there is clinical and metabolic evidence of malabsorption (Abu-Elmagd et al, 1992). Enteral feedings, through the jejunostomy tube, are usually initiated 1 to 2 weeks after the operation when GI motility recovers. An elemental, peptide-based diet is used starting at half strength at a rate of 10 to 25 mL/hour. The strength and rate of infusion are grad-

TABLE 11–5. NUTRITIONAL ASSESSMENT OF INTESTINAL GRAFT FUNCTION

Test	Rationale
D-xylose tolerance test	Evaluate carbohydrate absorption
Lactose tolerance test	
Sustacal (high-calorie nutritionally complete food) challenge test	
Schilling I test	Evaluate vitamin absorption
Serum vitamins A, D, E	
Serum triglyceride level	Measure essential fatty acids
Triene: tetraene ratio	
Skin-fold thickness	Measure body fat and muscle mass
Anthropometric measurements	
Serum zinc and magnesium	Determine intestinal absorptive
Iron studies	ability of allograft
72-hour fecal fat analysis	
Serum transferrin	Evaluate protein absorption
Serum albumin	
Serum total protein	
Daily weight	Evaluate daily caloric requirements
Daily calorie counts (total parenteral nutrition, tube feeding, and oral diet)	

(Adapted with permission from Funovits M, Altieri KA, Kovalak JA, Staschak-Chicko S (1993). Crit Care Clin North Am. *5:203–213.)*

ually increased as intestinal graft function and motility recover. The patient is gradually weaned from TPN during this period of graft adaptation.

Carbohydrate absorption recovers early in the postoperative period, followed by amino and fatty acid absorption. Fat malabsorption is most probably related to the lymphatic interruption at the time of transplantation. For this reason, administration of intravenous fat emulsion is generally recommended during the early postoperative period. High enteric output may be present even in the absence of a rejection episode. This phenomenon may be related to a hypersecretory phase, fat malabsorption, rapid transit time, or a gut hormonal imbalance. Rapid intestinal transit time is common soon after intestinal transplantation and is characteristic of adaptation of the graft. Medications to reduce transit times may be required by some patients (Reyes et al, 1993). Nursing Care Plan 11-4 (see p 357) details dietary and medication strategies that may help reduce and thicken enteric output, decrease intestinal transit time, and promote adequate nutritional intake.

The nurse, as part of a dietary support team, plays an integral role in nutritional support of these patients. The team should include a dietician, a clinical transplant coordinator, a staff nurse, and a pharmacist who meet formally with the patient. A formal dietary support program can assist patients in relearning and enjoying the art of eating.

Some adult patients, and almost all pediatric recipients, have demonstrated a reluctance to eat postoperatively. The cause of this phenomenon probably lies with the unpleasant experience patients had in association with food preoperatively or lack of experience with eating (Tzakis et al, 1992). At Children's Hospital of Pittsburgh, a dietician, clinical nurse specialist, and occupational therapist meet formally with pediatric patients on a weekly basis. These sessions include sharing a finger-food meal. It is hoped that by sharing a positive eating experience, the children will learn by imitation. If pediatric patients refuse to eat, tube feeding of modified Compleat B (high-fiber content) is given (Funovits et al, 1993).

Risk for Infection. Infection is the most important cause of morbidity and mortality among intestinal-transplant patients. General factors that predispose a patient to infection are the long-term use of TPN and the potential for associated sepsis; the abdominal operation itself; a debilitated preoperative state, a prolonged ICU stay; long-term immunosuppressive therapy; GI and vascular complications; and the potential for bacterial translocation from the transplanted intestine. Knowledge of risk factors associated with infection and adherence to infection control standards are of paramount importance in preventing infection in this patient population.

Assessment of intestinal-transplant patients for signs of infection is, unfortunately, difficult. As with any immunosuppressed patient, the signs may be subtle or masked altogether. Vital signs should be monitored every 4 hours. If the patient's temperature exceeds 38.5°C, specimens should be collected for panculture. Prednisone can mask an early fever; therefore, other signs of sepsis, such as tachycardia must be assessed (Staschak & Zamberlan, 1990). The development of opportunistic infections in immunocompromised patients is an important concern. Strict hand-washing before and after patient contact is imperative.

A patient who receives TPN is at high risk for recurrent bacteremia due to central-line sepsis. Contaminated enteral formulas can be responsible for gastroenteritis and sepsis. They are a superb microbiologic culture medium and are easily contaminated (Anderson et al, 1984). Adherence to strict aseptic techniques helps prevent transmission of infection.

Bacterial translocation may occur postoperatively. This phenomenon is caused by migration of pathogens from the transplanted intestinal lumen into the recipient's bloodstream. The predisposing factors are bacterial overgrowth inside the intestinal lumen, complete or segmental sloughing of the intestinal mucosa due to either preservation injury, or severe rejection (Abu-Elmagd et al, 1992). A high fever with chills and signs and symptoms of septic shock are frequent clinical manifestations. If there is evidence of rejection, cultures of more than 10^9 organisms accompanied by fever are particularly important because bacteria may translocate from the intestinal lumen through the damaged mucosa to the blood. Quantitative stool cultures are obtained weekly during the early postoperative period, and surveillance cultures are monitored on a routine basis. Patients usually undergo prophylactic intestinal decontamination for both gram-negative and gram-positive bacteria. Colistin, gentamycin, and nystatin are administered either orally or by nasogastric tube for 4 weeks postoperatively. They are restarted if sepsis, persistent rejection, or detection of pathogenic organisms in high concentration (>10⁹) occurs (Reyes et al, 1992). Systemic antibiotic therapy and augmentation of immunosuppression is initiated immediately if there is clinical evidence and histologic documentation of concomitant rejection (Funovits et al, 1993).

Herpes simplex virus (HSV), varicella-zoster virus (VZV), and Epstein-Barr virus (EBV) infections are common in the recipients of intestinal transplants. Cytomegalovirus (CMV) infection, however, is of greatest concern. Patients who are CMV seronegative before the transplant who receive a CMV seropositive organ are particularly at risk for CMV enteritis (Todo et al, 1993). Clinical manifestations of allograft CMV infection may include fever, nausea with vomiting, increased watery stomal output, anorexia with weight loss, fatigue, and malaise. To date, intravenous dihydroxy propoxymethyl quanine (ganciclovir) is the most effective drug to treat CMV. Transplantation of a CMV-positive intestinal graft to a CMV-negative recipient should be avoided. Currently, a prophylactic course (4 to 6 weeks) of ganciclovir is administered to all patients postoperatively. Administration of a 1- to 3-month course of ganciclovir is initiated whenever inclusion bodies are identified histologically or whenever the patient is serologically buffy-coat-positive and has symptoms. Oral acyclovir is administered for at least 6 months to all patients in an attempt to prevent viral infections.

Prophylactic therapy for the prevention of *Pneumocystis carinii* pneumonia is with trimethoprim–sulfamethoxozole. Oral candidiasis can be prevented by the use of an oral antifungal agent such as nystatin. Identification of risk factors, daily assessment for clinical signs of infection, adherence to strict aseptic technique, and meticulous hand-washing reduce the probability of infection in recipients of intestinal transplants.

Altered Comfort Related to Pain. Many recipients of intestinal grafts require maintenance narcotics for pain control when evaluated for transplantation. Chronic illness and previous multiple surgical procedures can lead to difficult narcotic withdrawal. Postoperative pain management frequently becomes a difficult problem for the patient, family members, and transplant team. Alterations in sleep patterns and corresponding thought processes, behavioral changes, and continued narcotic addiction are frequently observed in the posttransplant period. These patients may require larger doses of pain medication over a longer duration of time than most surgical patients. In addition, larger doses of narcotics may be needed postoperatively because of poor drug absorption secondary to GI malabsorption.

Nursing interventions should be aimed at identification of measures that are effective in pain management. Patient-controlled analgesia (PCA) and intermittent narcotic injections are used during the initial postoperative phase. Reduction and elimination of narcotics should be attempted when clinically indicated. A pain control consultation and, in some cases, a psychiatric consultation may be helpful in providing optimal support for the patient, family, and staff for patients who may experience narcotic withdrawal. Collaboration with the patient regarding noninvasive pain-relief methods may be helpful. Relaxation techniques, diversional therapy, and emotional support and reassurance may help to reduce the intensity of pain.

Follow-Up Phase and Discharge

Once the intestinal graft is adequately functioning and the patient is able to tolerate an oral diet, preparation for discharge is initiated, although teaching has been underway since the preoperative evaluation phase. The success of intestinal transplantation depends on the effectiveness of patient education. The ability of patients to understand their medications, independently continue record-keeping, and identify signs and symptoms of complications that require professional assistance affect the success of the follow-up phase. A systematic educational program is created for each patient on the basis of his or her individual learning needs. Patient education is provided by a clinical transplant coordinator, staff nurse, ostomy clinician, dietician, pharmacist, social worker, and psychiatric nurse liaison. A transplant booklet and formal postoperative classes are provided for the patient and family.

Once discharged from the hospital, patients are required to remain in the vicinity of the transplant center. Laboratory evaluation and clinic visits are required twice a week during the initial outpatient phase. The clinic visit is also a good time for reinforcement of patient education. Clinic visits are gradually decreased in frequency, and patients are discharged to home when their overall condition is deemed stable. Patients are once again cared for by their original providers with guidance from the transplant center.

Impaired Adjustment Related to Health Status Change. Patients may feel discouraged by their physical and emotional responses to the transplant process. For some, the need for continued short-term supportive nutritional therapy adds to their frustration. Postoperatively, both patients and their families may have high expectations. This transitional time can be fraught with stress and conflict between the expectations and the realities of recovery. A common cause of fear and anxiety is organ rejection. Patients may fear that their diet or activity level will precipitate a rejection episode. Recipients who live out-of-town also worry about their ability to return to the transplant center in time for treatment. Expert teaching and counseling are required to assist the patient and family in coping and adjusting to lifestyle changes associated with the transplant experience.

Alterations in Family Processes Related to an Ill Family Member. The psychosocial demands on patients and families who undergo intestinal transplantation are tremendous. Disruption of family routines, disturbances in body image, fear of rejection, financial concerns, and emotional changes among all family members are some of the stress factors that may aggravate the delicate psychologic balance of both the patient and family. Most of the psychiatric and psychosocial problems unique to small-intestinal transplantation are a function of the chronicity and severity of the patient's original disease, the extensive nature of the operation, and the protracted postoperative course with frequent setbacks and discomfort (Stenn et al, 1992).

After discharge, the patient and family may become more acutely aware of financial issues. Because of the evolving technologic nature of intestinal transplantation, Medicare and private insurance companies are reviewing reimbursement on a case-by-case basis. Fund-raising efforts and the uncertainty of financial approval can leave the patient and family physically, emotionally, and financially drained.

Knowledge of community and spiritual services should be made available to the family so that they may seek appropriate external resources when needed. While the patient and family are in the vicinity of the transplant center, a weekly transplant support group is one way to aid the patient and family in verbalizing their feelings and fears during this difficult adjustment period. At home, local chapters of national transplant support groups can provide long-term education and support.

Risk for Impaired Home Maintenance Management Related to Lack of Knowledge of Transplantation. Patient education is a primary nursing responsibility during all phases of the transplant process. Although it is ongoing, initiated at the pretransplant phase and continued throughout hospitalization and follow-up care, it is perhaps never more important than when the patient is ready for discharge from the hospital. Patient education should be multidisciplinary in nature. The nurse should assess the patient for learning needs, which may require the assistance of various consultation services. The patient and family must learn a great deal about intestinal transplantation and how it will affect their lives. This section presents information essential for the patient to learn before discharge.

Medications. Patient survival depends on compliance with the prescribed medication regimen. Formal medication teaching begins when the patient is able to participate, proceeds to independent administration at the time of discharge, and continues throughout the follow-up phase. The recipient must be instructed about the purpose, dosage, routes of administration, precautionary measures, and side effects of all medications. Continued function of the new intestine depends on strict adherence to prescribed immunosuppressive therapy. Therefore, it is imperative that the patient understands the life-threatening consequences of lack of compliance with the prescribed medication regimen.

Ostomy Care. Patients are discharged home with an ileostomy. Reversal of the ostomy does not occur until approximately 1 year after the transplant. Depending on the cause of short-bowel syndrome, some patients have not had an ileostomy before the transplant and may be anxious and fearful about how it will affect their lifestyle. The most commonly expressed fear is that of being offensive to themselves and others. Basic explanations of the anatomic structure and function of the GI tract, stoma pouching techniques, and the importance of taking prescribed bulking and antidiarrheal agents will help provide the patient with the necessary confidence to resolve the emotional issues related to having an ostomy. An ostomy clinician is instrumental in providing knowledge that will both decrease the patient's fear and facilitate ostomy self-care.

Jejunostomy Tube Care. A jejunostomy tube may be left in place if the patient requires short-term supportive nutritional therapy at the time of discharge from the hospital. Feedings of Peptamen nutritional supplement are generally administered over 8 to 10 hours at night, and the tube remains capped during the day. This intermittent schedule allows for consumption of small frequent meals while providing optimal nutritional intake for those who remain deficient in their oral diet during graft adaptation. The patient should be able to effectively demonstrate before discharge all procedures for self-administration of tube feedings. Recipients are instructed to notify the transplant team immediately if signs and symptoms of exit-site infection, such as redness, warmth, and drainage, develop. They are also instructed to report any intolerance to feedings, as evidenced by nausea and vomiting. Finally, the patient should be reassured that the feedings are short-term therapy. The jejunostomy tube is removed once adequate oral nutritional intake is achieved and maintained.

Infection. All patients must demonstrate before discharge knowledge of risk factors associated with risk for infection. The nurse must emphasize the seriousness of any infection because of the immunocompromised state. Evidence of infection in a recipient of an intestinal transplant is especially crucial and must be evaluated immediately. A stool bacterial count of more than 10^9 organisms may trigger a translocation episode. The patient must be taught to report immediately the development of fever, a sudden increase in ostomy or rectal output, or malodorous stool. These signs and symptoms may indicate the need for intestinal decontamination and systemic antibiotic therapy. Teaching should also include information about fever, exposure to communicable diseases, vaccinations, and contact with people who have episodic illnesses (Staschak-Zamberlan, 1990).

Rejection. Almost all patients experience one or more rejection episodes after intestinal transplantation. Although the chances of rejection diminish with time, it can occur at any time. Some patients may remain free of symptoms during mild cases of acute rejection, clinical signs and symptoms of rejection being seen only when intestinal rejection has progressed. Therefore, intestinal mucosal biopsy remains the standard for the definitive diagnosis of intestinal rejection. Once the stoma is closed, the intestinal mucosa is assessed by endoscopy or colonoscopy or both. Reversal of the ileostomy is not feasible in patients with active Crohn disease, a weak or diseased anal sphincter, no anal or rectal sphincter because it has been removed, or a previous abdominoperineal colonic resection. Routine surveillance biopsies are performed at 6-month intervals. The patient is reminded of the rationale for frequent ileoscopy with biopsy during the early follow-up phase and of the importance of long-term surveillance biopsies.

Follow-up Medical Care. Although laboratory evaluation assists in monitoring the overall health status of the patient, regular and timely outpatient visits provide an in-depth evaluation of the patient's progress. Adherence to follow-up laboratory evaluation and outpatient appointments should be stressed. Long-term steroid therapy requires routine eye examinations for the detection of cataracts and glaucoma. Women are encouraged to have annual pelvic examinations and Papanicolaou smears to detect any immunosuppressant-related tumor as well as any routine gynecologic problems. Patients should maintain good oral hygiene and receive regular dental care. Prophylactic antibiotics are advised before any dental procedure.

Graft-Versus-Host Disease. In addition to the list of complications unique to the intestinal-transplant population, a recipient may be at risk for development of graft-versus-host disease (GVHD). This complication may occur in an immuno-suppressed patient when donor T cells react against recipient tissue antigens (Burakoff et al, 1990). This phenomenon is most common after bone marrow trans-plantation; however, recipients of intestine also are at high risk because of the abun-dant amount of lymphoid tissue in the intestine, particularly in the ileum. It has been documented in patients who received either an isolated intestinal transplant or a liver-intestine transplant that migration of donor lymphocytes from the intestinal graft occurred during the first 5 to 6 weeks after transplantation, being totally replaced by recipient lymphocytes. Donor lymphocytes were detected circulating in the peripheral venous system of the recipient up to 60 days after intestinal trans-plantation (Iwaki et al, 1991). The fate of the donor lymphocytes is still not clearly understood. However, the assumption is that these cells settle in the recipient tis-sues as dormant cells and may reactivate with suboptimal immunosuppressant therapy (Todo et al, 1992). Pretreatment of the graft with irradiation, antilymphoid globulins, and muromonab-CD3 were previously used to sterilize the donor graft be-fore transplantation, but these measures did not successfully prevent GVHD (Starzl et al, 1991). No such pretreatment modalities have been used at our center (Funovits et al, 1993).

Gastrointestinal Dysmotility. Motility dysfunction of the patient's native GI tract and allograft occur in more than 50% of recipients of intestinal transplants. Disorders such as reflux esophagitis, pyloric spasm, and gastric hypomotility are frequently doc-umented early in the postoperative period. These disorders are temporary, and al-though recovery seems to be a slow process, these problems are completely resolved within 12 weeks after transplantation.

Diarrhea. Another possible postoperative complication is chronic diarrhea. The underlying cause is still unclear; however, the diarrhea may be attributed to a hypersecretory phase, fat malabsorption, rapid transit time, or a gut hormonal im-balance (Funovits et al, 1993). Intestinal denervation, ischemic damage, interrup-tion of lymphatics, and rejection also could be factors of cumulative impact (Todo, 1994). Successful management can be achieved by identifying the underlying cause for each patient. Medications such as camphorated tincture of opium (pare-goric), subcutaneous octreotide, or pectin can be effective in controlling diarrhea in most patients. A low-fat diet also may be helpful, especially in patients with fat malabsorption.

FUTURE CONCEPTS

Transplantation of the small intestine for short-bowel syndrome offers a new treat-ment option for patients who suffer from this catastrophic disease. Advances in immunosuppressive therapy combined with evolving surgical techniques indicate that intestinal transplantation has come of age.

Pioneering efforts in research laboratories has brought small-intestinal transplantation to its present status. Multidisciplinary teams of clinicians and scientists continue to join together to contribute their expertise in advancing this treatment. Advances resulting from tedious laboratory work are quickly realized for their clinical applicability. Laboratory trials for new and exotic drug combinations that will enhance patient survival, prevent rejection, and minimize side effects are underway. The hope for continued success lies in the development of these more specific and less toxic agents.

To increase the number of intestinal transplants, a more effective method for donor identification and procurement is needed. Cooperation among procurement and transplant centers is vital to help identify both donors and recipients. This can best be achieved by medical and public awareness through education.

Improvements in preservation techniques has lengthened cold ischemia time to beyond 12 hours. As techniques continue to improve, preparation and storage of the donor organ will extend beyond our current capabilities. Since the inception of our intestinal transplant program in May 1990, our patient survival rate has increased dramatically and is currently 86%. Additional advances in postoperative management, which includes identification of rejection and hemodynamic management, will extend graft survival and patient lives.

Multivisceral transplantation offers options for patients with celiac axis thrombosis who are not considered candidates for conventional liver transplantation. The current trend in small-intestinal transplantation is to include the ileocecal valve and at least the ascending colon in the graft in an attempt to decrease severe diarrhea and high stomal output and increase intestinal absorption. Enhanced intestinal absorption will prevent one of the most common complications of small-intestinal transplantation—dehydration.

SUMMARY

With the objectives more clearly defined—improved organ preservation techniques, effective immunosuppressive agents, and refined surgical techniques—tremendous strides have been made in small-intestinal transplantation since the 1960s. The crucial support and contributions of nursing staff, along with a dedicated multidisciplinary team approach, are essential to the successful outcome of small-intestinal transplantation.

ACKNOWLEDGMENTS

We would like to acknowledge the following individuals for their contribution in the preparation of this chapter: Kareem Abu-Elmagd, MD, Oscar Bronsther, MD, Saturu Todo, MD, Thomas E. Starzl, MD, PhD, David Van Thiel, MD, and Marianne Davis.

REFERENCES

Abu-Elmagd K, Fung J, Reyes J, et al (1992). Management of intestinal transplantation in humans. *Transplant Proc* 24:1243-1244.

Abu-Elmagd KM, Tzakis A, Todo S, et al (1993). Monitoring and treatment of intestinal allograft rejection in humans. *Transplant Proc* 25:1202-1203.

Anderson KR, Norris DJ, Godfrey MS (1984). Bacterial contamination of tube-feeding formulas. *JPEN* 8:673-678.

Burakoff SJ, Deeg HJ, Ferrara J, Atkinson K (1990). *Graft-vs-Host Disease: Immunology, Pathophysiology, and Treatment.* New York: Dekker.

Deltz E, Schroeder P, Gebhardt H, et al (1989). Successful clinical small bowel transplantation: Report of a case. *Clin Transplant* 3:89-91.

Edes T (1990). Clinical management of short bowel syndrome. *Postgrad Med.* 88:91-95.

Funovits M, Altieri KA, Kovalak JA, Staschak-Chiko S (1993). Small intestinal transplantation: A nursing perspective. *Crit Care Nurs Clin North Am* 5:203-213.

Grosfeld V, Rescorla F, West K (1986). Short bowel syndrome in infancy and childhood. *Am J Surg.* 151:4-46.

Hoffman AL, Makowka L, Banner B, et al (1990). The use of FK-506 for small intestine allotransplantation: Inhibition of acute rejection and prevention of fatal graft-versus-host disease. *Transplantation.* 49:483-490.

Iwaki Y, Starzl TE, Yagihashi A, et al (1991). Replacement of donor lymphoid tissue in human small bowel transplants under FK-506 immunosuppression. *Lancet.* 337:818-819.

Jain A, Venkataramanan R, Todo S, et al (1992). Intravenous, oral pharmacokinetics, and oral dosing of FK-506 in small bowel transplant patients. *Transplant Proc.* 24:1181-1182.

Kino T, Hatanaka H, Miyata S, et al (1987). FK-506: A novel immunosuppressant isolated from a streptomyces II immunosuppressive effect of FK-506 in vitro. *J Antibiot.* 40:1256-1265.

Lee KKW, Stangl MJ, Todo S, et al (1990). Successful orthotopic small bowel transplantation with short-term FK-506 immunosuppressive therapy. *Transplant Proc.* 22:78-79.

Lennard-Jones JE (1990). Indications and need for long-term parenteral nutrition: Implications for intestinal transplantation. *Transplant Proc.* 22:2427-2429.

Marsh JW, Gordon RD, Stieber A, et al (1988). Critical care of the liver transplant patient. In: Shomaker W, et al, eds. *The Society of Critical Care Medicine,* 2nd ed. Philadelphia: Saunders, 1329-1333.

McMichael J, Irish W, McCauley J, et al (1991). Evaluation of a novel "intelligent" dosing system for optimizing FK-506 therapy. *Transplant Proc.* 23:2780-2782.

Reyes J, Abu-Elmagd K, Tzakis A, et al (1992). Infectious complications after human small bowel transplantation. *Transplant Proc.* 24:1249-1250.

Reyes J, Tzakis AG, Todo S, et al (1993). Nutritional management of intestinal transplant recipients. *Transplant Proc.* 25:1200-1201.

Starzl TE, Todo S, Tzakis A, et al (1991). The many faces of multivisceral transplantation. *Surg Gynecol Obstet.* 172: 335-344.

Staschak S, Zamberlan K (1990). Liver transplantation: Nursing diagnosis and management. In: Sigardson-Poor KA, Haggerty LM, eds. *Nursing Care of the Transplant Recipient.* Philadelphia: Saunders, 140-179.

Staschak-Chicko S, Zamberlan K, Thomson AW (1992). An overview of FK-506 in transplantation and autoimmune disease. *Dial Transplant.* 21:500-531.

Steeves M, Abdallah R, Venkataramanan GJ, et al (1991). In-vitro interaction of a novel immunosuppressant, FK-506, and antacids. *J Pharm Pharmacol.* 43:574-577.

Stenn PG, Lammens P, Houle L, Grant D (1992). Psychiatric psychosocial and ethical aspects of small bowel transplantation. *Transplant Proc.* 24:1251-1252.

Thompson AW (1990). Profile of an important new immunosuppressant. *Transplant Rev.* 4:1-13.

Todo S, Tzakis A, Abu-Elmagd K, et al (1993). Clinical intestinal transplantation. *Transplant Proc.* 25:2195-2197.

Todo S, Tzakis A, Abu-Elmagd K, et al (1992). Intestinal transplantation in composite visceral grafts or alone. *Ann Surg.* 216:223-234.

Todo S, Tzakis A, Reyes J, et al (1994). *Transplantation.* Small intestinal transplantation in humans with or without colon. *Transplant Proc.* 57:840-848.

Todo S, Tzakis A, Reyes J, et al (1993). Intestinal transplantation in humans under FK-506. *Transplant Proc.* 25:1198-1199.

Tzakis A, Todo S, Reyes J, et al (1992). Clinical intestinal transplantation: Focus on complications. *Transplant Proc.* 24:1238-1240.

Wood R (1990). International symposium on small bowel transplantation. *Transplant Proc.* 22:2423-2426.

NURSING CARE PLAN 11–1. SMALL-INTESTINAL TRANSPLANTATION: ACUTE PHASE—THE INTENSIVE CARE UNIT

Nursing Diagnosis	Expected Outcomes	Nursing Interventions
Impaired Gas Exchange	• The patient maintains adequate oxygenation.	• Monitor for signs and symptoms of hypoxemia
Related to	• The patient is adequately monitored for hypoxemia and hypoventilation during weaning from mechanical ventilation.	• Monitor arterial blood gas results
• Prolonged anesthesia		• Check endotracheal cuff pressure as needed
• Intraoperative blood loss		
• Pain		• Monitor hemoglobin and hematocrit
• Premature weaning from mechanical ventilation		• Auscultate chest to assess breath sounds
• Prolonged mechanical ventilation		• Perform endotracheal suctioning every 2 hours and as needed
• Sepsis		• Reposition patient every 2 hours
Defining Characteristics		• Perform chest physical therapy
• Hypoxemia		• Monitor for signs and symptoms of sepsis
• Hypoventilation		
• Restlessness		• Provide for periods of rest
• Confusion		• Assess the need for analgesia and administer as ordered
• Dyspnea		
Altered Tissue Perfusion (Cardiopulmonary)	• The patient maintains adequate cardiac functioning and tissue perfusion.	• Monitor for changes in heart rate and rhythm
Related to	• The patient is adequately monitored for cardiac complications.	• Monitor for changes in arterial blood pressure
• Arrhythmia		• Monitor CVP and pulmonary artery pressures every 1–2 hours as ordered
• Hypovolemia		
• Fluid overload		• Perform cardiac output studies as ordered
• Electrolyte imbalances		

Defining Characteristics
- Abnormal electrocardiogram (ECG)
- Increased or decreased blood pressure (BP)
- Decreased cardiac output
- Increased or decreased pulmonary artery pressures
- Increased or decreased central venous pressure (CVP)

Impaired Tissue Integrity
Related to
- Ischemic injury to graft
- Stenosis, thrombosis of arterial or venous vasculature
- Intestinal anastamotic leak

Defining Characteristics
- Increased watery stomal output
- Bloody stomal output
- Pale stomal mucosa
- Abdominal distention and tenderness
- Increased white blood cell (WBC) count
- Endoscopic and histopathologic findings

High Risk for Fluid Volume Deficit or Excess
Related to
- Intraoperative fluid loss or administration
- Increased enteric losses
- Acute renal failure

- The patient is adequately monitored for signs and symptoms of graft ischemia and technical complications.
- Appropriate intervention is initiated.

- The patient retains homeostatic fluid and electrolyte balance.

- Monitor for excessive fluid losses from drains, jejunostomy, and ileostomy
- Monitor hemoglobin and hematocrit
- Administer fluid replacement as ordered
- Administer and titrate vasoactive medications as ordered

- Monitor and record enteric output and characteristics
- Assess and repeat changes in intestinal stoma characteristics
- Assess and report development of abdominal distention with tenderness
- Monitor vital signs for signs of hypovolemia
- Monitor hemoglobin, hematocrit, platelets, and coagulation times
- Follow endoscopic and histopathologic reports
- Provide patient and family emotional support if surgical procedure is necessary

- Monitor for signs and symptoms of hypovolemia or hypervolemia
- Maintain strict and accurate intake and output measurements

(continued)

NURSING CARE PLAN 11–1. SMALL-INTESTINAL TRANSPLANTATION: ACUTE PHASE—THE INTENSIVE CARE UNIT *(continued)*

Nursing Diagnosis	Expected Outcomes	Nursing Interventions
Defining Characteristics		
• Increased or decreased mean arterial pressure, CVP		• Monitor serum electrolyte levels as ordered
• Increased or decreased BP		• Administer or restrict fluids as ordered
• Increased or decreased urine output		• Replace electrolytes as ordered
• Abnormal serum electrolyte levels		
High Risk for Infection	• The patient is adequately monitored for signs of rejection or infection.	• Assess and report any symptoms of graft rejection or infection
Related to	• Appropriate therapy is administered as ordered.	• Administer immunosuppressive therapy and antimicrobial agents as ordered
• T- and B-cell activity	• The patient is adequately monitored for side effects of immunotherapy.	• Perform panculture for temperature >38.5°C
• Immunosuppressive therapy		• Adhere to strict aseptic techniques
• Implantation of a "dirty" organ		• Obtain quantitative stool cultures as ordered
• Multiple invasive lines, catheters, and drains, incisions		• Encourage coughing and deep breathing, use of incentive spirometer
• Anesthesia, mechanical ventilation		• Monitor for adverse effects of medications: (FK-506: decreased urine output, increased serum creatinine level, headache, nausea and vomiting, tremors, burning and tingling of lips, tongue, hands, feet)
• Bacterial translocation		• Provide patient teaching regarding rationale for evaluation and therapy
• Immobility		• Provide emotional support
Defining Characteristics		
• Abdominal distention		
• Diffuse abdominal pain		
• Decreased or absent bowel sounds		
• Edematous or dusky stomal mucosa		
• Increased watery stomal output		
• Fever, chills		
• Nausea, vomiting		
• Endoscopic and histologic findings		

Fluid Volume Deficit

Related to

- Intraoperative events (hemorrhage, hypotension)
- Hypovolemia
- Bacterial translocation
- Antibacterial and antifungal therapy
- FK-506 therapy

Defining Characteristics

- Decreased urine output
- Increased serum creatinine level, BUN
- Increased CVP
- Decreased hemoglobin and hematocrit
- Increased immunosuppressant and antibiotic blood levels
- Pulmonary edema

- The patient experiences satisfactory cardiopulmonary function and stable fluid volume.
- The patient stabilizes or corrects electrolyte and acid-base imbalances.

- Assess and report hourly output
- Monitor serum creatinine, BUN, and electrolyte levels
- Monitor vital signs as ordered and report substantial changes
- Maintain strict and accurate intake and output
- Auscultate lungs
- Obtain daily weights
- Administer IV therapy and medications as ordered to correct imbalances; evaluate for effectiveness
- Provide patient and family support and education if temporary dialysis is necessary

(continued)

349

NURSING CARE PLAN 11–1. SMALL-INTESTINAL TRANSPLANTATION: ACUTE PHASE—THE INTENSIVE CARE UNIT
(*continued*)

Nursing Diagnosis	Expected Outcomes	Nursing Interventions
Altered Nutrition: Less Than Body Requirements	• Patient has optimal nutritional intake.	• Obtain nutritional support consultation
Related to	• Patient has optimal health and healing in postoperative recovery.	• Administer total parenteral nutrition (TPN) and lipids as ordered
• Graft adaptation and preexisting malnutrition		• Monitor intake and output
• Poor absorptive ability of the intestinal allograft		• Monitor daily weights
• Fever, infection		• Monitor serum electrolyte levels
• Translocation		• Monitor for adverse reactions and intolerances to supplemental nutrition
• Secondary surgical procedures		
• Mechanical ventilation		
Defining Characteristics		
• Weight loss		
• Muscle wasting		
• Negative nitrogen balance		
• Impaired wound healing		
• Decreased resistance to infection		

Nursing Diagnosis	Expected Outcome	Nursing Interventions
High Risk for Fluid Volume Deficit	• The patient maintains an adequate fluid intake and serum electrolyte balance.	• Maintain strict and accurate measurements of intake and output
Related to		• Monitor for signs and symptoms of hypovolemia
• Abnormal fluid losses		• Monitor serum electrolyte levels as ordered
• Excessive enteric losses (ostomy, jejunostomy tube, nasogastric tube, vomiting)		• Replace fluids and electrolytes as ordered
• Abnormal drainage (wound, Jackson–Pratt drains)		• Obtain daily weights
• Increased metabolic rate (fever, infection)		• Monitor for fever and signs of infection
Defining Characteristics		
• Decreased urine output		
• Decreased central venous pressure (CVP)		
• Decreased blood pressure (BP)		
• Increased hemoglobin and hematocrit		
• Abnormal serum electrolyte levels		
High Risk for Impaired Skin Integrity	• Skin is free of excoriation or infection.	• Assess for risk of chemical tissue destruction
Related to		• Assure proper fit of ostomy appliance
• Chemical destruction		• Teach correct stoma pouching principles and skin-care techniques
• Poorly fitting ostomy appliances		• Use expertise of ostomy nurse specialist
• Uncontrolled fecal incontinence		• Devise method to contain intestinal incontinence
• Jejunostomy tube site drainage		• Use skin preparation products as needed

(continued)

351

NURSING CARE PLAN 11–2. SMALL-INTESTINAL TRANSPLANTATION: INTERMEDIATE PHASE—THE SURGICAL UNIT
(*continued*)

Nursing Diagnosis	Expected Outcome	Nursing Interventions
Defining Characteristics		
• Redness		
• Rash		
• Itching		
• Warmth		
• Swelling		
• Pain		
• Damage of Tissue		
Altered Immune Function	• The patient is adequately monitored for signs of rejection.	• Monitor for signs and symptoms of rejection
Related to	• Appropriate therapy is administered as ordered.	• Administer immunosuppressive medications as ordered
• T and B cell activity		• Monitor for adverse effects of medications
• Immunosuppressive therapy		• Obtain daily weights
Defining Characteristics		• Maintain strict and accurate intake and output records
• Abdominal distention		• Maintain complete daily caloric counts
• Diffuse abdominal pain		• Provide emotional support
• Decreased or absent bowel sounds		• Provide patient teaching regarding need for frequent biopsy
• Edematous or dusky stomal mucosa		
• Sudden increase in enteric output (>3 liters/24 hours)		
• Watery stomal output		
• Anorexia		
• Endoscopic and histologic findings		

Altered Nutrition: Less Than Body Requirements

Related to
- Poor absorptive ability of the intestinal graft
- Inadequate parenteral, jejunostomy, or oral intake

Defining Characteristics
- Weight loss
- Inadequate caloric intake
- Decreased serum albumin and total protein levels

- Patient has optimal nutritional health.
- Patient undergoes daily nutritional assessment and management.

- Obtain nutritional support consultation
- Administer total parenteral nutrition (TPN) and intravenous fat emulsion as ordered
- Administer enteral feedings as ordered
- Administer antidiarrheal and bulking agents as ordered
- Monitor for adverse reactions and intolerances to supplemental nutrition and antidiarrheal agents
- Monitor daily weights and calorie counts
- Monitor intake and output every 8 hours

High Risk for Infection

Related to
- Immunosuppression
- Risk for bacterial translocation
- Incisions, ostomy, skin breakdown
- Cellular susceptibility due to nutritional state
- Decreased mobility
- Long-term use of TPN (line sepsis)
- Invasive lines and catheters

Defining Characteristics
- Fever
- Chills
- Tachycardia
- Tachypnea

- The patient remains free of infection.
- Indication of infection is promptly recognized and reported, and appropriate therapy is initiated.

- Monitor vital signs every 4 hours
- Perform panculture for temperature elevation >38.5°C
- Wash hands before and after every patient contact
- Assess and report any changes in stomal output
- Assess and report development of abdominal pain, nausea and vomiting
- Obtain quantitative stool cultures as ordered
- Administer intestinal decontaminants as ordered
- Inspect mouth daily for oral candidiasis
- Monitor for side effects of antibiotics such as secondary infection, renal insufficiency

(*continued*)

NURSING CARE PLAN 11–2. SMALL-INTESTINAL TRANSPLANTATION: FOLLOW-UP PHASE AND DISCHARGE (*continued*)

Nursing Diagnosis	Expected Outcome	Nursing Interventions
• Abdominal pain • Nausea, vomiting • Increased watery stomal output • Anorexia and weight loss • Fatigue and malaise • Lesion eruption		
Pain *Related to* • Low pain tolerance due to chronic illness, previous multiple abdominal operations, pretransplant narcotic or analgesic addiction • Poor drug absorption secondary to gastrointestinal (GI) dysmotility *Defining Characteristics* • Alterations in sleep patterns and thought processes • Behavioral changes • Narcotic addiction	• The patient experiences minimal or no pain.	• Obtain pain control management or psychiatric consultation as needed • Encourage noninvasive pain measures as needed: relaxation techniques, diversional therapy, emotional support • Medicate with narcotics and analgesics as ordered • Ensure proper functioning of patient-controlled analgesia (PCA) pump • Assess effectiveness of pain measures • Reduce factors that may increase pain: anxiety, isolation, environmental, fatigue • Prepare the patient for procedures or activity that may cause or increase pain

NURSING CARE PLAN 11–3. SMALL-INTESTINAL TRANSPLANTATION: FOLLOW-UP PHASE AND DISCHARGE

Nursing Diagnosis	Expected Outcome	Nursing Interventions
Impaired Adjustment *Related to* • Health status change • Continued need for short-term nutritional therapy • Fear of organ rejection • Inadequate or unavailable support systems • Depression *Defining Characteristics* • Fear, anxiety, anger • Inability to become involved in problem-solving or goal-setting	• Patient identifies temporary and long-term post-operative recovery demands. • Patient demonstrates effective coping behaviors.	• Assess patient and family dynamics, perceptions, stress, and coping mechanisms • Explore goals and expectations • Begin health teaching when appropriate • Initiate referrals as indicated • Identify resources available (community, financial, counseling, transplant support groups)
Altered Family Processes *Related to* • Illness, operation, hospitalization • Change in family member's ability to function • Fear of rejection • Financial burdens • Change in family roles, disruption in routines • Emotional changes of all members *Defining Characteristics* • Fear, anxiety, anger • Absence of interaction	• The patient and family members verbalize feelings to the transplant team and to each other. • The family participates in care of ill family member. • The family maintains functional system of support for each member. • The family seeks appropriate external resources when needed.	• Provide a supportive hospital environment for family • Involve family members in care of ill member when appropriate • Facilitate communication and verbalization of feelings • Enlist consultation services when appropriate (social worker, psychologist, specialist) • Initiate health teaching and referrals to support groups as necessary *(continued)*

355

NURSING CARE PLAN 11–3. SMALL-INTESTINAL TRANSPLANTATION: FOLLOW-UP PHASE AND DISCHARGE (*continued*)

Nursing Diagnosis	Expected Outcome	Nursing Interventions
Impaired Home Maintenance Management *Related to* • Operation, ostomy • Impaired emotional functioning • Lack of knowledge of transplantation process, responsibilities for home management, and signs and symptoms of complications • Insufficient finances • Unavailable support system *Defining Characteristics* • Outward expressions of difficulty by patient or family • Lack of knowledge	• Patient and family members demonstrate ability to perform skills necessary to care for self and family member.	• Set priorities and goals with patient and family • Establish specific plan of teaching, utilizing internal and external resources as necessary • Record and communicate patient progress • Reinforce patient teaching throughout hospitalization and outpatient follow-up phase: medications; ostomy care; jejunostomy tube care; signs and symptoms complications; follow-up medical care

NURSING CARE PLAN 11–4. POSTOPERATIVE DIETARY AND MEDICATION STRATEGIES FOR INTESTINAL-TRANSPLANT RECIPIENTS

Strategy	Rationale	Nursing Interventions
Diet and Dietary Supplements		
• Total parenteral nutrition (TPN)	• To maintain or improve nutrition status as evidenced by body weight	• Consult a nutritional support team for all patients • Administer by infusion pump • Monitor glucose and electrolyte levels as ordered • Monitor daily weights • Monitor intake and output every 8 hours • Obtain daily calorie counts as ordered • Monitor for catheter-related infection and complications
• Fat emulsions	• To provide calories adjunctive to TPN • To prevent fatty acid deficiency	• Monitor serum lipids, hepatic function, and platelet count as ordered • Avoid rapid infusion or use of infusion pump • Monitor for adverse reactions, especially during first 30 minutes of infusion
• Peptamen (all recipients) • Modified Compleat B (pediatric recipients)	• To provide an elemental, peptide based, isotonic, low-residue supplemental diet • To provide a high-fiber content supplemental diet that is easily absorbed in the presence of impaired gastrointestinal (GI) function and malabsorption syndrome	• Administer by jejunostomy, gastrostomy, or oral routes • Deliver tube feedings by feeding pump • Increase strength and rate as ordered; monitor for intolerance • Monitor for abdominal distention, nausea, vomiting

(continued)

357

NURSING CARE PLAN 11–4. POSTOPERATIVE DIETARY AND MEDICATION STRATEGIES FOR INTESTINAL-TRANSPLANT RECIPIENTS *(continued)*

Strategy	Rationale	Nursing Interventions
• Small, frequent meals; low-fat diet	• To provide optimum intestinal absorption • To allow maturation of lymphatics	• Monitor calorie counts as ordered • Monitor for abdominal distention, nausea, vomiting • Monitor for food intolerances
Medications (doses highly variable and adjusted frequently)		• Be aware that risk of physical dependence increases with long-term use
• Opium tincture (deodorized) • Opium tincture (camphorated, paregoric) • Deodorized opiate morphine content 25 times greater than that of camphorated tincture	• To prevent diarrhea • To increase smooth-muscle tone in GI tract • To inhibit motility and propulsion • To diminish intestinal secretions	• Administer in food or in tube feedings • Monitor for opiate toxicity • Administer deodorized opium in drops • Administer paregoric opium in mL
• Diphenoxylate hydrochloride (Lomotil) • Dose of 2.5 mg is as effective as 5 mL of camphorated tincture of opium	• To prevent diarrhea • To increase smooth-muscle tone in GI tract • To inhibit motility and propulsion • To diminish intestinal secretions	• Be aware that risk for physical dependence increases with high dosage and long-term use (atropine sulfate included to discourage abuse) • Monitor for sedation, tachycardia, dry mouth, urine retention, and rash or pruritus
• Loperamide (imodium) • Antidiarrheal action similar to that of diphenoxylate but with fewer adverse effects on the central nervous system adverse effects	• To inhibit peristaltic activity • To prolong intestinal transit time	• Monitor for drowsiness, fatigue, dizziness, rash *(continued)*

358

- Octreotide acetate (sandostatin)

- To prevent diarrhea
- To mimic action of naturally occurring somatostatin

- Administer in subcutaneous injections
- Be aware drug may decrease FK-506 absorption (under investigation)
- Be aware half-life may be altered in patients with renal failure or undergoing dialysis
- Monitor closely for glucose imbalance
- Monitor for need of dose adjustments: drug may alter insulin or oral hypoglycemia needs

Bulking Agents (doses highly variable and adjusted frequently)

- Pectin
- Calcium polycarbophil

- To absorb water and increase bulk content of stool
- To absorb free fecal water, thereby thickening stool

- Inform patient that pectin can be purchased in grocery store
- Add to tube feedings or place in food or drink
- Inform patient that calcium tablets must be chewed before they are swallowed
- Monitor for abdominal fullness, increased flatus, and constipation

12

Ethical Issues in Transplantation

Marie T. Nolan

A front page article in *The Wall Street Journal* featured the story of Rex Voss, a 41-year-old father of four who died while awaiting a liver transplant (McCartney, 1993). The article noted that a liver was given to a less critically ill patient only 40 miles from Voss because of the current national organ allocation system, which gives preference to local transplant candidates. In the same year, Pennsylvania Governor William Casey received a heart-lung transplant after being on the transplant list less than 24 hours (Pa. governor, 1993). Although the Pennsylvania physicians followed previously established organ guidelines, which favored multiple organ recipients, they received a barrage of questions about whether the governor had improperly been given preference over other candidates.

The media attention given to issues of organ procurement and allocation reflect society's concern over the ethical dilemmas that surround transplantation. Nurses who serve as donor advocates, transplant coordinators, clinical nurse specialists, nurse managers, and clinical nurses should be aware of these dilemmas and be able to formulate a cogent ethical framework for addressing them. The purpose of this chapter is to briefly describe the major ethical frameworks and to review the ethical dilemmas associated with transplantation nursing.

ETHICAL FRAMEWORKS

Ethics is the study of the right and wrong of human actions. There are several ethical theories that may be called upon to resolve ethical dilemmas in transplantation care today. All are not equally good. The ideal theory is one that offers clear guidance in ethical decision making and respects those values that contribute to human flourishing and are therefore common across cultures.

Deontology and Principlism

Deontology is commonly known as a rule-based ethic. The Hippocratic Oath, which was influenced by Ancient Greek philosophy, represents one of the earliest forms of deontology in medicine. The Hippocratic ethic " . . . contains most of the genuinely ethical precepts, such as the obligations of beneficence, nonmaleficence, and confidentiality, as well as prohibitions against abortion, euthanasia, surgery, and sexual relationships with patients" (Pellegrino, 1993, p 1159).

Principlism involves the use of principles to guide moral reasoning. Beneficence (to act for the patient's good) and nonmaleficence (to do no harm) were called upon in the Hippocratic Oath and remain important principles today. The principles of autonomy and justice have more recently been added to discussions of health care ethics. The principle of autonomy directs that persons ought to be free to act without constraint by others, while the principle of justice directs that each person ought to be treated according to what is fair or owed. Often autonomy is pitted against beneficence when it may rightly be considered a component of beneficence. That is, to act for the patient's good is to respect the patient's autonomy.

Utilitarianism

Utilitarianism is the ethical system in which good is defined as that which achieves the greatest good for the greatest number (Beauchamp & Walters, 1989). A Utilitarian might seek to decrease the shortage of organs for transplantation by paying persons to donate organs to strangers for a fee. This would violate the principle of nonmaleficence, since to remove a healthy organ from one who will not significantly benefit from this action is to do harm. Also, if this donor is impoverished and is seeking to donate out of a desperate need for money, it is doubtful that the decision to donate is an autonomous one.

Casuistry

Casuistry is not an ethical theory but an approach to resolving ethical dilemmas. The casuist asserts that the right action is obvious in certain cases. These cases are "paradigm cases" and can be compared to cases of increasing complexity (Arras, 1991). For example, if we agree that a mother might rightly donate a section of her liver to save the life of her child, we can compare this case to other cases such as a mother who wishes to donate a section of her liver to an unknown recipient, in order to receive money to provide her child with food. Critics of casuistry point out that this method fails to recognize the need for a shared set of moral values prior to resolving ethical disputes (Kuczewski, 1994). To analyze this case, we would still be drawn back to the principles of nonmaleficence, beneficence, and autonomy.

Caring

During the past decade, several nurse authors have suggested that the concept of caring is central to the essence of nursing (Leininger, 1984; Watson, 1988; Benner &

Wrubel, 1989). This concept has also been suggested as a guide to ethical decision making (Fry, 1988; Valentine, 1989; Boykin & Schoenhofer, 1990). The weakness of caring as an ethical guide is that it remains ill defined. After a thorough review of the literature, Morse and associates (1990) stated, "There is no consensus in the literature regarding the definitions of caring, the components of care, or the process of caring" (p. 2). To some, caring is a relative concept to be defined by the patient (Valentine, 1989). In considering this view of caring, Nelson (1992) warns that since patients are identified as the exclusive choice makers and the nurse is charged only with carrying out patients' wishes, this negates any sense of personal responsibility on the part of the nurse.

Virtue

Virtue ethic is grounded in an understanding of what it is to be human. " . . . One is able to evaluate choices for actions as good or bad depending on how they harmonize with rational human beings" (O'Connell, 1991, p 2). This ethic serves as a companion to principlism. For example, the principle of autonomy flows from the nature of human beings as rational and self-determining individuals. Therefore, the virtuous person respects patient autonomy. But, unlike other ethical frameworks, autonomy is not always paramount. For example, we may accept the wishes of a mother to donate a lobe of her lung or liver to her child, but we would not allow a mother to donate her heart. This would be rejected because it is an act against a human good—the good of life. There are several basic human goods by which rational beings enjoy fulfillment. These include life, health, harmony with self, harmony with others, and appreciation of beauty. In resolving ethical conflicts, "the virtue of prudence, that is practical wisdom, enables us to arrive at the right and good ordering of principles and concrete facts in particular cases" (Pellegrino & Thomasma 1993, p 23).

ORGAN PROCUREMENT

Brain Death

The concept of brain death, defined as irreversible cessation of all brain function, has gained wide acceptance (Baldwin et al, 1993). A thorough description of its diagnosis is provided in the chapter on Organ and Tissue Donation. By 1991, 32 states had brain death laws in place (Norton, 1992). Despite consensus on the idea of brain death, confusion remains about the clinical application of this concept. In one study, one third of physicians surveyed were unable to identify and apply brain death criteria (Youngner et al, 1989). Also, in a retrospective study of the records of 52 infants who had been declared brain dead and went on to serve as donors, 12% did not meet the criteria for brain death in children (Ashwal, 1993).

One barrier to the identification of brain death is the risk involved in confirming this diagnosis. Many problems can occur during the apnea test, which is done to demonstrate that the patient has no spontaneous respiration in the presence of a Pa_{CO_2} of 60 mm Hg or higher. Arrhythmia, hypotension, and cardiac arrest are all potential side effects of the apnea test (Schwarz et al, 1992). Preoxygenation, coupled with the administration of oxygen during the test, will help to prevent hypoxia and protect the patient while still allowing for the buildup of $Paco_2$ levels which would meet the apnea criteria (Marks & Zisfein, 1990; Ashwal & Schneider, 1991).

Persons in a Permanent Vegetative State as Donors

Using patients who are in a permanent vegetative state (PVS) is currently being considered. Robert Veach calls the whole-brain-oriented definition of death "old fashioned" and suggests that for human life to be present, integrated functioning of mind and body must be present (Veach, 1993). Ethicist, J. Downie (1990) notes the utilitarian appeal of using PVS patients as organ donors. " . . . Thousands of organs could become available for those requiring transplantation to stay alive . . . and we would not incur the cost of maintaining [PVS] patients for a number of years" (p 995). Downie goes on, however, to provide three compelling reasons for rejecting PVS patients as organ donors. First, the diagnosis of PVS is not reliable enough to prevent the possibility of a patient who is not in a PVS being mistakenly killed to obtain organs for transplantation. Second, "If we allow the killing of PVS patients for organ harvesting, we will inevitably allow the killing of demented patients, the mentally handicapped, and any other group deemed unfit for continued existence" (Downie, 1990, p 995). And third, designating PVS patients as dead will further confuse the public, contributing to fear that patients will not be dead before their organs are removed (Downie, 1990). It has been shown that this fear already exists and serves as a barrier to organ donation (Dominguez-Roldan et al, 1992).

Another negative consequence of using PVS patients as organ donors is cited by Keatings (1990). He cautions that if we redesign death to include those patients in PVS. "This definition must be absolute since it is not our practice to care for and nurture the dead" (p 998). Therefore, all patients who are in PVS would have to have care withdrawn, not just those who indicated a desire to serve as an organ donor.

Anencephalic Infants as Donors

The consideration of anencephalic infants is similarly fraught with ethical conflicts. Truog and Fletcher propose that using anencephalic infants as donors could decrease shortage of transplantable organs (1989). Although they concede that these infants do not meet the criteria for brain death, they state that anencephalic infants lack integrative brain function in the same manner that brain dead patients do. Shewmon and co-workers (1989) counter by stating, "Whether those [anencephalic infants] with relatively intact brain stems have any subjective awareness associated with their responsiveness to the environment is inherently unverifiable, but what is known about the functional capabilities of the brain stem, particularly in newborns, suggests at least keeping an open mind" (p. 1776).

Medearis and Holmes (1989) note important clinical features of anencephaly. "Evidence indicates that anencephaly is a heterogeneous condition anatomically and functionally, that the diagnosis of anencephaly cannot be made with sufficient accuracy, and that the condition cannot be distinguished well enough from other severe intracranial disorders to justify changing the law. Anencephalic infants are alive and the length of their lives cannot be predicted accurately" (p 393). Capron (1993) adds,

"Classifying anencephalic infants as dead denies their humanity and treats them solely as a means (without their consent) to others' ends" (p S375).

Since the natural cause of death in anencephaly is ultimately hypoventilation, which renders vital organs unsuitable for transplantation, ventilatory support is required until the infant deteriorates to the point of brain death (Shewmon et al, 1989). Physicians at Loma Linda Hospital in California developed a protocol to provide this type of ventilatory support for anencephalic infants who were designated as potential organ donors (Peabody et al, 1989). When after 7 months of the protocol, only 2 of 12 infants met the criteria for brain death, the protocol was suspended. Physicians in the Loma Linda protocol noted with amazement the number of infants with less severe anomalies referred to them as potential organ donors. These included infants with hydrocephaly, and infants born without kidneys, but with a normal brain. Dr. Joyce Peabody, Chief of Neonatology at Loma Linda said, "I have become educated by the experience . . . the slippery slope is real" (Shewmon et al, 1989, p 1775).

Fetuses as Donors

The transplantation of tissue from fetuses was first undertaken as a treatment for patients with Parkinson disease, while later experiments included patients with Alzheimer disease and diabetes (Sanders et al, 1993). Although initially the federal government placed a ban on experimentation with fetal tissue obtained from elective abortions, it established fetal tissue banks that stored the donated tissues of spontaneously aborted fetuses. Under the Clinton administration the ban was lifted, raising ethical issues about the link between experimentation with fetal tissue and elective abortion.

Some of the ethical issues surrounding the use of fetuses as donors are similar to those involving the use of anencephalic infants as donors. The same slippery slope argument applies. That is, if we classify the fetus as a type of human unworthy of protection, other types of humans such as the elderly or the handicapped may soon be similarly classified.

Also, as with the anencephalic infant, donation does not serve the good of the fetus. Moreover, "consent from women who have chosen to abort is mortally problematic because of their dual role in causing the death and determining the disposition of the remains" (Nolan, 1990, p 1029).

Barry and Kesler (1990) provided a thorough review of the scientific literature on fetal tissue transplantation and concluded that studies of fetal tissue transplantation have shown little promise. They also present scientific advances in other areas that have demonstrated greater success in achieving the therapeutic objectives of fetal tissue transplantation. Martin (1993) also concludes that "advocates have referred to the potential benefits of fetal tissue transplantation as an ethical justification for it, yet the benefit remains a hope and not a reality" (p 1). Ahlskog (1993) predicted that instead of fetal tissue transplantation, ". . . advances in molecular biology may allow for transplantation of genetically engineered cells or modification of existing brain cells" (p 591).

Hillebrecht (1989) warned of the emergence of a for-profit fetal transplant industry if fetal transplantation is successful. Those who are predicted to benefit from this type of transplant are 1.5 million people with Parkinson disease, 3 million persons with Alzheimer disease, and 6 million persons with diabetes. Since about 1.5 million abortions are performed in the United States each year, the demand for fetal tissue would quickly outstrip the supply. Hillebrecht predicts that economic incentives could lead women in poverty to become pregnant and abort for cash. Dr. Kathleen Nolan concludes, "Parenting is an incredible act of creation and to plan the destruction of this new identity, even at the early stage, is to turn one of humanity's most intimate and wonderful activities into an objectifying and mechanical pharmaceutical production mechanism." (1990, p 1029).

Minority Donors

Among adults, there is an inadequate number of donors to serve the minority population. While African Americans comprise 12.3% of the total population, they account for 30% of the population with end-stage renal disease (ESRD) (Reitz & Callender, 1993). Despite this overrepresentation, African Americans receive renal transplants at half the rate of white Americans (Norris, 1991). One reason for this disparity is an insufficient number of African American donors. Due to differences in HLA antigens, 20% of African Americans would have greater transplant success by having an African American donor (Reitz & Callender, 1993). Waiting times are long for this 20% of African Americans because African Americans make up fewer than 10% of organ donors nationally (Norris, 1991).

Reasons influencing the reluctance of African Americans to donate organs were described by Reitz and Callender (1993, p 354):

1. Lack of awareness of transplantation.
2. Religious beliefs and misperceptions.
3. Distrust of the medical community.
4. Poor access to medical care.
5. Lack of an organ procurement specialist.
6. Intrafamilial relationships.

Creecy and colleagues (1992) studied factors associated with willingness to consider cadaveric kidney donation in African Americans. They found that African Americans most likely to consider organ donation are female and young, have obtained knowledge about transplantation from the newspaper or friends, and believe that organ donation is a way of honoring God. Hong and associates (1994) described a community-specific program using African American community educators and organ requesters for African American families. This program increased African American organ donation from 7% of the total donor population to 20% of the total donor population. The investigators plan to conduct interviews with African American families who were approached for donation to determine what factors are most important to the donation process.

To offset the scarcity of African American donors, some investigators have suggested reformulating the existing allocation system to give preference to those less likely to find an HLA match (Gaston et al, 1993). Others oppose this and defend the "race-correlated but prejudice-free technique of HLA matching" as the state of the science (Wolicki, 1994, p 270). Finally, others, including Dr. Thomas Starzl, contend that tissue matching criteria is only marginally relevant to outcome and should be reexamined. Starzl explained that cell interactions that occur after transplantation, resulting in "clonal silencing" of both donor and recipient immunocytes, warrant further study and may ultimately prove tissue matching to be unnecessary (Starzl et al, 1993, p 2451).

Living Related Donors

Living related donation has occurred for years in bone marrow and renal transplantation and, more recently, in liver and lung transplantation. Five categories of living donation were identified by Daar, Salahudeen, Pingle, and Woods (1990): living related, emotionally related, altruistic donation, rewarded gifting, and rampant commercialism. Living related refers to a genetically related donor, while emotionally related refers to a close family member such as a spouse or friend who is genetically unrelated. In altruistic donation, the donor does not necessarily know the recipient and expects no material reward of any sort. Rewarded gifting is similar to altruistic donation except that the donor is compensated for the inconvenience of hospitalization and loss of income associated with donation. In rampant commercialism, the focus is on financial gain from organ donation rather than on the health and safety of the donor and recipient.

Rewarded gifting and rampant commercialism have not been condoned in the United States; however, commercialism in organs has been reported in other countries. Daar and associates (1990) reported that 130 patients from their dialysis units in the United Arab Emirates and Oman had undergone transplantation in Bombay after purchasing kidneys from living nonrelated donors there. Johny, Nesim, Namboori, and Gupta (1990) reported that 53 patients from their renal transplant program in Kuwait received organs from unrelated donors in India (49), Egypt (2), the Philippines (1), and Iraq (1). The majority of the patients from Kuwait viewed their transplant physicians as competent. However, 15 of the patients felt that the physicians' motivation was commercial. In Japan, the country's society for transplantation has adopted a policy that living unrelated renal transplantation may be permitted if certain criteria are met such as the lack of cadaveric or living related donors (Hiraga et al, 1992).

In considering living related donation, the transplant team may be guided by the principles of beneficence, nonmaleficence, and autonomy. Clearly, the team is obligated to act for the good of the recipient, but what are their obligations toward the donor? Nonmaleficence directs health professionals to do no harm. Harm is minimized by selection criteria that require donors to be in a good state of health prior to donation. For example, a parent without a smoking history was chosen over a parent with a smoking history for partial lung donation (Kirchner, 1991). Despite these precautions, however, donors incur some risks. The mortality for renal donors was reported as .06%, and the mortality associated with liver donation was estimated as 1% to 2% (Busuttil, 1991). Respect for patient autonomy allows us to permit the donor to take on some risk if we can be reasonably sure that a donor's decision is informed, free from coercion, and truly autonomous.

Ashley and O'Rourke (1989) propose four criteria that should be met prior to permitting living donation:

1. There is a serious need on the part of the recipient that cannot be fulfilled in any other way.
2. The functional integrity of the donor as a human person will not be impaired, even though anatomic integrity may suffer.
3. The risk taken by the donor as an act of charity is proportionate to the good resulting for the recipient.
4. The donor's consent is free and informed (p 308).

Donors should be informed not only of the risks for physical harm but also the risks for psychologic harm. Russel and Jacob (1993) described two suicides and one suicide attempt among renal donors who became despondent following the graft rejection and death of the organ recipients. They also describe several cases where the spouses of donors were upset by the donation, "as if giving an organ to someone outside of the nuclear family threatened its boundaries" (p 92). Nurses who work closely with the family, donor, and recipient during the recovery period should assess for psychologic distress relating to the transplant. Psychiatric intervention prior to and after transplantation should be provided if it appears that donors or their families are experiencing any psychologic turmoil.

Assuring that the potential donor is free from coercion may be difficult. Concerning liver transplantation, Busuttil (1991) asked, "How can a parent be expected to make an informed, uncoerced, free choice when asked to consider donating an organ to his/her dying child?" (p 44). Dennison, Azoulay, and Maddern (1993) stated that directly approaching a potential donor should not be permitted unless the recipient is critically ill and in urgent need of transplantation. They propose that the family should be informed of the donor problem and the transplant team should then await a spontaneous volunteer.

At the University of Chicago, Singer and associates (1989) proposed that liver transplant from a living donor would be offered only to recipients with a higher chance of survival. They employed a two-step process for obtaining donor consent and assigned a consultant in internal medicine to act as a consent advocate for the donor. Others have also supported the concept of a consent advocate to protect the donor's interests (Shaw et al, 1991). Spital and Spital (1990), however, criticized the University of Chicago team for choosing only donors whose family members had a high chance of survival. They claimed that this process might deprive some people of the chance to donate an organ in the hope of saving a loved one and asked, "how can physicians tell a parent how much risk is too much?" (p 550).

Caplan (1993) resolves the tension between the autonomy of the donor and the nonmaleficent desires of the transplant team by advising that " . . . transplant centers must make sure that unreasonable risks are not presented to those who could not possibly refuse to accept them lest they see themselves as failing their moral duties to families or friends" (p 1999). Caplan concludes, "Medical ethics can accommodate the imposition of risk upon a patient to benefit another, but only if the person bearing the risk has a full understanding of exactly what is being asked, what the alternatives are, and what the realistic chances are for achieving a success-ful liver transplant" (p 2000).

Future Developments in Transplantation

Since there are many ethical concerns over many issues in transplantation, we are ob-ligated to continue to seek out other ways to restore health to persons with organ fail-ure. Each issue of *The International Journal of Artificial Organs* provides new research concerning the development of artificial means to replace organs. Some heart transplants could become unnecessary if cardiomyoplasty proves to be effective. This new surgical procedure involves wrapping a skeletal muscle around the heart and stimulating it to augment ventricular function (Zabala et al, 1992). Several investiga-tors have reported success in transplanting kidneys from non-heart beating donors (Koyama, et al, 1992; Watanabe et al, 1992; Alvarez, et al, 1992). Although it is diffi-cult to estimate the potential impact, some families may consent to donation from a non-heart beating family member more readily than they would from a brain dead fam-ily member. Finally, at The University of Pennsylvania, investigators have demon-strated that transplanting adult mouse hepatocytes into mice with failing livers can result in up to 80% of the liver being regenerated. Scientists still need to conduct fur-ther studies using this animal model before the technique can be adopted in humans (Hopkin, 1994).

ORGAN ALLOCATION

Severity of Illness

The current method of ordering patients on the waiting list for a cadaveric donor in the United States takes into consideration the patient's severity of illness, blood type, body size, and length of time on the waiting list (Mudge et al, 1993). Location is also important as local organ procurement organizations will allocate organs to local re-cipients prior to making the organs available nationally. This policy is an attempt to balance fairness, efficacy, and urgency (Ubel et al, 1993). Yet the weight given to each of these three variables is contested. Giving priority to more critically ill patients is viewed by some as an injudicious use of a scarce healthcare resource because more critically ill patients have higher mortality rates after transplantation. For example, Mudge and associates (1993) reported that critically ill heart transplant patients have an operative mortality rate of 14% compared with 6% for transplant patients in stable condition prior to surgery. Nevertheless, Stevenson and associates (1991) note that when the entire cardiac recipient pool is taken into account, survival is maximized by giving priority to those most likely to die without transplant. These investigators esti-mate that postoperative mortality rate would have to approach 50% to offset the ben-efit of transplanting the most critically ill patients.

Moral Virtue of the Recipient

In the case of liver transplantation, some support transplanting the most critically ill patient but would give a lower priority to patients who acquired their end-stage liver disease through alcoholism. Initially, alcoholics may have been excluded from liver transplant programs because of a belief that a high rate of relapse would be inevitable and survival limited. In contrast, Starzl and associates (1988) reported that survival rates of liver transplant patients with alcohol-related end-stage liver disease were no different from those of patients with other sources of end-stage liver disease. Nevertheless, Moss and Siegler (1991) argue that, "it is only fair that patients who have not assumed equal responsibility for maintaining their health should be treated differently" (p 1298). The authors also point out that since alcoholism is present in all socioeconomic levels, it is not discrimination against the poor when patients with alcohol-related liver disease are left off of the list. Killeen (1993) counters this by asserting that patients from lower socioeconomic strata with alcohol-related liver disease are at a greater disadvantage because of an inability to afford treatment for their disorder (p 8).

Cohen and Benjamin (1991) also argue against penalizing those with alcohol-related end-stage liver disease by stating, "We could rightly preclude alcoholics from transplantation only if we assume that qualifications for a new organ requires some level of moral virtue" (p 1299). The authors note that we do not attempt to determine whether transplant candidates are abusive parents, cheat on their income tax, or lie. Because it would be impossible to fairly judge the moral character of all in need of a transplant, Cohen and Benjamin (1991) suggest that it is fair to treat all in need of scarce resources by the same standard. "Public confidence in medical practice in general, and in organ transplantation in particular, depends on the scientific validity and moral integrity of the policies adopted" (p. 1301).

Efficacy

Retransplantation. Another challenge to this policy of giving the most severely ill patients priority in transplantation arises when a patient is in need of a second or third transplant. Ubel, Arnold, and Caplan (1993) note that 10% to 20% of hearts and livers donated for transplantation are used to retransplant patients. They cite three issues that affect the decision to have a patient undergo two or more transplantations. First, the obligation of the team not to abandon patients on whom they have already performed a transplant; second, the fairness of allowing patients to get multiple transplants while others die awaiting their first; and third, the difference in efficacy between primary transplantation and retransplantation. Ubel and co-workers (1993) dismiss the transplant team's obligation not to abandon a transplant patient as feelings of attachment that should not alter allocation priorities.

While Ubel and associates (1993) make an important point, that allocation of scarce resources should not be based on emotion, they may not have given proper weight to the obligation of the transplant team to act for the good of the patient. Patients rightly expect that their physician or nurse will act for their good and not as a double agent acting on the behalf of all of society. With their obligation to a particular patient in mind, it is understandable that the team may seek a second, third, or more transplants if to do so would benefit this patient.

On the issue of fairness, Ubel and associates (1993) hold that allowing only one transplant per person requires a very narrow view of healthcare. They point out that other factors affect health such as income, education, and access to primary care and these are not fairly distributed among transplant patients. They conclude that only the difference in efficacy justifies giving preference to primary transplant recipients. In one study, primary liver transplant recipients demonstrated survival rates that were 21% greater than secondary liver transplant recipients (Shaw, Gordon, Iwatsuki, & Starzl, 1985). In a study of heart transplant recipients, one-year survival for primary transplant recipients was 81% compared with 44% for secondary transplant recipients (Dein et al, 1989). Ubel and co-workers (1993) concluded that if we are to continue to limit access to transplant by referring to factors related to efficacy such as blood type, we must also consider the decreased efficacy of retransplantation as justification for limiting access to transplantation.

Racial Factors. Whether efficacy should be a deciding factor in organ allocation is now questioned in view of the previously mentioned differences in waiting times of minority transplant candidates. In addition to the need to match 20% of African American recipients with an African American donor, there are other reasons for this disparity. African Americans choose transplantation only half as often as whites (Callender, 1989). Also, African Americans have not been as available for transplantation when contacted. During a one-year period at a multi-center organ procurement organization, 11 of 57 African American candidates (19.3%) were unavailable for transplantation when called. Five refused to come, three were ill, and three could not be located. In contrast, only 2 of the 61 white transplant candidates (3.3%) were unavailable (Cunningham, 1992).

Further investigation should be undertaken regarding each variable influencing minority transplantation. African Americans may choose transplantation less often for reasons similar to those given for declining organ donation: lack of knowledge of transplantation, distrust of the medical community, and poor access to medical care (Reitz & Callender, 1993). Causes of unavailability at the time of transplantation may be similar.

Futility. One final concern regarding the efficacy of transplantation deals with the dilemma of when to stop treatment. It is generally assumed that patients who consent to transplantation are consenting to an aggressive venture. Although the science of transplantation has advanced rapidly in the past decade, some problems remain insurmountable. Informed consent is routinely obtained from patients at the outset of transplantation. It is less frequently confirmed throughout the transplant experience.

One mother recounted the experience of her 13-year-old daughter undergoing bone marrow transplantation. Although she and her daughter had hopes for a cure at the start of treatment, in the end, these hopes were unrealized. The side effects, setbacks, and disappointments led this mother to write after her daughter's death, "Consumers of health services generally believe doctors honor their own code 'To Do No

Harm.' It is my contention that the failure rate in bone marrow transplants does not merit this assumption by consumers" (Connell, 1990, p 956).

Nurses are in an ideal position to monitor the patient's and family's response to treatment. Sensitivity and immediate attention to the amelioration of side effects can help make the transplant experience more tolerable. But respect and support should be given to the patient who chooses to stop treatment.

Nurses who practice in the area of transplantation will continue to experience sorrow in the death of fathers like Rex Voss due to the organ shortage, and joy in the life of Governor Casey, who survived. The contributions nurses make to education, care of patients and families, advancement of the science, and establishment of policy regarding transplantation give witness to their commitment to human flourishing and the ethic of virtue, which is the heart of nursing.

REFERENCES

Ahlskog JE (1993). Cerebral transplantation for Parkinson's Disease: Current progress and future prospects. *Mayo Clin Proc*. 68(6):578–591.

Alvarez J, Gomez M, Arias J, et al (1992). One-year experience in renal transplantation with kidneys from asystolic donors. *Transplant Proc*. 24(1):34.

Arras JD (1991). Getting down to cases: The revival of casuistry in bioethics. *J Med Philosophy*. 16:29–51.

Ashley BM, O'Rourke KD (1989). Reconstructing human beings. In: Ashley BM, O'Rourke KD. *Health Care Ethics: A Theological Analysis*. St. Louis: The Catholic Health Association of the United States.

Ashwal S (1993). Brain death in early infancy. *J Heart Lung Transplant*. 12(6), part 2: S176–S178.

Ashwal S, Schneider S (1991). Pediatric brain death: Current perspectives. In: Barness LA, ed. *Advances in Pediatrics*. Chicago: Mosby-Year Book; 181–202.

Baldwin JC, Anderson JL, Boucek MM, et al (1993). Cardiac transplantation task force 2: Donor guide lines. *J Am Col Cardiol*. 22(1):15–20.

Barry R, Kesler D (1990). Pharaoh's magicians: The ethics and efficacy of human fetal tissue transplants. *The Thomist*. 54(4):575–608.

Beauchamp TL, Walters L (1989). Ethical theory and bioethics. In: Beauchamp T, Walters L, eds. *Contemporary Issues in Bioethics*. Belmont, Ca: Wadsworth Inc; 1–43.

Benner P, Wrubel J (1989). *The Primacy of Caring: Stress and Coping in Health and Illness*. Menlo Park, Ca: Addison Wesley.

Boykin A, Schoenhofer S (1990). Caring in nursing: Analysis of extant theory. *Nurs Sci Q*. 4:149–155.

Busuttil RW (1991). Living-related liver donation: Con. *Transplant Proc*. 23(1):43–45.

Callender CO (1989). The results of transplantation in blacks: Just the tip of the iceberg. *Transplant Proc*. 21:3407–3410.

Caplan A (1993). Must I be my brother's keeper? Ethical issues in the use of living donors as sources of liver and other solid organs. *Transplant Proc*. 25(2):1997–2000.

Capron AM (1993). The criteria for determining brain death should not be revised to place anencephalic infants into the category of dead bodies. *J Heart Lung Transplant*. 12(6) part 2:S374–S378.

Cohen C, Benjamin M (1991). Alcoholics and liver transplantation. *JAMA*. 265(10):1299–1301.

Connell SG (1990). An experimental bone marrow transplant experience. *Transplant Proc.* 22 (3):955–956.

Creecy RF, Wright R, Berg WE (1992). Discriminators of willingness to consider cadaveric kidney donation among black Americans. *Social Work in Health Care.* 18(1):93–105.

Cunningham PRG (1992). Differences in waiting time of minority transplant candidates in the United States. *J Transplant Coordination.* 2(2):78–79.

Daar AS, Salahudeen AK, Pingle A, Woods HF (1990). Ethics and commerce in live donor renal transplantation: Classification of the issues. *Transplant Proc.* 22(3):922–924.

Dein JR, Oyer PE, Stinson EB, et al (1989). Cardiac retransplantation in the cyclosporine era. *Ann Thorac Surg.* 48:350–355.

Dennison AR, Azoulay D, Maddern GJ (1993). Living related hepatic donation: Prometheus or Pandora's box? *Austral NZ J Surg.* 63:835–839.

Dominguez-Roldan JM, Murillo-Cabezas F, Perez-San-Gregorio MA (1992). Psychological aspects leading to refusal of organ donation in southwest Spain. *Transplant Proc.* 21(1):25–26.

Downie J (1990). The biology of the persistent vegetative state: Legal, ethical and philosophical implications for transplantation. *Transplant Proc.* 22(3):955–996.

Fry S (1988). The ethic of caring: Can it survive in nursing? *Nurs Outlook.* 1:48.

Gaston RS, Ayers I, Dooley LG, Diethelm AG (1993). Racial equity in renal transplantation: The disparate impact of HLA-based allocation. *JAMA.* 270:1352–1356.

Hillebrecht JM (1989). Regulating the clinical uses of fetal tissue: A proposal for legislation. *J Legal Med.* 10(2):269–322.

Hiraga S, Tanaka K, Watanabe J, et al (1992). Living unrelated donor renal transplantation. *Transplant Proc.* 24(4):1320–1322.

Hong BA, Kappel DF, Whitlock M, et al (1994). Using race-specific community programs to increase organ donation among blacks. *Am J Public Health.* 84(2):314–315.

Hopkin K (1994). Transplanted adult hepatocytes replace diseased liver. *J NIH Res.* 6(5):50–52.

Johny KV, Nesim J, Namboori N, Gupta RK (1990). Values gained and lost in live unrelated renal transplantation. *Transplant Proc.* 22(3):915–917.

Keatings M (1990). The biology of the persistent vegetative state, legal and ethical implications for transplantation: Viewpoints from nursing. *Transplant Proc.* 22(3):977–998.

Killeen T (1993). Alcoholism and liver transplantation: Ethical and nursing implications. *Perspectives in Psychiatric Care.* 29(1):7–12.

Kirchner SA (1991). Living related lung transplantation. *AORN J.* 54(4):703–714.

Koyama I, Taguchi Y, Watanabe T, et al (1992). Development of a reliable method for procurement of warm ischemic kidneys from non-heart-beating donors. *Transplant Proc.* 24 (4):1327–1328.

Kuczewski MG (1994). Casuistry and its communitarian critics. *Kennedy Institute of Ethics J.* 4(2):99–116.

Leininger MM (1984). Care: The essence of nursing and health. In: Leininger MM, ed. *Care: The Essence of Nursing and Health.* Thorofare, NJ: Slack.

Marks SJ, Zisfein J (1990). Apneic oxygenation in apnea tests for brain death: A controlled trial. *Arch Neurol.* 47:1066–1068.

Martin DK (1993). Abortion and fetal tissue transplantation. *IRB.* 15(3):1–4.

McCartney S (1993, April 1). Agonizing choices: People most needing transplantable livers now often miss out. *The Wall Street Journal*, pp A-1, A-8.

Medearis DN, Holmes LB (1989). On the use of anencephalic infants as organ donors. *N Engl J Med.* 321(6):391–393.

Morse JM, Solberg SM, Neander WL, et al (1990). Concepts of caring and caring as a concept. *Adv Nurs Sci.* 1:1–14.

Moss AH, Siegler M (1991). Should alcoholics compete equally for liver transplantation? *JAMA*. 265(10):1295–1298.

Mudge GH, Goldstein S, Addonizio LJ, et al (1993). Recipient guidelines/prioritization. *J Am Col Cardiol*. 22(1):21–31.

Nelson HL (1992). Against caring. *J Clin Ethics*. 3(1):8–15.

Nolan K (1990). The use of embryo or fetus in transplantation: What there is to lose. *Transplant Proc*. 22(3):1028–1029.

Norris MK (1991). Disparities for minorities in transplantation: The challenge to critical care nurses. *Heart Lung*. 20(4):419–420.

Norton DJ (1992). Clinical applications of brain death protocols. *J Neurosci Nurs*. 24 (6):354–358.

O'Connell DA (1991). Ethical implications of organ transplantation. *Crit Care Nurs Q*. 13 (4):1–7.

Pa. governor got rapid transplants by unique listing. (June 1992). *The Baltimore Sun*, p 19A.

Peabody JL, Emery JR, Ashwal S (1989). Experience with anencephalic infants as prospective organ donors. *N Engl J Med*. 321:344–350.

Pellegrino ED (1993). The metamorphosis of medical ethics: A 30-year retrospective. *JAMA*. 269 (9):1158–1162.

Pellegrino ED, Thomasma DC (1993). The link between virtues, principles, and duties. In: Pellegrino ED, Thomasma DD. *The Virtues in Medical Practice*. New York: Oxford University Press; 18–30.

Reitz NN, Callender CO (1993). Organ donation in the African-American population: A fresh perspective with a simple solution. *J Natl Med Assoc*. 85(5):353–358.

Russel S, Jacob RG (1993). Living-related organ donation: The donor's dilemma. *Patient Educ Counsel*. 21:89–99.

Sanders LM, Giudice L, Raffin TA (1993). Ethics of fetal tissue transplantation. *West J Med*. 159 (3):400–407.

Schwarz G, Litscher G, Pfurtscheller G, et al (1992). Brain death: Timing of apnea testing in primary brain stem lesion. *Intensive Care Med*. 18:315–316.

Shaw BW, Gordon RD, Iwatsuki S, Starzl TE (1985). Hepatic retransplantation. *Transplant Proc*. 17:264–271.

Shaw LR, Miller JD, Slutsky AS, et al (1991). Ethics of lung transplantation with live donors. *Lancet*. 338:678–681.

Shewmon DA, Capron AM, Warwick LLB, Peacock J, Schulman BL (1989). The use of Anencephalic infants as organ sources. *JAMA*. 261(12):1773–1781.

Singer PA, Siegler M, Whitington PF, et al (1989). Ethics of liver transplantation with living donors. *N Engl J Med*. 321(9):620–621.

Spital A, Spital M (1990). The ethics of liver transplantation from a living donor. *N Engl J Med*. 322(8):549–550.

Starzl TE, Demetris AJ, Trucco M (1993). Matching the black recipient. *Transplant Proc*. 25 (4):2450–2451.

Starzl TE, Van Thiel D, Tzakis AG, et al (1988). Orthotopic liver transplantation for alcoholic cirrhosis. *JAMA*. 260:2542–2544.

Stevenson LW, Warner SL, Hamilton MA, et al (1991). Distribution of donor hearts to maximize transplant candidate survival. *Circulation*. S-4(suppl II):II-352.

Truog RD, Fletcher JC (1989). Anencephalic newborns: Can organs be transplanted before brain death? *N Engl J Med*. 321(6):388–390.

Ubel PA, Arnold RM, Caplan AL (1993). Rationing failure: The ethical lessons of the retransplantation of scarce vital organs. *JAMA*. 270(20):2469–2474.

Valentine K (1989). Caring is more than kindness: Modeling its complexities. *J Nurs Admin* 11:28–34.

Veach RM (1993). The impending collapse of the whole-brain definitions of death. *Hastings Center Rep.* 23(4):18–24.

Watanabe T, Koyama I, Taguchi Y, et al (1992). Salvage of warm ischemic pancreas from non-heart-beating donors by a core-cooling method with cardiopulmonary bypass. *Transplant Proc.* 24(4):1331–1332.

Watson J (1988). *Nursing: Human Science and Human Care, a Theory of Nursing.* New York: National League for Nursing.

Wolicki KT (1994). Race and allocation of kidneys for transplantation. [Letter to the editor]. *JAMA.* 271(4):270.

Youngner SJ, Landefeld CS, Coulton CJ, Juknialis M (1989). Brain death and organ retrieval—a cross-sectional survey of knowledge and concepts among health professionals. *JAMA.* 261 (15):2205–2210.

Zabala MS, Herreros J, Gil OI, et al (1992). Dynamic cardiomyoplasty in a patient with end-stage cardiomyopathy. *Int J Artificial Organs.* 15(8):488–492.

13

The Legal Regulation
of Transplantation

Fred H. Cate

Human organ and tissue transplantation has historically been subject to little regulation. This is surprising given both the importance of legal issues, such as consent and the definition of death, to transplantation and the tendency of the government to regulate activities, such as transplantation, that involve public funding. The absence of regulation is changing rapidly, however; the federal government in particular is playing a larger role in transplantation. This chapter examines expanding state and federal regulation of clinical transplantation and the role of regulation in the future.

EARLY REGULATION BY STATES

State legislatures adopted the earliest regulatory measures to facilitate transplantation. As advances in medical technology made the widespread transplantation of hearts and kidneys feasible, these institutions sought to encourage the donation of organs and to provide a legal framework for organ donation and transplantation.

The Uniform Anatomical Gift Act

In the 1960s, the National Conference of Commissioners on Uniform State Laws began the process of formulating a model organ donation act. In 1968 the Conference adopted the Uniform Anatomical Gift Act (UAGA) and by 1972 some version of the UAGA had been adopted in every state and in the District of Columbia.

The UAGA provides that any person who is at least 18 years old may make or refuse to make an anatomical gift. When a decedent has neither executed an anatomical gift nor indicated opposition to such a gift, the UAGA provides that certain people may authorize a gift of all or part of the decedent's body. Those people must fall within one of six classes of individuals who the statute provides can authorize donation: spouse, adult son or daughter, parent, adult sibling, guardian, or any other person authorized or under obligation to dispose of the body. A person in one class may authorize the gift only if no member of a prior class is available at the time of death and there has not been actual notice of opposition by any member of the same or a prior class.

According to the UAGA, "[a]n anatomical gift that is not revoked by the donor before death is irrevocable and does not require the consent or concurrence of any person after the donor's death." The donation of a specific body part is not presumed to be a refusal to give other parts, should the next-of-kin consent. Similarly, the revocation by the donor of an anatomical gift is not presumed to be a refusal of the donor to make a subsequent anatomical gift, should the next-of-kin consent.

The UAGA defines who may receive human body part donations and for what purposes:

1. A hospital, physician, surgeon, or procurement organization for transplantation, therapy, medical or dental education, research, or advancement of medical or dental science
2. An accredited medical or dental school, college, or university for education, research, advancement of medical or dental science
3. A designated individual for transplantation or therapy needed by that individual.

The UAGA provides that human body parts may be donated through a will or by other document. If the gift is through a will, it becomes effective upon death and does not have to wait for probate. If the donation is by other document, most commonly a donor card, the document must be signed in the presence of two witness, but it does not have to be delivered during the lifetime of the donor. Under UAGA, a donor may, but is not obligated to, specify a recipient of the anatomical gift. The donor may revoke a gift at any time, even if notice of the intent to donate has been given to a specified donee. When donation does take place, the UAGA requires that the organ or tissue must be taken without unnecessary mutilation and that the decedent's body must be returned to the family or other person under obligation to dispose of the body.

Any person who acts in good faith in accordance with the terms of the UAGA or of any state's or nation's anatomical gift laws is not liable for civil damages or subject to criminal prosecution for his or her act.

In 1984, the Executive Committee of the National Conference of Commissioners on Uniform State Laws began the process of drafting a new UAGA in response to the increasingly visible inadequacies of the 1968 Act. In 1987 the Conference approved the new UAGA; the Act was approved by the American Bar Association (ABA) in 1988.

The 1987 UAGA contains an entirely new section, entitled "Routine Inquiry and Required Request; Search and Notification." This section requires that a patient, upon admission to hospital, be asked: "Are you an organ or tissue donor?" If the answer is positive, the hospital is to request a copy of the document of gift. If the answer is negative, the hospital, with the consent of the attending physician, "shall discuss with the patient the option to make or refuse to make an anatomical gift." In the event the patient is at or near death and there is no medical record that the patient has made or refused to make an anatomical gift, the hospital is directed to consider approaching the next-of-kin about donation of human body parts.

The section obligates law enforcement officers, firemen, paramedics, other emergency rescuers, and hospital personnel to "make a reasonable search for a document of gift or other information identifying the bearer as a donor or as an individual who has refused to make an anatomical gift." The penalty for failing to comply with the section is neither criminal nor civil liability, but rather "appropriate administrative sanctions." The first two states to pass required request legislation were New York and Oregon in 1985. By January 1992, 46 states and the District of Columbia had enacted some form of required request legislation.

The 1987 UAGA also forbids the purchase or sale of a body part for transplantation or therapy for "valuable consideration," "if removal of the part is intended to occur after the death of the decedent." The Act defines "valuable consideration," consistent with the National Organ Transplant Act, discussed later, to exclude "reasonable payment for the removal, processing, disposal, preservation, quality control, storage, transportation, or implantation of a part."

The new UAGA also simplifies the process by which a donor makes an anatomical gift and requires that the intentions of the donor be followed. For example, witnesses to the donor's signature on the gift document are no longer required.

Determination of Death

A second area for early state regulation of transplantation was the definition of death. For organs to be viable for transplantation, both circulation and respiration must have been maintained in the host body. Death must therefore be determined by the absence of all brain activity. Before 1970, no state had a statutory definition that permitted such a determination of death. Doctors and hospitals were at legal risk if they removed artificial life support systems from a body based on the absence of brain activity and lack of response to stimuli. The UAGA contained no definition of "brain death," because the drafters were concerned that the controversy surrounding the issue of brain death in the 1960s would delay passage of the Act by states. Instead, the UAGA merely provided that death shall be determined by a physician who will not participate in the removal or transplantation of any of the decedent's body parts.

In 1980, however, the National Conference of Commissioners on Uniform State Laws promulgated its Uniform Determination of Death Act (UDDA) and it was approved by both the ABA and the American Medical Association (AMA) the following year. Recommended by the President's Commission for the Study of Ethical Problems in Medicine and Biomedical and Behavioral Research, the UDDA provides:

> An individual who has sustained either (1) irreversible cessation of circulatory and respiratory functions, or (2) irreversible cessation of all functions of the entire brain, including the brain stem, is dead. A determination of death must be made in accordance with accepted medical standards.

Forty-four states and the District of Columbia have enacted statutes that recognize irreversible cessation of all brain function as an acceptable method for determining death for legal as well as medical purposes. Six states—Arizona, Massachusetts, Nebraska, New Jersey, New York, and Washington—recognize "brain death" by judicial determination rather than by statute.

THE GROWTH OF FEDERAL REGULATION

The National Organ Transplant Act

Cotton and Sandler observed in 1986 that "[t]he most striking aspect of the legal environment surrounding the procurement and transplantation of human organs is the virtual absence of federal regulation." The primary federal regulation stems from the National Organ Transplant Act (NOTA), which was passed by Congress and signed by President Reagan in 1984.

The NOTA was the product of a series of hearings conducted by House and Senate committees of the 98th Congress. In June 1983, Surgeon General Koop convened a workshop entitled "Solid Organ Procurement for Transplantation: Educating the Physician and the Public." Legislation regulating organ procurement and transplantation was subsequently introduced in both the House and the Senate. House and Senate conferees met in October of 1984 and produced a compromise measure that was enacted as the NOTA.

The NOTA has six principal provisions. The Act:

1. Established a 25-member task force on Organ Procurement and Transplantation, responsible for examining a broad range of "medical, legal, ethical, economic, and social issues presented by human organ procurement and transplantation"
2. Required the Secretary of Health and Human Services to convene a conference on the feasibility of establishing a national registry of voluntary bone marrow donors
3. Established the Division of Organ Transplantation
4. Empowered the Secretary to make grants for the planning, establishment, initial operation, and expansion of organ procurement organizations (OPOs)
5. Required the Secretary to contract for an Organ Procurement and Transplantation Network (OPTN)
6. Prohibited the purchase and sale of human organs.

The latter four requirements have proved to be of the most lasting consequence.

Division of Organ Transplantation

The NOTA mandated the establishment of "an identifiable administrative unit in the Public Health Service" to administer the Act, coordinate organ procurement activities, encourage organ donation, and report to Congress about the status of organ procurement and transplantation. The Secretary of Health and Human Services responded by creating the Division of Organ Transplantation. Today the Division is responsible for the OPTN and Scientific Registry contracts and grants to OPOs. The two branches of the Division of Organ Transplantation—the Operations and Analysis Branch and the Public and Professional Education Branch—have expanded their public, news media, and professional education activities, oversight of both the OPTN and the Scientific Registry, and exploration of current issues in transplantation, such as participation by minority communities and better coordination among organ and tissue organizations.

Organ Procurement Organizations

The NOTA enshrined OPOs as the backbone of the organ procurement and distribution system. First established in a 1968 pilot program in Boston and Los Angeles, OPOs flourished with the establishment of the End-Stage Renal Disease Program of the federal government, through which federal funds became available for kidney procurement and distribution. The NOTA authorized $25 million for grants to "qualified" OPOs. The Health Resources and Services Administration has awarded grants each year, beginning in 1986. Between the End-Stage Renal Disease Program and the OPO grant program, OPOs, although private organizations, receive substantial federal funding. Because of this, OPOs have become increasingly subject to federal regulations. In the Omnibus Budget Reconciliation Act of 1986, Congress expanded federal regulation of OPOs by subjecting all OPOs to the authority of the Secretary of Health and Human Services and requiring all OPOs, as a condition of participating in Medicare, to be members of, and agree to abide by the rules of, the OPTN.

Organ Procurement and Transplantation Network

In a compromise provision of the NOTA, Congress opted for the establishment of a private organization to maintain the list of people waiting for organs. Whereas delegating that task to a government entity would likely have guaranteed federal oversight of organ procurement and distribution generally, the Reagan administration objected to any measure that might produce more government bureaucracy. Congress therefore established the OPTN as a private monopoly, funded by taxpayer dollars and user fees, and required that it be operated only by organizations working exclusively in transplantation.

According to the Act, the OPTN is designed to establish a national list of people who need organs and a national computer system to match available organs with patients on that list. The Network also is to maintain a 24-hour telephone service to assist with the matching process, adopt standards of quality for the acquisition and transportation of donated organs, and collect and distribute information on organ donation and transplantation. The NOTA provided that no more than $2 million per fiscal year be spent to support the Network.

On September 30, 1986, the Secretary awarded a $379,000 1-year contract for the Network to the United Network for Organ Sharing (UNOS). On September 30, 1987, the contract was renewed for 3 years, in the amount of $1.1 million for fiscal year 1987, $1.2 million for fiscal year 1988, and approximately $1.5 million for fiscal year

1989. The contract was renewed again for 3 years on September 30, 1990. Additional funds for operation of the Network are raised by charging waiting list registration fees.

In the Transplant Amendments Act of 1990, Congress expanded the function of the Network and the types of organizations who could participate in its operation. For example, the operator of the Network is no longer required to be an organization "which is not engaged in any activity unrelated to organ procurement," but instead may be any organization "that has expertise in organ procurement and transplantation." The Act also requires the Network to assist in the nationwide and equitable distribution of organs, work actively to increase the supply of organs, and report annually to the Department of Health and Human Services on the comparative costs and patient outcomes at each transplant center.

The Omnibus Budget Reconciliation Act of 1986 required all hospitals that perform transplants, as a condition of participation in Medicare and Medicaid (and OPOs, as discussed earlier) to be members of, and agree to abide by the rules of, the OPTN. As a result of this development, the question was raised whether Congress' provision for the required membership of transplant centers and OPOs in the private OPTN (and the required compliance by these entities with the Network's rules) vested in the OPTN federal regulatory power. In the Health Omnibus Programs Extension of 1988, Congress amended Section 372 of the NOTA to provide that the Secretary of Health and Human Services must establish procedures for receiving and evaluating comments from the public on the manner in which the Network is carrying out its statutory responsibilities. In September 1989, Acting Surgeon General James Mason notified Robert Corry, then President of UNOS, that UNOS rules and sanctions would be subject to approval by the Department of Health and Human Services.

DOT renewed the OPTN contract with UNOS for 3 years beginning September 30, 1993. The new OPTN contract reimburses only 15 percent—$2.37 million over 3 years—of the cost of operating the network; other funds are raised through fees charged to patients for being registered on the organ waiting lists, although these are paid primarily by the Health Care Financing Administration. The contract contains new, detailed requirements concerning the operation of the OPTN and its relation with the federal government. For example, the contract mandates establishment of a data committee, random waiting list audits, 24-hour electronic access to UNOS policies and bylaws and electronic access for the Health Resources and Services Administration to OPTN data, a communications plan, and professional education activities that target trauma physicians and surgeons, emergency room nurses, and coroners and medical examiners. The contract also imposes limits on registration fees for the computer waiting lists.

Prohibition on Sale

The final important provision of the NOTA was the prohibition on buying or selling organs for "valuable consideration." The term "valuable consideration" is defined to exclude

> the reasonable payments associated with the removal, transportation, implantation, processing, preservation, quality control, and storage of a human

organ or the expenses of travel, housing, and lost wages incurred by the
donor of a human organ in connection with the donation of the organ.

Congress was apparently galvanized into action banning the sale of human organs
and tissues in response to a plan by H. Barry Jacobs, who established a company in
Virginia to broker human kidneys. According to press reports, Jacobs, whose license
to practice medicine had been revoked in 1977 after a mail-fraud conviction involving Medicare and Medicaid reimbursement, intended to broker kidneys from healthy,
living donors at an agreed-upon price, to which Jacobs would add $2000 to $5000 for
his services. Jacobs testified before Congress that he also intended to bring Third
World indigents to the United States so that they could sell their kidneys. Congress responded by banning the sale of human organs and tissues.

This provision acts as a positive prohibition on the use of financial incentives to
encourage organ donation, even in the face of a dramatic shortage of organs and increasing waiting lists. It was adopted without study of the possible consequences and
without justification for why financial incentives should be excluded from this one
area of medical practice. Moreover, the text of the prohibition allows everyone involved in the transplant process to be paid except for the donor and his or her family. The government's determination not to allow payment for organs and tissues has
restricted the development of any type of financial incentive for enhancing the supply of organs, despite the widely recognized fact that the supply of transplantable organs falls far short of the need.

Perhaps the most notable feature of the NOTA is what it does not do. Given the
wealth of regulation that surrounds the dispensing of prescription drugs or the provision of medical care, the 1984 NOTA stands in stark contrast with its bare skeletal
nature, the relatively small funding authorized to carry out its programs, and the Con-
gressional willingness evidenced by the NOTA to depend on private industry to stan-
dardize and regulate organ procurement, distribution, and transplantation.

Pending Organ Transplant Legislation and Regulations

Bills to reauthorize the NOTA have been pending in both House and Senate for almost
a year. Although their precise terms differ, the two most important bills would substantially increase federal regulation of organ transplantation. For example, the bills
would require the creation of a single national list for United States citizens and permanent residents and a single national list for foreign nationals. The OPTN would no
longer be free to allocate organs based on the consensus of medical professionals. Similarly, the bills would require each OPO to maintain a single waiting list. The bills
would centralize the waiting lists for organs and the lists of potential bone marrow
donors. The pending legislation is likely to require the Secretary of Health and Human
Services to issue the comprehensive regulations governing organ procurement and
distribution promised in 1989. The pending legislation subjects OPTN user fees to approval by the Secretary. The bills would also initiate a General Accounting Office investigation into procurement and distribution practices.

Whereas the NOTA focused on transplant-related institutions (the OPTN, OPOs,
transplanting hospitals), the pending legislation focuses instead on individuals in-

volved in the transplant process as donors, people on the waiting list, recipients, and their families. For example, the bills would reduce the OPTN board of directors from 32 to 21 members and require that at least one-third of both the UNOS board and OPO boards be recipients, recipient families, donor families, people waiting for organs, and their families.

Tissue Regulations and Pending Legislation

This same trend of greater government involvement is also reflected in tissue regulation. Initially, the United States Food and Drug Administration (FDA) avoided announcing a policy on tissue and then, in 1987, stated that the agency was satisfied to use its medical device regulatory authority to passively monitor tissue banking and transplantation. However, after incidents involving the transmission of infectious diseases through transplants, Congress, the FDA, and the Centers for Disease Control and Prevention are taking new interest in tissue regulation.

The FDA issued interim rules on December 14, 1993, that regulate the sale of tissues for transplant. The rules, which took effect immediately, require testing of tissues, donor screening for disease risk factors, and give the FDA the authority to recall tissues that do not meet quality control standards. The agency has promised future regulations to require all groups that handle tissue to register with the government, set standards for obtaining consent for tissue donation, and establish standards and enforcement mechanisms for ensuring tissue quality. Legislation to regulate human tissue banks and banking practices is currently pending in both the Senate and the House of Representatives.

THE ROLE OF LAW IN TRANSPLANTATION

The Failure of Transplantation

Clinical transplantation has been influenced and in many places definitively guided by the resolution of legal issues. For example, cadaveric transplantation was not feasible as a practical treatment until the concept of defining death by absence of brain function was adopted into law. Similarly, the UAGA is essential to obtaining consent for organ donation in every state and the District of Columbia. Without these laws, the more than 150,000 organ transplants performed in the United States would have been impossible.

It is ironic that law also plays a role in the failings of transplantation. Despite impressive successes, transplantation has been sharply curtailed by a shortage of donated organs and tissues. The number of people who either die of conditions for which transplantation is indicated or are maintained on suboptimal therapies in the absence of a transplant, far exceeds the number of transplants performed. For example, in 1990, 18,592 people were in need of a kidney (only half received one); 40,959 needed a heart (only 1 in 20 received one); 14,751 needed a liver (only 1 in 5 received one); 4108 needed a pancreas (only 1 in 8 received one); and 4618 needed a combination heart-lung transplant (fewer than 1 in 85 received one) (Evans, 1991).

Not all people who would benefit from a transplant are actually on the waiting list. Nonetheless, the number of registrations on the national list both far exceeds the current supply and is increasing. As of December 31, 1993, there were 24,973 registrations for a kidney; 2834 for a heart; 2997 for a liver; 1106 for a pancreas or combination kidney-pancreas transplant; 1240 for a lung; and 202 for a combination heart-lung transplant. In short, the demand for organs is far outstripping the supply, and the gap is widening; more than 33,000 people are on the waiting list. In the case of life-saving organs such as hearts, this means that one-third or more of patients waiting die before an organ is found. Every 4 hours a person dies while waiting.

The Response of the Legal System

The legal regime governing transplantation is at least partly to blame. In the case of organ donation, transplant law offers no incentives for people to donate or for health professionals and institutions to facilitate donation. On the contrary, the law largely impedes donation. For example, despite overwhelming public support for transplantation, current law assumes that no one wishes to donate organs or tissues upon death. According to a 1990 Gallup poll, 94% of Americans report having heard or read about organ transplants; 84% believe that transplants are successful in prolonging and improving the quality of life; and 89% say they are likely to honor the request of a loved one that his or her organs be donated after that person's death (Gallup Organization, 1990). Still, the law presumes an unwillingness to donate.

The law provides two avenues around this presumption. First, a person may sign a donor card or otherwise indicate willingness to donate. There are, however, many impediments to a donor card's having any effect. Most important, even if a valid donor card is found, medical professionals and hospitals fear professional criticism and legal liability if they procure organs against the wishes of the next-of-kin. Donor cards are legally binding in 48 states (Florida and New York grant certain family members the right to veto the deceased's decision to donate organs), and health professionals who act on them are immune from liability under the UAGA in every state, but the cards have proved useless unless next-of-kin approve the donation (Developments, 1990).

The second and by far more important means to obtain consent is from next-of-kin, who, under state and federal required request and routine inquiry laws, must be approached about organ donation in medically appropriate situations. These laws, however, have proved ineffective. One study found that 30% of the families of medically appropriate potential donors were never asked to donate, despite the legal obligation that they be asked (Association of Organ Procurement Organizations, 1989). Another study found that 47% of medically suitable patients were "overlooked" by hospital personnel (Ross et al, 1990). To date, there is no reported case of a government agency seeking to enforce routine inquiry or required request laws.

The law thus presumes that a person does not want to donate and then minimizes the likelihood that a donor's legally expressed desire to donate will be respected. Laws that encourage transplantation, such as "required request" statutes, frequently receive inadequate resources to assure their implementation and little if any enforcement. In short, the legal framework is a deterrent to donation.

Legal Issues in the Future

The legal system is not without options for addressing some of the problems in transplantation to which it has contributed. Alternatives to the voluntary consent and required request systems are currently being tried in various states and foreign countries. Examples are "presumed consent," under which the law would presume that the decedent did want to donate human body parts, or the use of financial incentives, currently prohibited by the NOTA. Important medical advances may help reduce the shortage of organs. Examples are improvements in measuring the absence of brain activity to determine death; the use of living donors, both related and unrelated; xenotransplantation—the use of animal organs and cells; the transplantation of organ segments; and the removal of kidneys from cadaveric donors in which the hearts are not beating. Each of these advances, like transplantation itself, raises serious legal issues. The question is whether there is sufficient political will to investigate and, when appropriate, implement those alternatives and to alter when necessary the existing legal structure to make it possible to do so.

The most important role for law, however, is guaranteeing the integrity of the organ procurement, distribution, and transplantation system. If transplantation is to be truly successful, the public—as citizens and as potential donors—must have confidence in the fairness and accuracy of the systems that regulate transplantation in this country. A Caucasian on the kidney waiting list has a 1 in 6 chance of receiving a transplant within 1 year of being placed on the list. An African American has a 1 in 13 chance. On average, African Americans wait twice as long as Caucasians. The organ distribution system does not appear to be fair. Not surprisingly, studies show that African Americans and other minorities are far less likely than Caucasians to donate (Perez et al, 1988).

Similarly, no one is placed on the national waiting list for an organ unless he or she demonstrates the ability to pay for transplantation—the so-called green screen. Transplants are very expensive, in many cases more than $100,000. In addition, permanent maintenance on immunosuppressive drugs and other medical care associated with the transplant may cost between $17,000 and $68,000 annually (Evans, 1991). According to Evans, organ acquisition charges are increasing far above inflation (64% for hearts and 62% for livers since 1985) and vary widely ($11,289 to $24,161 for a kidney). The efficiency of OPOs in obtaining organs varies as well; OPOs obtain organs from 25–90% of potential donors. "Some transplant hospitals routinely mark up by as much as 200 percent the charges that are billed by organ procurement organizations" (Evans, 1993).

Although Medicare pays for most kidney transplants and Medicare, Medicaid, and private insurers now cover most other transplants, an estimated 60 million people do not have insurance that covers transplants. They can give organs and tissues but are virtually ineligible to receive them. Approximately 37 million Americans have no effective access to health care. Nonetheless, although they are denied access to transplantation and even to basic health services, we do not hesitate to ask for their organs. "It becomes," in the words of Harvard immunologist Terry Strom, "the rich buying health at the expense of the poor" (Swedlow & Cate, 1990). The law has an important role to play in addressing these inequities, both perceived and real, in the transplant system.

CONCLUSION

The attitude of both state and federal governments toward transplantation could aptly be described as schizophrenic. The UAGA and the UDDA laid the essential groundwork for widespread clinical transplantation. Yet states have resisted enforcing the requirements contained in these laws, such as routine inquiry and required request. Similarly, Congress' establishment of the national OPTN and of OPOs served vital needs in the procurement and distribution of organs yet reflected an apparent reluctance to commit adequate government resources or funds to these important tasks. Since passage of the NOTA in 1984, Congress and the Department of Health and Human Services have steadily increased the regulatory mandate of the OPTN and regulation of the OPTN, OPOs, and transplanting hospitals, while waiting more than 4 years (as of this writing) to actually issue the regulations with which transplant-related organizations must comply. Congress has emphasized consensus decision-making and the important role of patients, donors, and their families while pushing for increased centralization.

As was the case more than 20 years ago when lawmakers were debating the legal definition of death and the ways in which a person could consent to donation, transplantation today is confronted with issues that require, at least in part, a regulatory response. Administering the transplant system fairly and efficiently, allocating scarce organs, and increasing the supply of organs for transplantation all urgently demand the attention of lawmakers and regulators. In a very real sense, transplantation today is constrained not by medical issues but by legal ones, and their resolution is essential to save lives and reduce human suffering.

REFERENCES

Association of Organ Procurement Organizations (1989). OPO Directors Survey.

Cotton R, Sandler A (1986). The regulation of organ procurement and transplantation in the United States. *Leg Med.* 7:55.

Developments—Medical Technology and the Law (1990). *Harvard Law Rev.* 103:1520.

Evans R (1991). *Executive Summary: The National Cooperative Transplantation Study*. BHARC-100-91-020. Seattle: Battelle-Seattle Research Center, June.

Evans R (1993). Organ procurement expenditures and the role of financial incentives. *JAMA*. 269:3113.

Gallup Organization (1990). *The U.S. public's attitudes toward organ transplants/organ donation*. Princeton: The Gallup Organization.

Health Omnibus Programs Extension of 1988. Pub. L. No. 100-607, 102 Stat. 3048, § 403 (codified at 42 U.S.C.A. §§ 273-274g [West 1991]).

Human Tissue Intended for Transplantation. 58 Fed. Reg. 65,514 (HHS, PHS, FDA Dec. 14, 1993) (interim rule).

Human Tissue for Transplantation Act of 1993 (S. 1706). 103rd Cong., 1st Sess., 139 Cong. Rec. S16,432 (1993).

Human Tissue for Transplantation Act of 1993 (H.R. 3547). 103rd Cong., 1st Sess., 139 Cong. Rec. H10,300 (1993).

National Organ Transplant Act. Pub. L. No. 98-507, 98 Stat. 2339 (1984) (codified at 42 U.S.C.A. §§ 273-274g [West 1991]).

Omnibus Budget Reconciliation Act of 1986. Pub. L. No. 99-509, 100 Stat. 1874, § 9318 (codified at 42 U.S.C.A. §§ 273-74, 1320b-8 [West 1991]).

Organ and Bone Marrow Transplantation Amendments of 1993 (H.R. 2659). 103rd Cong., 1st Sess., 139 Cong. Rec. H4756 (1993).

Organ Transplant Program Reauthorization Act of 1993 (S. 1597). 103rd Cong., 1st Sess., 139 Cong. Rec. S14,529 (1993).

Perez, et al (1988). Organ donation in three major American cities with large Latino and black populations. *Transplantation*. 46:557.

Ross, Nathan, O'Malley (1990). Impact of a required request law on vital organ procurement. *J Trauma*. 30:820.

Social Security Amendments of 1972. Pub. L. No. 92-603, 86 Stat. 1329, § 299I (codified at 42 U.S.C.A. §§ 426[e]-[g] [West 1991]).

Swedlow J, Cate F (1990). Why transplants don't happen. *Atlantic* xx:99.

Transplant Amendments Act of 1990. Pub. L. No. 101-616, 104 Stat. 3279, §§ 201-207 (codified at 42 U.S.C.A. §§ 273-274g [West 1991]).

National Conference of Commissioners on Uniform State Laws, Uniform Anatomical Gift Act (1987).

National Conference of Commissioners on Uniform State Laws, Uniform Determination of Death Act (1980).

14

Nursing Research in Transplantation

Marie T. Nolan

Now is an exciting time for nurses in the field of transplantation. Although they have collaborated in multidisciplinary studies since the inception of this field, nurses have only recently begun to establish a scientific base for practice in transplantation care. By examining recent nursing research findings, nurses gain perspective on their unique contributions to the field of transplantation and what challenges lie ahead. The purpose of this chapter is to provide an overview of recent nursing research in transplantation and to outline future challenges. Strategies for conducting research are presented.

OVERVIEW OF NURSING RESEARCH IN TRANSPLANTATION

An automated search of The Nursing and Allied Health (CINAHL) database was conducted to retrieve recent research in transplantation nursing. This database includes material related to nursing and allied health disciplines from more than 900 journals. To limit the review to recent research, only the literature from 1989 to the present was included. Forty-three studies fell into one of five categories: physiologic needs, patient psychosocial needs, family psychosocial needs, organ procurement issues, and ethical issues. Table 14-1 lists the number of studies undertaken within each category. Together, the categories of patient psychosocial needs and family psychosocial needs accounted for 26 articles, or more than half of the nursing studies published. Table 14-2 lists the journals in which the studies appeared. Three journals accounted for the majority of the studies published: *Heart & Lung, ANNA Journal,* and *Oncology Nursing Forum.*

TABLE 14–1. GROUPING OF TOPIC AREAS

Topic Areas	No. of Articles
Patient Psychosocial Needs	19
Quality of life	
Stress and coping	
Hope	
Family Psychosocial Needs	7
Stress and coping	
Informational needs	
Physiologic Needs	9
Symptom distress	
Infection prevention	
Rejection	
Weight control	
Blood transfusion	
Weight gain	
Organ Procurement Issues	6
Nursing attitude, knowledge	
Family attitude, knowledge	
Ethical Issues	2
Anencephalic infant donors	
Do not resuscitate orders	
Total Number of Articles	43

Summaries of the nursing research articles have been organized by the type of transplantation studied. This should enable the reader to obtain a quick overview of the research in a particular area of transplantation nursing.

Physiologic Needs

Physical issues in transplantation were the subject of nine studies. Four of the studies dealt with heart-transplant patients; one dealt with liver transplantation; and four dealt with bone marrow transplantation.

Heart Transplantation. Symptom distress in 175 heart-transplant candidates was described by Grady and associates (1992). The most frequent and distressing symptoms cited were tiredness, difficulty breathing, difficulty sleeping, and generalized weakness. Higher symptom distress was related to lower life satisfaction and quality of life and greater functional disability. The second study described nursing inter-

TABLE 14–2. PERCENTAGE OF TRANSPLANTATION NURSING RESEARCH STUDIES BY JOURNAL APPEARANCE (n = 43)

Journal	n	Percent
Heart & Lung	9	21
ANNA Journal	8	19
Oncology Nursing Forum	6	14
Cancer Nursing	3	7
Journal of Pediatric Nursing	2	15
Other	15	35

ventions used to prevent infection in patients who have undergone heart transplantation (Lange et al, 1992). The investigators surveyed 68 transplant centers and found a great diversity in infection control practices. Older and larger transplant programs tended to use fewer precautions. Survival rates were not related to the number of precautions used.

In the third study, the effectiveness of the drug muromonab-CD3 in reversing acute rejection was reported in a study of 10 cardiac transplant patients (Rogers et al, 1989). Investigators found that the drug reversed the rejection episodes without major side effects. The fourth and final physiologic study described weight changes in 91 patients who had undergone heart transplantation. Only 37% of the patients weighed more after transplantation than before transplantation. It was surprising that no difference was found between patients who gained weight and patients who did not gain weight in terms of fat intake and exercise (Rubin et al, 1991).

Liver Transplantation. One physiologic study focused on patients who had undergone liver transplantation (Vehrenkamp et al, 1992). In this study, investigators retrospectively reviewed 263 adult patients to determine the relation of prothrombin time (PT) and activated partial thromboplastin time (APTT) to the amount of blood transfused after reperfusion of the liver. They found a positive relation between PT and the amount of blood transfused. The investigators provide recommendations regarding transfusion after liver transplantation.

Bone Marrow Transplantation. Four physiologic studies focused on recipients of bone marrow transplants. A comparison of perceived symptoms of patients undergoing bone marrow transplantation and the nurses caring for them was the focus of the first study (Larson et al, 1993). Thirty patients and 28 nurses responded to questions about symptom distress. Patients perceived significantly more distress from their symptoms than their nurses perceived that they were experiencing. In the second study, 78 nurses were surveyed regarding their knowledge of graft-versus-host disease (GVHD). Nurses who read journal articles and attended continuing education programs had more knowledge than those who did not engage in these activities

(Copel & Smith, 1989). In the third study, 17 patients were asked about their pain and psychologic distress. Patients reported low-grade, persistent pain along with mild to moderate anxiety and depression (Gaston-Johansson et al, 1992). In the fourth study, the relation of oral mucositis to medical treatment variables was studied in 20 patients (Zerbe et al, 1992). Investigators reported that patients who had received total body irradiation experienced more severe mucositis than patients who received the chemotherapeutic agent busulfan. The onset of mucositis occurred between day 4 and day 8 after transplantation, the peak severity occurring between day 5 and day 12 after transplantation.

Patient Psychosocial Needs

Studies that examined patient psychosocial needs dealt with how patients coped with the stress of transplantation and with their quality of life after transplantation.

Heart Transplantation. In a study of the quality of life of 41 patients who were awaiting heart transplantation, Muirhead and associates (1992) found patients experienced a moderate dissatisfaction with their quality of life. In spite of this dissatisfaction, the investigators found that patients maintained a positive psychologic and social adjustment.

The stress of the pretransplantation period was described in a retrospective study of three heart-transplant patients (Porter et al, 1991). Porter and associates found that the most common stressors were fear of financial burdens, deteriorating health, loss of control, and receiving erroneous signals on the pager meant to alert the patient that a donor had been found. The investigators noted, however, that it was difficult to keep the patients focused on the stressors of the waiting period, because at the time of the interview, they were enmeshed in the stressors of the posttransplant period. Subsequently, these investigators did a prospective study of pretransplantation stress and coping among 39 cardiac transplantation patients who were on the waiting list for transplantation at the time they were interviewed. The three most common stressors identified by these patients were recognition that their heart disease was terminal, discovery of the need for heart transplantation, and knowing that they caused family members to worry. Patients used optimistic coping strategies such as thinking positive and having a sense of humor (Porter et al, 1994).

Nursing interventions patients perceived to be helpful were studied in 175 patients undergoing heart transplantation (Grady et al, 1993). Provision of information, self-care teaching, and emotionally supportive interventions were the types of interventions most valued by patients. The specific interventions deemed most helpful were explanation of the reasons for tests, the evaluation process for heart transplantation, and the heart transplant itself.

The quality of life of patients who had undergone heart transplantation 6 months previously was compared with the quality of life of a similar group of cardiac patients who had not undergone transplantation and were being treated medically (Walden et al, 1989). Both groups were similar in psychosocial functioning: patients who received medical therapy reported greater dysfunction in social activities. There were no differences in exercise tolerance and employment.

In another study of the psychologic functioning of cardiac patients, the pretransplant status of 44 patients was compared with their status 6 months after transplantation (Bohachick et al, 1992). Most patients showed improvement in emotional, social, sexual, and job functioning. However, 25% of the patients experienced deterioration in psychosocial adjustment during this time period.

Renal Transplantation. Pretransplant stressors among 14 renal-transplant patients were described in a retrospective study by Weems and Patterson (1989). Two common feelings patients expressed were uncertainty and ambivalence. Patients were uncertain about whether or when they would receive a kidney and were ambivalent about whether a transplant would improve their quality of life. In another study of pretransplantation perceptions, Hathaway and associates (1990) interviewed 57 renal-transplant recipients and their nurses. Patients and nurses viewed transplantation as a way of attaining a higher quality of life, but nurses anticipated more positive in addition to negative changes than did the patients.

An instrument to identify the stressors experienced by renal-transplant patients in the early postoperative period was described by Hayward and colleagues (1989). Sixty patients who had undergone renal transplantation were asked to rate the severity of 44 possible stressors. The possibility of rejection was rated as the most stressful factor. Similar concerns were expressed by renal-transplant patients in another study (White et al, 1990). Uncertainty about whether the transplant would be a success was one of the most stressful factors identified in this group.

Changes in the quality of life of 48 renal-transplant patients 6 and 12 months after the operation were described by Hathaway and associates. Investigators found that patients experienced favorable quality-of-life changes. Nevertheless, when employment was studied in another group of renal-transplant patients, the outcome was not as favorable (McNatt & White, 1992). Of the 83 patients studied, 63% reported working full or part time after transplantation. Variables found to be positively related to being employed after transplantation were having a job before transplantation, viewing one's health as good, and the absence of diabetes.

Liver Transplantation. Stress and coping after transplantation were studied in liver-transplant patients (Thomas, 1993a; Thomas, 1993b). A group of liver-transplant patients sought to gain control over their illness and treatment by adjusting the times of their immunosuppressive medications. Although this placed them at risk for rejection, patients described this action as a method of gaining control (Thomas, 1993a). Another group of liver-transplant patients reported that returning to work was a great source of stress. They feared that by returning to work they might lose both disability and health insurance benefits (Thomas, 1993b).

Hicks and colleagues (1992) found no difference in the quality of life of patients 1 year after liver transplantation when compared with the quality of life of patients 2 years after liver transplantation. High levels of life satisfaction were noted in both groups, suggesting that patients were coping well with their posttransplant limitations.

The quality of life of 20 school-age children after liver transplantation was described by Zamberlan (1992). All children were in school and perceived their quality of life as good or excellent. Some problems with self-concept and cognitive delays were identified, but the investigator noted that further study would be required to explore to what extent these problems were associated with having a chronic illness, the transplant experience, and the posttransplant medications.

Bone Marrow Transplantation. Mixed feelings about undergoing transplantation were described by Ersek (1992) in her study of 20 leukemia patients facing bone marrow transplantation. Ersek recounted how these patients maintained a sense of hope, even while acknowledging the threats of their illness and its treatment. Steeves (1992) found that the dependency experienced in prolonged hospitalization was stressful for a group of patients undergoing bone marrow transplantation. These patients described the need to renegotiate their social position as they interacted with the staff caring for them. Calculating the odds of recovery and having a belief in God were two coping methods used in facing their dependency.

Two studies examined the quality of life of patients after bone marrow transplantation. When Ferrell and associates (1992) asked 119 of these patients how transplantation had affected their quality of life, several concerns emerged. Experiencing side effects of the treatment such as weakness and hair loss was cited as stressful. Limiting work activities was another negative factor identified. Positive effects of transplantation also were described; these included an increase in spirituality and an increased appreciation for life. Similarly, most of the 24 bone marrow transplantation patients Belic (1992) studied, rated their quality of life as acceptable. Many patients reported that having faced a life-threatening illness they were now leading more meaningful lives.

Family Psychosocial Needs

Heart Transplantation. The impact of the transplant experience on the family was the focus of a classic study by Mishel and Murdaugh (1987). These investigators labeled the process of family adjustment to heart transplantation as "redesigning the dream." Working with 20 patients, the investigators identified three phases in the adjustment process: immersion, passage, and negotiation. During the first phase, immersion, which occurs before transplantation, the family member is immersed in the needs of the transplant patient. New roles previously belonging to the patient, such as managing family finances, may be taken on by the family member. After the operation, in the passage phase, the family member becomes focused on adjusting to the changes in the health of the patient and gradually realizes that whereas the patient's quality of life may have improved, a return to the preillness state of health is impossible. During the negotiation phase, the family member relinquishes some of the roles taken on during the immersion phase.

A study of family stress and coping during the pretransplantation phase included 38 family members who had loved ones on the waiting list for heart transplantation (Nolan et al, 1992). Family members reported moderate and low levels of stress and reported using positive coping strategies such as facing problems head on and seeking the support of friends. The investigators concluded that the high number of coping strategies used and the low levels of stress reported by family members indicated that the strategies used were effective in mediating the stress. They also noted that the family members' preference for active rather than passive coping strategies may have been reflective of the transplant selection criteria that included a supportive, dependable family.

The impact of heart transplantation on the spouse's life was the focus of a study by Buse and Pieper (1990). Studying 26 wives and 4 husbands, the investigators found that spouses viewed the pretransplant experience more negatively than the post-transplant experience. Fear of loss of spouse was identified as one of the most important factors in the pretransplant period, whereas the need to learn more about transplantation was an important factor in the posttransplant period.

Finally, the impact of pediatric heart transplantation on parents was described by Uzark and Crowley (1989). The investigators interviewed parents of 10 children who had undergone heart transplantation 3 to 24 months after the operation. The most important stressors identified by the parents were the uncertainty of the child's future health and well-being, role strain, social isolation, and financial burdens.

Liver Transplantation.   Only one study described the impact of liver transplantation on the family. Weichler (1990) interviewed 8 mothers 2 to 3 weeks after their child's liver transplant. The mothers were asked to describe what type of information was valuable to them. They identified knowledge of liver laboratory values, indications of rejection and infection, and ways to support their child emotionally as the information of greatest importance to them.

Renal Transplantation.   The information needs of parents following their child's renal or liver transplant was studied by Weichler (1993). Parents ranked the importance of information needed before and after transplantation. Information about rejection was the most important information needed in the pretransplant phase. The need to be kept well informed about the child's progress was the most important information during the operative phase of transplantation. Knowing how the organ was functioning was most important during the intensive care unit (ICU) phase. Learning the signs and symptoms of rejection was most important during the recovery phase. When asked how well they had been prepared for the transplantation experience, all subjects indicated that they would have preferred more information in advance about transplantation. Stressors identified by family members of renal transplant patients in the first 6 months after transplantation were described by Voepel-Lewis and associates (1990). Health-related factors were the most stressful, and work-related factors were the least stressful.

Organ Procurement Issues

Seven studies reviewed nurses' attitudes toward organ procurement or the role of the nurse in organ procurement. Kiberd and Kiberd (1992) surveyed 102 nurses about their feelings about organ donation. Perceived transplant success and support for organ procurement were related to the nurse's decision to sign a donor card or driver's license indicating consent to be an organ donor. Nurses in specialties such as dialysis, who were familiar with the benefits of transplantation, perceived transplantation as successful and were more likely to report signing an organ card than nurses in other areas. In a similar study, Bidigare and Oermann (1991) surveyed 60 nurses about their attitudes and knowledge of organ procurement. A positive attitude toward donation and comfort with obtaining consent to donate were positively related to knowledge of organ procurement.

The knowledge of 50 pediatric nurses concerning organ procurement was measured by Martin (1993). The investigator gave the nurses three case studies and asked them to determine if the child in each case was a potential organ donor. Most of the nurses had a positive attitude toward donation, but anencephalic infants were incorrectly identified as donors by 86% of the nurses. Martin emphasized the need for further education about organ donation. Knowledge of donor criteria was also noted to be related to the setting in which a nurse practices. Stoeckle (1990) surveyed 44 nurses. Some of the nurses were from hospitals with trauma centers and others were from hospitals without trauma centers. Nurses from hospitals with trauma centers demonstrated greater knowledge concerning the identification and management of organ donors than nurses from hospitals without trauma centers.

Exposure of nurses to education regarding organ donation was noted to be related to the likelihood of the nurse to approach a family about donation. Driscoll (1992) questioned 69 critical care nurses about their experiences approaching potential donor families. She also noted that attitudes toward donation were positively related to years of critical care experience.

Knowledge was also noted to be a factor in identifying potential organ donors in a study of 969 registered nurses in New Jersey and Pennsylvania (Adams et al, 1993). Pennsylvania nurses were more knowledgeable than New Jersey nurses about organ procurement and were more frequently involved in organ procurement. Investigators concluded that providing nurses with education about organ procurement could increase the number of organ donors in an institution.

Ethical Issues

Because patients who have consented to transplantation have indicated a wish to pursue an aggressive type of therapy, it is sometimes difficult to decide when to discontinue treatment. A study of variables involved when instituting a do-not-resuscitate (DNR) order for patients undergoing bone marrow transplantation was described by Kern and associates (1992). A retrospective review was conducted of the medical records for 40 patients who had died while being treated in a transplantation unit. Six patients did not have a DNR order at the time of death and 34 patients did have a DNR order at the time of death. Twenty-six percent of those with a DNR order had issued it themselves, whereas the other patients had a DNR order signed by a family member. Patients who died without a DNR order had life-threatening complications early in the course of transplantation. Investigators suggested that for this group of patients, issuing a DNR order may have been considered inappropriate because complications may have been viewed as reversible and death may not have been anticipated.

The use of anencephalic infants as donors has been rejected in the United States. However, Loma Linda Medical Center in California briefly sponsored a program to maintain these infants on ventilator support until whole-brain death could be established and heart valves and corneas could be retrieved. Van Cleve (1993) studied the experience, attitudes and concerns of 110 nurses practicing on the unit with the anencephalic organ donors. Fifty-one percent of the nurses were uncomfortable providing care for the donor infants. Nurses expressed concern about whether this program respected the dignity of the life of the infants and wondered if the infants felt pain. As feelings of conflict intensified, some nurses asked not to be assigned to care for these infants.

FUTURE NEEDS IN NURSING TRANSPLANTATION RESEARCH

There are many opportunities for research in transplantation nursing. Suggestions for additional areas of study may be found in the discussions or conclusions of most of the articles described in this chapter. To examine the research needs for the entire profession of nursing, the National Institute for Nursing Research (NINR), one of the National Institutes of Health (NIH), has established a national nursing research agenda. One of the research priorities that may be of particular interest to nurses caring for transplant patients is the assessment and management of symptoms. For example, the study of symptom distress in 175 heart transplant patients by Grady and associates (1992) is a study that should be replicated with other transplant populations. Grady and colleagues noted that higher symptom distress was related to lower life satisfaction and quality of life. Once the symptoms common to a particular transplant population have been identified, interventions to manage these symptoms may be tested.

Advances in technology and pharmacology also require nursing research to evaluate their impact on patient outcomes. New immunosuppressive agents and genetic engineering hold great promise for reducing the donor shortage by allowing for successful xenographic transplantation. However, the question arises that if obtaining a donor organ is no longer considered a problem, will patients comply with prescribed posttransplant medication, diet, and exercise regimens?

The timing and content of patient teaching are another important area to be examined. Parents whose children had undergone liver or kidney transplantation indicated that they would have preferred more information in advance about transplantation (Weichler, 1993). This seems to conflict with the findings of Buse and Pieper (1990), who found that spouses of heart transplant patients felt that learning about heart transplantation was more important in the posttransplant phase than in the pretransplant phase, when they were overwhelmed with the fear that their spouse might not survive until a donor organ could be found. A randomized clinical trial to examine the effect of the timing and content of patient education on patient anxiety and patient satisfaction could help establish educational standards for particular transplant populations.

Patient education may be an effective method of allaying patient and family anxiety throughout the transplantation experience, but other nursing interventions should also be tested. Individual care given by a psychiatric clinical nurse specialist, support groups, and partnering with a patient or family member who has successfully managed the transplant experience in the past are three other methods of decreasing patient anxiety.

Finally, many ethical areas in transplantation are in need of study. Because living-related donation is new in liver and lung transplantation, the effects of this treatment on the donor and the recipient should be examined. Boone and associates (1992) have identified the role of the transplant nurse caring for living-related donors as one of educator, communicator, and source of emotional support. It must be determined what types of education and support these donors require. After the operation, one must ask if the donor feels the education received before consenting to donation accurately reflected the experience of donation and the benefits of transplantation for the recipient. One must ask if unreasonable pressures were placed on the donors by family members or health professionals. It is also important to understand the long-term effects of this type of surgery on the donor when the transplant is unsuccessful and the recipient dies. Information obtained from a careful study of living-related donation would be useful in establishing standards for patient education to ensure informed consent and to decrease anxiety.

A final ethical issue in need of study is the impact of donation on the lives of children who were conceived to serve as bone marrow donors for siblings. Jecker (1990) suggests that this violates the principle of respect for people because it involves using a child as a means to another's end. Parents who abort a fetus in utero who has been identified as unsuitable as a bone marrow donor for a sibling violate this same principle. The psychologic sequelae experienced by parents who have requested one or several abortions for this reason must be identified. The impact of this decision on the child who is to be the bone marrow recipient or on other siblings must be determined. Only VanCleve's (1993) study of the use of anencephalic infants as organ donors has discussed these ethical issues in transplantation. Nurses who form close relationships with patients and families are in the ideal position to carry out these ethical studies and to use research findings to evaluate standards in transplantation.

Steps in Conducting a Transplantation Research Project

Many nurses caring for transplant patients have an area of patient care they would like to study but are uncertain about how to initiate a research project. Many resources are available to assist nurses to conduct research. A few suggestions are provided here on how to access these resources at each stage of the research process.

Refining the Question. The first step is determining what is a researchable question. A research question should be posed only after a thorough review of the literature. Also, it is helpful to discuss the question with nursing colleagues and other members of the transplant team. Input from a variety of these sources allows the investigator to narrow the focus of the study and to concentrate on topics that hold the greatest promise for influencing practice. The question should also guide the study design.

Building the Research Team. A doctorally prepared nurse researcher is the ideal person to have on the research team. If the institution does not have a nurse researcher, this assistance many be found at other institutions in the area, such as a teaching hospital or school of nursing. Often doctorally prepared nursing faculty are interested in serving as research consultants to gain access to a clinical setting in which to carry out their own research. A clinical nurse researcher at a teaching hospital may be interested in providing assistance in exchange for the opportunity to develop a network of nurses interested in participating in multi-institutional studies in the future. Some researchers charge a fee for consultation. Others may not charge a consultation fee but expect to be included as a co-investigator and co-author if a long-term commitment is required in serving as a member of the research team. Mutual expectations can be clarified at the first meeting.

Professional organizations provide another source of research consultation. Sigma Theta Tau publishes a directory of nurse researchers and their area of expertise. Other avenues for obtaining consultants and useful questions to ask the consultants are outlined in an editorial by Rempusheski (1992).

The investigator should consider adding other team members with varied expertise. A dietitian would be an ideal team member on a project examining nutritional needs of transplant patients. A medical team member and perhaps an exercise physiologist would be valuable in examining patterns of activity tolerance in patients in the rehabilitation period after transplantation. A social worker and child life specialist could greatly contribute to a study of the adjustment of children to school after a long absence associated with transplantation. Finally, a statistician may be an important team member if the study involves complex data analysis. Involving the statistician in the planning phase is helpful because he or she may present several options among statistical methods to be used. Also, the statistician or nurse researcher can help decide how large the study sample should be if the investigators are to be confident that the findings are statistically significant and not based on chance.

Selecting a Study Design. Research designs range from descriptive to experimental. Descriptive studies, which describe phenomena of interest, require the least amount of control, whereas experimental studies that test hypotheses about causal relations between variables require the greatest amount of control.

In addition to different types of research design, there are two main approaches to research: qualitative and quantitative. The quantitative approach involves seeking data in an objective and controlled manner. A qualitative approach involves descriptive and subjective data. An example of a quantitative approach to studying family stress and coping with transplantation is found in the study by Nolan and associates (1992). Transplant family members were asked to examine a list of stressors and indicate whether the stress was present. A stress score was compiled for each individual to indicate whether the family member was experiencing mild, moderate, or severe stress. An example of a qualitative approach to studying the same topic is found in the study by Mishel and Murdaugh (1987). These investigators conducted semistructured interviews with family in which they asked about the transplant experience. The responses of the subjects were compiled, and common themes were identified. These common themes suggested a process of coping with transplant stress that the investigators labeled "redesigning the dream" or coming to terms with the stressors surrounding cardiac transplantation.

Obtaining a Sample. The easiest sample to obtain should include patients who are part of the current practice. By studying patients with whose care the investigator is familiar, the investigator avoids frustrating delays that occur when barriers to research that exist in every patient care setting are not anticipated. Another way of obtaining a sample is to use secondary data. Secondary data are data that were originally collected for another purpose (Reed, 1992). Gleit and Graham (1989) describe how secondary data may be used. Another way to obtain a sample is to add a nursing research study to a planned clinical trial. Hill and Schron (1992) point out that nurses have previously been involved in clinical trials as study coordinators or research nurses. The authors encourage nurse investigators to design studies that involve the concurrent collection of data along with a related clinical trial.

Not every study must have a large sample. Single case studies can contribute to the research literature. Single case-study reports are of great value in transplantation nursing because this area of nursing practice is changing so rapidly. An example of a single case-study report involved a 22-year old female patient who, having successfully undergone a heart transplant 4 years before, was seeking advice about becoming pregnant (Jordan & Pugh, in press). Johnson (1992) discussed how to write a case study to strengthen this approach. McLaughlin and Marascuilo (1990) discuss ways to analyze data when multiple interventions are tested on a single subject.

Selecting Study Instruments. One method of finding valid and reliable study instruments is to use instruments used in previous studies. The investigator can contact the author of a study article to obtain further information about an instrument and ultimately, permission to use the instrument if the author is the creator of the tool. If not, the author can refer the investigator to the creator of the tool to obtain permission to use the instrument.

Another source of study instruments are books and catalogs that describe or contain study instruments. An excellent book that describes instruments used to measure 24 different areas of concern in nursing is *Instruments for Clinical Nursing Research* (Frank-Stromborg, 1988). This book provides reliability and validity information on a large number of instruments used widely in nursing research. A catalog of psychologic instruments is published by Psychological Assessment Resources Inc. (1993). This publication includes hundreds of instruments that measure stress, neuropsychologic functioning, behavior, and personality factors.

Obtaining Funding. Many resources are available to fund nursing research. The North American Transplant Coordinators Organization (NATCO) sponsors an annual award to fund transplantation research. Many of the nursing specialty organizations such as The American Association of Critical Care Nurses (AACN) and the American Nephrology Nurses Association (ANNA) provide research grants for studies that con-

TABLE 14–3. RESEARCH GRANT SOURCES

Name of Grant	Budget Maximum	Number of Grants Available	Description of Grant
Sigma Theta Tau Small Grant	$3000	10–15	No specific focus. Pilot, multidisciplinary and international research is encouraged.
Sigma Theta Tau American Nurses Foundation Grant	$6000	1	Clinical topic
Sigma Theta Tau/American Association of Critical Care Nurses Critical Care Grant	$10,000	1	Critical care nursing
Sigma Theta Tau/Oncology Nursing Society Grant	$10,000	1	Oncology nursing
American Nurses Association Virginia Kelley Award	$2700	1	Women's health care
American Association of Critical Care Nurses Grant	$15,000	1	Critical care nursing
Oncology Nursing Society Grants	$4250–$10,000	11	Oncology nursing
American Heart Association Nation's Capital Affiliate	$5000	1	Cardiac nursing in Washington, DC (check local affiliate)

Based on information from each organization available on April 20, 1994.

tribute to the scientific base of their practice. Table 14-3 provides information about some of these types of grants. Contacting the funding organization directly to discuss the idea is an excellent way to determine if the organization is appropriate for the project and to obtain advice on writing the proposal. The investigator should ask for copies of previously funded proposals.

Publication of Study Findings. Careful consideration should be given to where the findings will be published. Authors should send their manuscripts to journals that will be read by those whose practice they are seeking to influence. An overview of 92 nursing journals was provided by Swanson and associates (1991). These authors categorized the journals by specialty practice areas and provided information about the circulation, frequency of publication, and percentage of research articles in each journal. An excellent source for help in writing the research manuscript was written by Tornquist (1986). In addition to providing a guide to composing a research manuscript, Tornquist offers advice on when or whether an investigator should send editors a query letter before submitting a manuscript.

SUMMARY

Nurses have met the challenges of providing care to transplant patients since the introduction of the field. A great deal of progress has been made, especially since 1989, in creating a scientific base for transplantation nursing practice. Just as nurses will rise to the continuing demand of medical and technologic innovations in transplant care, research will enable us to parallel these advances with innovations in the practice of transplantation nursing.

REFERENCES

Adams EF, Just G, DeYoung S, Temmler L (1993). Organ donation: Comparison of nurses' participation in two states. *J Crit Care.* 2:310–316.

Belic RH (1992). Quality of life: Perceptions of long-term survivors of bone marrow transplantation. *Oncol Nurs Forum.* 19:31–37.

Bidigare SA, Oermann MH (1991). Attitudes and knowledge of nurses regarding organ procurement. *Heart Lung.* 20:20–24.

Bohachick P, Anton BB, Wooldridge PJ, et al (1992). Psychosocial outcome six months after heart transplant surgery: A preliminary report. *Res Nurs. Health.* 15:165–173.

Boone P, Kelly S, Smith CD (1992). Liver transplantation: Living-related donations. *Crit Care Nurs Clin North Am.* 4:243–248.

Buse SM, Pieper B. (1990). Impact of cardiac transplantation of the spouse's life. *Heart Lung.* 19:641–648.

Copel LC, Smith ME (1989). Oncology nurses' knowledge of graft-versus host disease in bone marrow transplant patients. *Cancer Nurs.* 12:243–249.

Driscoll E (1992). The emotions experienced by critical care nurses when approaching potential organ/tissue donor families. *Heart Lung.* 21:288.

Ersek M (1992). The process of maintaining hope in adults undergoing bone marrow transplantation for leukemia. *Oncol Nurs Forum.* 19:883–889.

Ferrell B, Grant M, Schmidt GM, et al (1992). The meaning of quality of life for bone marrow transplant survivors. *Cancer Nurs.* 15:153–160.

Frank-Stromborg M (1988). *Instruments for Clinical Nursing Research.* Norwalk: Appleton & Lange.

Gaston-Johansson F, Franco T, Zimmerman L (1992). Pain and psychological distress in patients undergoing autologous bone marrow transplantation. *Oncol Nurs. Forum.* 19:41–48.

Gleit C, Graham B (1989). Secondary data analysis: A valuable resource. *Nurs Res.* 38:380–381.

Grady KL, Jalowiec A, Grusk BB, et al (1992). Symptom distress in cardiac transplant candidates. *Heart Lung.* 21:434–439.

Grady KL, Jalowiec A, White-Williams C, et al (1993). Heart transplant candidates' perception of helpfulness of health care provider interventions. *Cardiovascular Nurs.* 29:33–38.

Hathaway D, Hartwig M, Winsett RP, Gaber AO (1992). Quality of life 6–12 months after renal transplant (abstract). *ANNA J.* 19:152.

Hathaway D, Strong M, Ganza M (1990). Posttransplant quality of life expectations. *ANNA J.* 17:433-439.

Hayward MB, Kish JP, Frey GM, et al (1989). An instrument to identify stressors in renal transplant recipients. *ANNA J.* 16:81-84.

Hicks FD, Larson JL, Ferrans CE (1992). Quality of life after liver transplant. *Res Nurs Health.* 15:111-119.

Hill MN, Schron EB (1992). Opportunities for nurse researchers in clinical trials. *Nurs Res.* 41:114-115.

Jecker NS (1990). Conceiving a child to save a child: reproductive and filial ethics. *J Clin Ethics.* 1:99-103.

Johnson SH (1992). Strengthening your case study approach. *Nurse Auth Ed.* 2:1-7.

Jordan E, Pugh L (1994). Pregnancy after cardiac transplantation: Principles of nursing care. *JOGNN.* In press.

Kern D, Kettner P, Albrizio M (1992). An exploration of the variables involved when instituting a do-not-resuscitate order for patients undergoing bone marrow transplantation. *Oncol Nurs Forum.* 19:635-640.

Kiberd MC, Kiberd BA (1992). Nursing attitudes towards organ donation, procurement, and transplantation. *Heart Lung.* 21:106-111.

Lange SS, Prevost S, Lewis P, Fadol A (1992). Infection control practices in cardiac transplant recipients. *Heart Lung.* 21:101-105.

Larson PJ, Viele CS, Coleman S, et al (1993). Comparison of perceived symptoms of patients undergoing bone marrow transplant and the nurses caring for them. *Oncol Nurs Forum.* 20:81-88.

Martin S (1993). Pediatric critical care nurses' perceptions and understanding of cadaver organ procurement. *Crit Care Nurse.* 13:74-81.

McLaughlin FE, Marascuilo LA (1990). Single subject research. In: *Advanced Nursing and Health Care Research: Quantification Approaches.* Philadelphia: Saunders, 317-332.

McNatt G, White M (1992). Return to work in renal transplant recipients (abstract). *ANNA J.* 19:151.

Mishel MH, Murdaugh CL (1987). Family adjustment to heart transplantation: Redesigning the dream. *Nurs Res.* 36:332-338.

Muirhead J, Meyerowitz BE, Leedham B, et al (1992). Quality of life and coping in patients awaiting heart transplantation. *J Heart Lung Transplant.* 11:265-272.

Nolan MT, Cupples SA, Brown M, et al (1992). Perceived stress and coping strategies among families of cardiac transplant candidates during the organ waiting period. *Heart Lung.* 21:540-547.

Porter RR, Bailey C, Bennett GM, et al (1991). Stress during the waiting period: A review of pretransplantation fears. *Crit Care Nurs Q* 13:25-31.

Porter RR, Krout L, Parks V, et al (1994). Perceived stress and coping strategies among candidates for heart transplantation during the organ waiting period. *J Heart Lung Transplant.* 13:102-107.

Psychological Assessment Resources Incorporated (1993). *Testing Resources for the Professional.* Odessa, Fla: Psychological Assessment.

Reed J (1992). Secondary data in nursing research. *Journal of Advanced Nursing.* 17:877-883.

Rempusheski VF (1992). A researcher as resource, mentor, and preceptor. *Appl Nurs Res.* 5:105-107.

Rogers KR, Sinnott JT, Ferguson JE (1989). Using OKT3 to reverse cardiac allograft rejection. *Heart Lung.* 18:490-496.

Rubin S, Dale J, Santamaria C, Tomalty J (1991). Weight change in cardiac transplant patients. *Can J Cardiovasc Nurs.* 2:9–13.

Steeves R (1992). Patients who have undergone bone marrow transplantation: Their quest for meaning. *Oncol Nurs Forum.* 19:899–905.

Stoeckle ML (1990). Attitudes of critical care nurses toward organ donation. *DCCN.* 9:354–361.

Swanson EA, McCloskey JC, Bodensteiner A (1991). Publishing opportunities for nurses: A comparison of 92 U.S. Journals. *Image.* 23:33–38.

Thomas DJ (1993a). Risking infection: An issue of control for liver transplant recipients. *AACN Clin Issues Crit Care Nurs.* 4:471–474.

Thomas DJ (1993b). Returning to work after liver transplant: Experiencing the roadblocks. Presented at The American Nurses Association Council of Nurse Researchers Meeting, November 13, 1993, Washington DC.

Tornquist EM (1986). *From Proposal to Publication: An Informal Guide to Writing about Nursing Research.* Menlo Park: Ca: Addison-Wesley.

Uzark K, Crowley D (1989). Family stresses after pediatric heart transplantation. *Prog Cardiovasc Nurs.* 4:23–27.

Van Cleve L (1993). Nurses' experience caring for anencephalic infants who are potential organ donors. *J Pediatr Nurs.* 8:79–84.

Vehrenkamp DM, Rettke SR, Sittipong R, Ilstrup DM (1992). Association of coagulation tests with blood use during liver transplantation. *Nurse Anesth.* 3:166–172.

Voepel-Lewis T, Ketefian S, Starr A, White MJ (1990). Stress, coping, and quality of life in family members of kidney transplant recipients. *ANNA J.* 17:427–431.

Walden JA, Stevenson LW, Dracup K, et al (1989). Heart transplantation may not improve quality of life for patients with stable heart failure. *Heart Lung.* 18:497–506.

Weems J, Patterson ET (1989). Coping with uncertainty and ambivalence while awaiting a cadaveric renal transplant. *ANNA J.* 16:27–31.

Weichler N (1990). The expressed informational needs of mothers of children following liver transplantation. *J Ped Nurs.* 5:88–96.

Weichler NK (1993). Caretakers' informational needs after their children's renal or liver transplant. *ANNA J.* 20:135–140.

White MJ, Ketefian S, Starr AJ, Voepel-Lewis T (1990). Stress, coping, and quality of life in adult kidney transplant recipients. *ANNA J.* 17:421–424.

Zamberlan KE (1992). Quality of life in school-age children following liver transplantation. *Mat Child Nurs J.* 19:185–186.

Zerbe MB, Parkerson SG, Ortlieb ML, Spitzer T (1992). Relationships between oral mucositis and treatment variables in bone marrow transplant patients. *Cancer Nurs.* 15:196–205.

Index